INTRODUCTION TO
RESEARCH
IN THE
HEALTH SCIENCES

To the memory of Dr George Varnai and Dr George Polgar

To Liam, Kali, Taran, Rani, Collette and June

For Elsevier:

Commissioning Editor: Steven Black
Development Editor: Catherine Jackson
Project Manager: Gail Wright
Designer: Charles Gray
Illustrations Manager: Gillian Richards
Illustrator: Hardlines Studio

INTRODUCTION TO
RESEARCH
IN THE
HEALTH SCIENCES

FIFTH EDITION

Stephen Polgar
BSc(Hons) MSc
Senior Lecturer, School of Public Health,
Faculty of Health Sciences, La Trobe University,
Melbourne, Australia

Shane A. Thomas
DipPubPol PhD MAPS
Director of Primary Care Research, Faculty of
Medicine, Nursing and Health Sciences, Monash
University, Melbourne, Australia

CHURCHILL
LIVINGSTONE
ELSEVIER

EDINBURGH LONDON NEW YORK OXFORD PHILADELPHIA ST LOUIS SYDNEY TORONTO 2008

CHURCHILL
LIVINGSTONE
ELSEVIER

First edition 1988
Second edition 1991
Third edition 1995
Fourth edition 2000
Fifth edition 2008
  Reprinted 2008 (twice)

ISBN: 978-0-443-07429-5

British Library Cataloguing in Publication Data
A catalogue record for this book is available from the British Library

Library of Congress Cataloging in Publication Data
A catalog record for this book is available from the Library of Congress

Notice
Knowledge and best practice in this field are constantly changing. As new research and experience broaden our knowledge, changes in practice, treatment and drug therapy may become necessary or appropriate. Readers are advised to check the most current information provided (i) on procedures featured or (ii) by the manufacturer of each product to be administered, to verify the recommended dose or formula, the method and duration of administration, and contraindications. It is the responsibility of the practitioner, relying on their own experience and knowledge of the patient, to make diagnoses, to determine dosages and the best treatment for each individual patient, and to take all appropriate safety precautions. To the fullest extent of the law, neither the Publisher nor the Authors assume any liability for any injury and/or damage to persons or property arising out of or related to any use of the material contained in this book.

The Publisher

ELSEVIER your source for books,
journals and multimedia
in the health sciences
www.elsevierhealth.com

Working together to grow
libraries in developing countries
www.elsevier.com | www.bookaid.org | www.sabre.org

ELSEVIER   BOOK AID International   Sabre Foundation

The
Publisher's
policy is to use
**paper manufactured
from sustainable forests**

Printed in China

Contents

Preface

Consistent with previous versions, the 5th edition of this textbook has two overall aims:

1. To introduce the fundamental principles of research methodology and explain how these principles are applied for conducting research in the health sciences.
2. To demonstrate how evidence produced through research is applied to solving problems in every-day health care.

It is widely recognized that the advancement of knowledge and practice in an area of health care depends on the education of individuals who are competent in undertaking health research and evaluations. We recognize that only a relatively small proportion of health sciences professionals have the interest or the opportunity to undertake full-blown research. At the same time, all contemporary health professionals participate in a 'culture' which privileges knowledge based on the critical review of scientific evidence. This textbook will enable students to participate in discussions concerning health problems and scientific approaches to treatment.

It must be emphasized that, in its 5th edition, *Introduction to Research in the Health Sciences* remains an introductory textbook. In order to retain the simplicity and readability of the text we have made the following changes:

- Inclusion of an additional chapter which focuses on the use of qualitative methods in health research.
- Inclusion of a new chapter for discussing systematic reviews and meta-analyses.
- More revision questions, in particular ones which emphasize the utilization of research for the solution of health problems.
- Revised and updated clinically relevant research designs such as single case studies and focus groups.
- Expanded discussion of effect size and clinical significance of quantitative data.
- Improvements in the presentation and formatting of the text, in particular by updating the figures and diagrams.

We would like to acknowledge our colleagues who have contributed in various ways to the development of this book since it was first published in 1988. We are grateful to our readers and students who have made helpful comments, making this book relevant for introducing students to health research. We are particularly grateful to Joanna Ng for her hard work and dedication in organizing the text for this 5th edition.

Melbourne 2007

Stephen Polgar
Shane A. Thomas

Section One

The scientific method

In this section we will examine some of the basic characteristics of the scientific method. A 'method', in the present context, refers to a system for acquiring knowledge and establishing its truth. Health providers justify their theories and practices on the grounds that they are 'scientific', that is, based on scientific methodology. The scientific method is essential for conducting research and evaluation aimed at producing evidence, improving the effectiveness and cost-effectiveness of health services.

A common view of the scientific method is that it enables us to describe, predict, explain and perhaps to control events in the world. As an example, consider how researchers and practitioners in the health care system responded to the outbreak of the acquired immuno-deficiency syndrome (AIDS) epidemic in the early 1980s. One of the first signs of this epidemic was the clinical observation that young men presented with a deadly cancer (Kaposi's sarcoma) which was previously found only in the elderly. This was the initial evidence which indicated that further facts and explanations were required. It was hypothesized that the premature failure of the immune system was responsible for the disorder. Subsequent clinical evidence supported this hypothesis, leading to

a clear definition of the disease as 'AIDS'. As more cases of AIDS were identified it became evident that some groups in the population were most at risk: persons who were involved in multiple homosexual relationships or who were intravenous drug users, or those who required blood products, for example, for haemophilia. An important development was the confirmation of the hypothesis that the disease was caused by a specific virus labelled 'HIV' (human immuno-deficiency virus). On the basis of the above clinical, epidemiological and virological evidence it was hypothesized that the HIV was transmitted through body fluids such as blood or semen. In this way it became possible to predict which practices in the population involved a high level of risk for transmitting the virus.

The above findings and hypotheses contributed to constructing theories of AIDS, providing systematic and integrated conceptual frameworks for explaining the transmission and the clinical features of the disorder. These theories also inform current practices aimed at controlling the epidemic, such as testing blood products for HIV, or promoting 'safe sex' behaviours. The effectiveness of these practices (at least in some countries) for containing the epidemic provided evidence confirming the accuracy

1

of our understanding of the problem. At the same time, we remain sceptical about certain aspects of our theories, recognizing that there are as yet no vaccines or pharmacological cures for AIDS.

You might have recognized that the above brief account of attempting to contain AIDS is deficient in an essential way: it excludes evidence concerning the personal experiences and actions of persons at risk of or having HIV. The above account represented a quantitative approach to the scientific method aiming to provide a mechanistic or reductionistic explanation of health and illness. This method is not appropriate for researching and theorizing how persons, their families and the community respond to health-related issues and problems. Research methods should also include qualitative or interpretive approaches to discover the personal meanings involved in being at risk of or suffering from diseases or disabilities. Qualitative methods are also appropriate for researching the cultural context and social construction of a disorder; for instance, discovering the images of AIDS sufferers communicated by the media in a given community.

The position taken in the present book is that the scientific method, as applied to health care, must include both quantitative and qualitative methods. These methods are used to produce evidence for solving health-related problems. Regardless of controversies regarding the nature of science and its methodology, there is a broad consensus concerning the principles and rules for producing scientific evidence. Our goal is to convey these principles and rules to our readers.

Chapter One

Methods and health research

1

CHAPTER CONTENTS

Introduction

Health research is a systematic and principled way of obtaining evidence (data, information) for solving health care problems and investigating health issues. Research is *systematic* in that researchers tend to follow a sequential process (Fig. 1.1) and *principled* in that research is generally carried out according to explicit rules. These rules or principles constitute the method.

The primary aim of this chapter is to outline the key characteristics of methods for conducting enquiry. Special emphasis is placed on method as a means for conducting applied research and producing the best possible evidence for solving health problems.

The general aims of this chapter are to:

1. Define what is meant by a method, and outline some common methods of enquiry.
2. Draw attention to some controversies concerning the nature of scientific method.
3. Compare qualitative and quantitative approaches to research.
4. Discuss how method is applied to conducting health sciences research.

Methods and knowledge

Patient care involves the acquisition of a set of specific skills, the practice of which is justified in

Figure 1.1 • The research process.

terms of a body of professional knowledge. This body of knowledge is based on the use of appropriate methods. In general the term 'method' refers to a systematic procedure for carrying out an activity and in the present context implies a set of rules which specify:

1. How knowledge should be acquired.
2. The form in which knowledge should be stated.
3. How the 'truth' or validity of the knowledge should be established.

Before we begin a discussion of the scientific method it is useful, as a means of contrast, to look at some of the other methodological approaches.

Authority

According to this method, knowledge is considered true because of tradition, or because an experienced and distinguished clinician says that it is true. As a student, you are often asked to accept statements as true because your teachers and clinical supervisors say they are true. To maintain their authority, the 'sources' of knowledge acquire and cultivate various signs of expertise, such as the appellation of 'Professor', or encourage the performance of status rituals. For example, consider the 'Consultant' who sweeps into a hospital ward followed by a retinue of students, registrars and nurses. Who would dare to question the truth of any of the consultant's sacred utterances? However, there are problems with the method of authority: what happens when the statements arising from one authority are contradicted by those made by an equally prestigious authority? For example, say Authority X claims that in their experience psychoanalysis is effective, while Authority Y states that the technique is useless. How can we resolve such conflicting claims? In practice, unless objective and acceptable criteria for resolution can be found, we will have unending arguments, *ad hominem* (personal) attacks, or in instances of some religious or political disagreements, violence. That is, the controversy is resolved by denigrating or silencing the dissenting authority. In contrast, the scientific method emphasizes the evaluation of the evidence for establishing the truth of conflicting statements.

Reasoning

Reasoning is commonly used to arrive at true knowledge. It is assumed that if the rules of logic are applied correctly, then the conclusions are guaranteed to be valid. As an example, let us look at the following syllogism:

1. All persons suffering from heart disease are males.
2. Person X has heart disease.
3. Therefore, person X is a male.

Logic guarantees that the conclusion (3) is true, provided that the syllogism is in a valid form and the premises (1) and (2) are true. Clearly, the limitation of formal (that is, 'content-independent') reasoning is that it works in practice only if we have means for establishing the factual truth of the premises. In the above example, conclusion

(3) might be empirically false, given that the premise (1) is factually false.

Logic and mathematics are very much a part of science but we require strong evidence to support the effective logic and mathematical operations.

Intuition

Knowledge is sometimes acquired by sudden insights which arise without conscious reasoning. Truth is judged by the clarity of the experience and its emotional content (the 'Eureka!' experience). For example, after working with a patient without success, you might have a sudden insight about how to change your treatment programme. Sometimes these insights lead to new theories and treatments. Unfortunately, even the strongest intuitions are sometimes proven false by cold, boring facts. Newton has referred to the disappointment that occurs when a beautiful hypothesis is destroyed by an ugly fact.

Discoveries are sometimes resisted because they seem counterintuitive. Ignaz Semmelweis, a perceptive and humane 19th-century physician, noticed appalling levels of puerperal (child birth-related) fever and maternal death at his hospital. He argued that the infection was spread by medical students and staff who went to delivery rooms from the morgue without adequately washing their hands. In 1848, Semmelweis introduced antiseptic procedures in his wards and demonstrated a substantial reduction in mortality from puerperal fever. However, his colleagues were offended by the notion that physicians were carriers of disease. Semmelweis was dismissed from his post, ostracized by the medical establishment and died in pitiful circumstances. Clearly, in the light of contemporary knowledge we can say that Semmelweis' insights were correct, while his colleagues' intuitions were mistaken. Authority, logic and intuition all have their places in health care and research. In a general way the scientific method can be contrasted with other methods in that it emphasizes the need for evidence. What constitutes scientific evidence and what the evidence indicates are complex matters that are being addressed in this book.

The scientific method and positivism

The scientific method has crystallized over a period of several centuries, concomitantly with the growth of scientific research. The beginnings of modern Western science are generally traced to the 16th century, a time in which Europe experienced profound social changes and a resurgence of great artists, thinkers and philosophers. Gradually, scholars' interests shifted from theology and armchair speculation to systematically describing, explaining and attempting to control natural phenomena. These changed circumstances allowed philosophers such as Descartes and Francis Bacon to challenge tenets of medieval thinking, and scientists such as Galileo, Newton and Harvey to propose new models of natural phenomena.

The approaches of such great thinkers had three basic elements, which are the basis of scientific method:

1. *Empiricism.* The notion that enquiry ought to be conducted through observation and knowledge verified through evidence.
2. *Determinism.* The notion that events in the world occur according to regular laws and causes. The aims of research are to discover these rules and causes.
3. *Scepticism.* The notion that any proposition or statement, even those by great authorities, is open to analysis and critique.

The scientific method is represented in a simple form in Figure 1.2. This representation is consistent with a view of natural science methodology called 'positivism' by the 19th-century philosopher Comte, as well as 'reductionism'. Both these terms have acquired multiple meanings in the area of philosophy of science. Our interpretation of Figure 1.2 is explained below.

Figure 1.2 • The scientific method.

Observations, description and measurement

Considering Figure 1.2, let us start with observations. The description of phenomena involving the precise, unbiased recording of observations of aspects of persons, objects and events forms the empirical basis of all branches of science. Observations can be expressed as either verbal descriptions or sets of measurements (see Section 4). The perceptions of the investigator must be transformed into descriptive statements and measurements that can be understood and replicated by other investigators. Some research is based on observation made with instruments (such as recording electrodes, microscopes and standardized clinical tests), while other research calls for observation unaided by instruments. Although advances in instrumentation have contributed enormously to scientific knowledge, the use of complex instrumentation is not a necessary feature of scientific observation. Rather, the key attributes of scientific observation are accuracy and replicability by other scientists. When observations are appropriately summarized and are confirmed by others, they form the factual bases of scientific knowledge.

Generalization and induction

Statements representing observations or measurements are integrated into explanatory systems called hypotheses and theories. The logic underlying scientific generalizations is called induction. Induction involves asserting general propositions (hypotheses, theories) about a class of phenomena on the basis of a limited number of observations of select elements. For example, having observed that penicillin is useful for curing pneumonia in a limited set of patients, we make the generalization 'The administration of penicillin cures pneumonia (in all patients)'.

Hypotheses

The statement 'The administration of penicillin cures pneumonia' is an example of a hypothesis. Scientific hypotheses are statements that specify the expected nature of the relationship between two or more sets of variables. In this instance, the first variable relates to the administration of penicillin and the second variable is related to changes in clinical observations or measurements concerning pneumonia. As we shall see in subsequent sections, an important feature of scientific hypotheses is that the terms used must have clear-cut, observable referents. When these hypotheses acquire strong empirical support, they may be called laws.

Theories

Scientific theories are essentially conjectures representing our current state of knowledge about the world. Hypotheses are integrated into more general explanatory systems called theories. A theory will clarify the relationships between diverse classes of observations and hypotheses. For example, a theory to explain why drugs called antibiotics are effective in curing some infectious diseases integrates evidence from diverse sources such as microbiology, pharmacology, cell physiology and clinical medicine. Other examples of theories are the heliocentric theory of the solar system, the DNA theory of genetic inheritance, and the neuronal theory of central nervous system functioning. It is an essential feature of scientific theories that they are statements based on the correct use of language and logic. Some theories entail a model (see Fig. D1.1, p. 16), which is a mathematical or physical representation of how the theory works. In this way, theories specify the causes of events and provide conceptual means for predicting and influencing these events. In health care, theories are important for explaining the causes of health and illness and predicting the probable effectiveness of treatment outcomes.

Deduction

A scientific theory should lead to a set of empirically verifiable statements or hypotheses. In addition to being generalizations based on evidence, hypotheses are also deduced logically from the statements and/or mathematical models which specify the causal relationships postulated by the theories. For example, if we hold the theory that the patterns of activity of a set of neurones in the occipital lobe mediate visual sensation in humans, then the hypothesis follows that the activation of these neurones (say, by electrical stimulation) will lead to the report of visual sensations. Such hypotheses have been the bases for subsequent spectacular clinical advances such as artificial vision through cortically implanted electrodes.

Controlled observation

It is desirable that hypotheses are tested under controlled conditions. The aim of control is to discount other competing hypotheses for explaining the predicted phenomenon. For example, if we intend to show that occipital lobe stimulation causes the visual sensations, we must show that we are controlling for any type of brain stimulation causing such changes. Conversely, we would need to show that occipital lobe stimulation does not lead to a host of other types of sensations. Only by discounting alternative explanations through control can we have confidence in the relevance of our observations for our research hypothesis. Of course control must be ethical, as we shall see in later chapters.

Verification and falsification

An essential characteristic of a scientific proposition is that it should be 'falsifiable'. That is, there should be a clear empirical outcome that could, if found, show that the proposition was false. For example, consider Einstein's hypothesis that $E = mc^2$. If laboratory researchers found that the energy locked up in matter corresponded to, say, $E = mc^3$, then Einstein's hypothesis would be shown to be false. This seems not to have happened yet, so that $E = mc^2$ is falsifiable but not false. After the evidence has been collected, the investigator decides whether or not the findings are consistent with the predictions of the hypothesis. If the hypothesis is supported by the evidence, then the theory from which the hypothesis was deduced is strengthened or verified. However, when the data do not support the hypothesis, the related theory is falsified. If a theory can no longer predict or explain evidence in its empirical domain, it becomes less useful and is usually later discarded in favour of new,

more powerful theories. Therefore, scientific theories are not held to be absolute truths, but rather as provisional explanations of available evidence.

The application of the above process has contributed to the spectacular growth of scientific knowledge. Observation and measurement, facilitated by new instrumentation, resulted in the discovery of an enormous number of accurate and reproducible facts about health and illness. New facts both challenge existing theories and call for the creation of novel, more powerful theories. The new theories serve as impetus for more research, resulting in new instrumentation and observations. Advances in scientific knowledge have been applied to creating new technologies, which in turn contribute to new discoveries and advances in scientific knowledge. For example, the invention of computers was possible because of advances in electronics, chemistry and mathematics. In turn, the use of computers is now contributing to making and summarizing scientific observations or formulating explanatory models. In addition, the use of computers as information-processing systems has generated useful metaphors for theoretical advances, such as explaining the human brain and mental functioning. In this way, the scientific method contributes to advancing theory and practice, helping us to describe, explain, predict and sometimes control the world in which we live.

Controversies concerning the nature of method: post-positivism

The above description is not the only interpretation of scientific method. Rather, there are good reasons why the positivist view of the scientific method was challenged in the second half of the 20th century.

First, the scientific method is a set of rules devised and applied by philosophers and scientists. They are not eternal truths, but conventions believed to be useful for conducting scientific enquiry. In this way, not only the content but also the methodology of science is open to criticism, debate and change.

Second, the interpretation of what constitutes the scientific method is an activity pursued by philosophers of science and epistemologists. In exploring different conceptual frameworks (realism, instrumentalism, anarchism, idealism, etc.) concerning the nature of reality and knowledge, philosophers generate unending controversies over the nature of the scientific method.

Third, advances in science contributed to changes to our methods and the ways in which we explain the world. For example 'quantum theory' and the 'theory of relativity' challenged the mechanistic, clockwork-like view of reality. Modern theories of physical reality are fuzzier and more probabilistic and the observers are not seen as being outside the phenomena they are studying.

The following ideas represent key aspects of the post-positivist view of scientific methodology.

The theory-dependence of observation

Critics such as Chalmers (1976) argued that it is simplistic to believe that observations are made independently of theoretical notions held by the observer. The observer is selective with regard to what is recorded as evidence. Our observations and facts are 'theory-dosed', that is, theories specify what observations are of importance and what aspects of these observations should be recorded or ignored. Schatzman & Strauss (1973) put this point elegantly when they stated that the researcher 'harbours, wittingly or not, many expectations, conjectures and hypotheses which provide him with thought and directives on what to look for and what to ask about'. For instance, in observing the electroencephalogram (EEG) of an epileptic patient, our perception is guided by theories of the electrical activity of the brain and the nature of brain pathology. We will also hold ideas about how the EEG machine works (for example, electrode sensitivity, amplification, etc.) and identify artefacts in the evidence. What is observed as evidence of epilepsy by an expert could be perceived as meaningless squiggles by a naive observer. We shall take account of this point later in this book, when we discuss the reliability and validity of measurement.

The validity of induction

Philosophers of science have questioned the logical validity of making general claims on the basis of a limited set of observations. To quote Chalmers (1976): 'any observational evidence will consist of a finite number of observation statements, whereas a universal statement makes claims about an infinite number of possible situations'.

For example, we might have observed that the administration of penicillin cured pneumonia in 100 000 patients. This does not necessarily guarantee the logical 'truth' of the universal statement 'penicillin cures pneumonia', or that patient number 100 001 will be cured. We will look at the theories-related issue of generalization from samples in this book. Scientific theories are seen as probabilistic, in the sense that new, inconsistent evidence might emerge in the future, challenging the generality of the theory. Also, it has been argued by some philosophers of science that hypotheses *need not* be based on induction, but may arise from any source, provided that they have falsifiable empirical consequences.

What constitutes falsification?

It was stated earlier that when novel empirical evidence is inconsistent with the predictions of a theory, the theory is 'falsified' and is eventually modified or discarded. Commentators such as Lakatos (1970) argued that theories are not, in practice, so readily modified or discarded by scientists. Rather, they are structures which have an inner hard core of propositions protected by an outer belt of auxiliary, modifiable hypotheses. Evidence inconsistent with predictions based on the theory results in the modification of auxiliary hypotheses, rather than discarding the 'core'. Consider, for example, the 'germ' theory of infectious disease, on the basis of which one would predict that penicillin (which kills germs) will cure bacterial infections. Suppose that we administer penicillin to a number of patients with an infectious disease and find, contrary to what was predicted, no clinically useful changes. On the basis of this falsification, will we discard the germ theory of disease? No. Rather, we will utilize an auxiliary hypothesis to explain our findings, such as 'the development of penicillin-resistant bacteria'. The methodological issue which remains controversial is the logical basis for discarding one theory and accepting its rival (see Feyerabend 1975). As we shall see, we judge the outcome of a research programme in the context of an overall pattern of related findings and theories.

Science and the cultural context

Science as a human activity

An important aspect of post-positivism has been the recognition that human values are an integral part of scientific inquiry. Scientific enquiry is conducted in particular social settings, by individuals with personal aims and values. Some more recent formulations of methodology take into account the social and interpersonal conditions which influence scientists' professional activities (Feyerabend 1975, Kuhn 1970). In this text, we will pay attention to social values, in the context of ethical considerations for designing and conducting research (Ch. 2). Also, we recognize that the formulation of hypotheses and theories are creative acts, rather than the outcomes of the automatic application of induction. In this way, the questions asked by health researchers and the ways in which they explain their findings are influenced in subtle ways by the cultures in which they live and work.

To understand the nature of scientific research in general, and health research in particular, it is useful to examine how they fit into an overall social context. That is, the way in which persons living in a society view health and illness and the ways in which health workers carry out their professional roles influence the range and scope of health care research (e.g. Taylor 1979). Until recently, the 'medical model' was by far the most dominant approach to understanding illness in Western society. Briefly, in terms of the medical model, illness is represented by a particular lesion or dysfunction within the human body. The role of the health professional is to identify the location and nature of the lesion or the clinical imbalance and to implement appropriate measures to correct the problem. The patient is assigned a rather passive role in this process, being the 'locus' of the lesion or imbalance and a person complying with the health professionals' recommendations. In the context of the medical model, the most appropriate research is seen as that which improves the technical effectiveness and, therefore, the social power of the health professional.

In Western society the medical model has been, and will continue to be, an influential model for guiding clinical practice and health research. Nevertheless, there have been gradual changes in health care that require the questioning of the generality of the medical model for the following reasons:

1. There have been important changes in the roles and status of health professionals such as nurses, occupational therapists, physiotherapists, speech pathologists and podiatrists. Rather than taking an ancillary, paramedical position, these individuals are becoming directly and independently responsible for a broad range of health care functions, including prevention, assessment, therapy and rehabilitation. However, the perspectives and practices of these health professionals are at times quite different from those involved in the medical model and may require quite different approaches to research and theory. The gradual establishment of university-based education for these professionals has provided an increased opportunity for relevant research, which is not necessarily guided by the medical model.

2. From the 1970s onwards it had become evident that there had been a significant increase in the cost of health care, in part due to the adoption of very expensive diagnostic procedures and the increasing trend for specialization among medical practitioners (Taylor 1979). Attempts to contain health care costs have resulted in several lines of approach, including:

   (a) increased focus on preventive health care, as shown by anti-smoking campaigns, or drink driving legislation to contain the incidence of road trauma

   (b) increased efforts to enhance the cost-effectiveness of current treatment strategies; for example, by improving communications between clinicians and patients or managing patients' fears concerning treatments through the application of psychological techniques

   (c) increased support for self-help groups and community-managed health centres with a more active involvement of individuals in understanding and managing their own health.

3. Preventive and educational approaches require somewhat different views of the client and the professional to that implicit in the medical model. In turn, research is required which can clarify the relationships between community lifestyles, individual behaviours, health and illness and general economic and social circumstances (e.g. Gardner 1989).

The more holistic approach, which also informs health care research, is called the *psychosocial* or *biopsychosocial* model (Engel 1977), and currently has had considerable influence in how we conceptualize health care and how we plan and carry out research. At the same time, the medical model strongly based on positivist thinking remains influential in research aimed at understanding the workings of the human body and improving the technical aspects of health care.

Pragmatism: the combined use of quantitative and qualitative methods

Not all scholars agreed with the notion that qualitative and quantitative methods could be logically combined. The controversy was resolved on pragmatic grounds; both methods are needed to solve applied problems in areas such as health care (McGartland & Polgar 1994).

Pragmatism is a system of philosophy that avoids speculation about nebulous abstractions such as 'The Truth'; rather it defines truth as what works (Tashakkori & Teddlie 1998). A pragmatic, problem-solving approach is followed in the present book, emphasizing the need for both qualitative and quantitative methods for effectively solving health problems.

The introduction of a biopsychosocial approach has raised questions about the combination of methodologies relevant to health sciences research. We perceive patients or clients in two different but interrelated frameworks: first, as broken down or malfunctioning biological systems; and second, as persons, like ourselves, living in a society and who

are attempting to make sense of and cope with their particular health care problems.

As argued earlier, the first view informs a reductionist or *quantitative* approach to research and knowledge. That is, we view our patients objectively, as natural objects, and attempt to identify and measure important variables which represent the causes and expressions of a clinical condition. We develop models and theoretical frameworks which systematically explain how these variables are interrelated and undertake therapeutic actions which serve to diminish the variables representing illness or disability. Our therapeutic actions are the technical applications for our scientific theories; their outcomes and effectiveness should be tested under controlled conditions.

The second view informs a *qualitative* or interpretive approach to research and knowledge. We view our patients as persons and attempt to gain insights into their subjective experiences and the reasons for their actions in particular situations. We develop theories for interpreting the nature and development of their personal points of view, and to inform our therapeutic actions so that they seem meaningful and appropriate to our patients.

Take, as an illustration of the above approaches, a patient with cancer. In a quantitative analysis we attempt to quantify the problem by using appropriate instrumentation which measures variables such as the size and location of the tumour and the extent of its spread within the organism. Consistent with current theories of the nature of cancer, various techniques such as surgery, radiology or chemotherapy might be brought into play, the effectiveness of which will be judged in terms of controlling specific variables associated with the condition, such as levels of pain, weight or time of survival of the patient.

With a qualitative perspective, we may address the meaning of the condition from the patient's personal point of view, within the context of his or her family setting and social circumstances. That is, the patient's value systems must be clarified and understood before actions such as assessments and therapeutic actions are undertaken. Enquiry might uncover conflicting values, for instance, concerning the implementation of a programme of chemotherapy. From the clinician's point of view, a radical programme of chemotherapy might seem appropriate, as probably quantitatively extending the patient's life by several years. However, from the patient's point of view, the quality of life under chemotherapy might seem inadequate, and also they might not wish to be a burden on their families. Clearly, both in clinical practice and in related research, evidence from both quantitative and qualitative enquiries should be integrated to ensure effective health care.

Although there are differences in how health scientists approach problems, Figure 1.1 shows the sequence of procedures commonly involved in quantitative research. You will find that the organization of this book follows the sequential stages of the research process, as outlined below.

1. *Research problems and questions.* The first step in problem solving is to state, clearly and unambiguously, the problem which we are attempting to solve. In general, research problems reflect both the unmet health care needs of patients and opportunities created by new theoretical and technological advancements for improving health care. Having identified a problem (or opportunity) our next step is to ask the 'right' question. A well-formulated research question will guide the research project for producing the evidence to answer the question and solve the research problem.

2. *Planning.* As we shall show in Section 2, research planning involves selecting appropriate strategies and measurements to answer questions or to test hypotheses. It will be argued in Chapter 2 that planning must take into consideration previous research evidence as well as ethical and economic factors before the appropriate research strategy and measurement are selected, and the precise research hypothesis or aim is stated.

3. *Research design.* The usefulness of research depends on plans specifying appropriate sampling methods for ensuring the generalizability of the results. Appropriate designs are selected to ensure controlled observation in order to demonstrate causal relationships.

4. *Data collection.* The next step in the research process is collection of data. We will examine data collection methods commonly employed in qualitative and quantitative health research and the appropriate ways of carrying out measurements, and different types of measurement scales available for research and clinical assessment.

5. *Organization and presentation of the data.* Section 5 introduces descriptive statistics representing the conventions for summarizing and describing the data. Chapters 13–16 examine basic concepts in this area, outlining how graphs and various descriptive statistics are used to condense and communicate research and clinical findings. The presentation and analysis of qualitative data will be discussed in this text.

6. *Data analysis.* Data analysis involves applying the principles of probability for calculating confidence intervals and testing hypotheses. The area of inferential statistics, involving decisions concerning whether the data support experimental hypotheses, is outlined in this text.

7. *Interpretation of the evidence.* The final step in any research project involves interpreting one's findings. The findings may support existing theories or practices, suggest that new techniques may be more effective, or suggest new theoretical notions that are more able to explain phenomena. It is rare that the findings from any single research project are completely definitive, and often the results may suggest the need for further investigation in related subject areas or contexts. This issue will be examined in Sections 6 and 7.

8. *Publication.* For research to be scientifically meaningful, investigators must present their results in professional journals and at conferences. Research findings become part of scientific knowledge only if they stand up to methodological critique and replication. We will discuss conventions for preparing publications and outline steps for critically evaluating published research. Finally, in this text we will see how evidence from various related publications can be synthesized for guiding evidence-based practices.

Research and clinical practice

Research methods cover a wide variety of skills and techniques aimed at the methodologically valid investigation of questions of interest to the researcher. These methods of enquiry are not restricted to research laboratories, nor need they involve expensive equipment or large research teams. Rather, these methods imply an approach to stating and answering questions in any setting.

Applied research in the health sciences focuses on issues such as the prevalence and causes of illness, the usefulness and accuracy of assessment techniques, or the effectiveness of treatments. Applied research which is published aims at producing findings that are of general interest to groups of professionals working in the health field.

Research methods interact with health practices in multiple and mutually productive ways. An important general aim of this textbook is to discuss the relationships between theories, practices and the ways in which research methods contribute to improvments in health care. The term 'evidence-based medicine' has been defined by Sackett et al (2000) as '. . . the integration of best research evidence with clinical expertise and patient values'. Evidence-based health care (EBHC) is a contemporary movement aimed at ensuring that health services are based on the best available scientific and clinical evidence. The fundamental question which is explored in this book is 'what constitutes best research evidence?' The evidence is, of course, produced by applied health research conducted in accordance with the principles of the scientific method. Clearly if you expect to participate in the programme of EBHC you will need to understand research methods sufficiently for making informed and critical judgments concerning the quality of the available evidence.

Finally, we need to keep in mind that the research is produced by the hard work of men and women who were undergraduate students, just like you. Ultimately it will be up to you (as nurses, podiatrists, physiotherapists, speech pathologists and occupational therapists) to carry out the research which underpins the effectiveness, advancement and prestige of your profession. If not you, then who?

Summary

There are several common methods used for acquiring, stating and establishing knowledge. The scientific method is one of these and it underpins the validity of diagnoses and clinical interventions in Western health care systems. The scientific method is concerned with applying a set of rules or conventions that will allow us to produce scientifically valid knowledge. These rules specify how observations should be made, and how theories and hypotheses should be stated and evaluated.

Theories and hypotheses obtained and verified through scientific enquiry are not held to be absolutely 'true'. An inherent part of the scientific approach is scepticism regarding both the contents of knowledge and the underlying methodology. We have pointed out that there are controversies concerning what constitutes scientific methodology. It was argued that the scientific method is directly applicable to conducting research in the health sciences. In general, the stages for research include planning, stating aims or hypotheses, and formulating designs; collecting, summarizing and analysing the data; and drawing conclusions. This process can be applied to ensuring advances in health care and to problem solving in specific clinical settings. EBHC is a current approach to using best available research evidence for delivering health care. There is a close relationship between professional practices and health sciences research. The rest of the book is organized to follow the stages involved in performing and applying health research.

Self-assessment

Explain the meaning of the following terms:

authority
data
deduction
determinism
empiricism
evidence-based health care
falsification
hypothesis
induction
intuition
observation
positivism
post-positivism
pragmatism
qualitative
quantitative
rationalism
research programmes
scepticism
theory

True or false

1. A 'method' specifies how knowledge should be acquired, stated and tested.
2. Very strong intuitions always turn out to be true.
3. The method of authority depends on the status and credibility of the source.
4. When a syllogism is in a valid form, the conclusions should be factually true provided the premises are true.
5. Rationalism calls for correct reasoning for acquiring truth.
6. The case of Ignaz Semmelweis illustrates that medical decisions are based on the scientific method.
7. Scepticism refers to the notion that all knowledge is false.
8. Empiricism refers to the notion that events in the world occur according to regular laws and causes.
9. Scientific observations are different from ordinary observations because they depend on the use of instruments.
10. Scientific observations must be recorded as numbers.
11. Hypotheses are unproven theories.
12. Hypotheses are statements which specify the nature of the relationship between two or more sets of observations.
13. The logic underlying scientific generalization is called induction.
14. Scientific theories represent notions of natural events and their causes.
15. A good scientific theory is one that, in principle, cannot be falsified.
16. Controlled observation aims to identify the causes of events.
17. Scientific theories should enable the deduction of empirically verifiable hypotheses.
18. When the empirical evidence is found to be consistent with the implications of a hypothesis, we can say that the theory from which the hypothesis was deduced is absolutely true.
19. When we say that a theory was falsified, we mean that hypotheses deduced from it were not supported by empirical evidence.
20. We can question the content but not the methodology of science.

Multiple choice

1. A scientific theory is a set of statements:
   a conforming to the rules of logic
   b explaining the relationships which pertain among apparently diverse phenomena
   c which lead to empirically testable hypotheses
   d all of the above.
2. The statement 'Persons who are highly anxious do not perform well on learning tasks' is:
   a a theory
   b a hypothesis
   c false
   d in principle empirically untestable.
3. A scientific hypothesis:
   a should be verified through the use of logic and disputation
   b should be open to empirical verification
   c cannot arise through intuition
   d a and c.
4. The results of scientific research:
   a should be made available for critique and replication
   b should not be used to support existing theories
   c must be obtained under controlled laboratory settings
   d must conform to public expectations about the outcome.
5. Descriptive statistics:
   a are based on the principles of probability
   b represent conventions for planning research
   c represent conventions for summarizing and organizing data
   d specify the selection of appropriate measurement scales.
6. The scientific method is a set of rules specifying how:
   a scientific knowledge should be acquired, stated and tested
   b scientists should conduct their life
   c society should conduct its affairs
   d all of the above.
7. Authority, as a method, is:
   a no longer relevant to the conduct of health care
   b the fundamental source of the scientific method
   c neither a nor b
   d both a and b.

8. A therapist without formal medical qualifications treated cancer patients using an 'alternative' regimen of herbs, massage and meditation. Say that there is no scientific evidence available that such a treatment is effective. It follows that:
   a the treatment was ineffective because it lacks scientific evidence
   b the treatment was ineffective because the practitioner was unqualified
   c both a and b
   d neither a nor b.

9. As evidence for the effectiveness of the treatment, the therapist provides 100 signed statements from current or former patients claiming that they were satisfied with the treatment. One reason such evidence lacks scientific validity is that:
   a the opinions of patients cannot, in principle, constitute scientific evidence
   b it was not acquired in a manner consistent with the principles of scientific observation
   c we cannot, in principle, generalize from only 100 observations
   d it pertains to an 'alternative', non-scientific treatment regimen.

10. In the context of the scientific method, evidence which would be most indicative of the effectiveness of the treatment would be:
    a the support of medically qualified people
    b the argument that each patient has the right to select their own form of treatment
    c that the survival times of the patients were better than those of equivalent patients being treated with conventional therapies
    d that the patients were willing to pay money to receive the treatment.

11. The statement 'If my theory of schizophrenia is true, then the sun will rise tomorrow morning' is:
    a probably based on the invalid use of deduction
    b untestable
    c based on the method of authority
    d a and b.

12. According to an astrologer, people who were born under a particular star sign are 'basically kind and very intelligent, although because of their modesty, not sufficiently appreciated by others'. To test the truth of this statement, the astrologer asks a group of individuals if this description fits their personality; 95% of the sample agrees that the description is accurate. One of the problems with this enquiry is that:
    a astrology is inherently false, therefore the evidence must be wrong
    b 'personality' is inherently a misunderstood concept
    c in this case a 100% agreement is required for acceptable evidence
    d it is contrary to the principles of controlled observation.

13. The notion that facts are 'theory-dependent' implies that:
    a what is recorded as evidence is independent of the event being studied
    b theories and hypothesis have no relationship to empirical observations
    c what is recorded as evidence can be influenced by the theoretical notions of the observer
    d only our minds exist, rather than a material world.

14. Lakatos argued that:
    a theories are discarded only when their 'hard core' of propositions are falsified
    b a 'belt' of auxiliary hypotheses protect the fundamental 'hard core' propositions of a theory
    c theories cannot be refuted or falsified on the basis of empirical evidence
    d both a and b.

15. Which is the least controversial statement concerning the scientific method?
    a There is only one acceptable form of the scientific method independent of the phenomenon being investigated.
    b Scientific theories are derived from the use of induction, rather than creative insights.
    c The principles of the scientific method can be usefully applied to conducting health research.
    d Scientific enquiry is conducted independently of the personal values and social environment of scientists.

16. Which of the following problems might be best approached through the scientific method?
    a The clinical effectiveness of a new instrument needs to be evaluated.
    b The hospital budget is cut by 10%.
    c Personnel refuse to staff an abortion clinic on moral grounds.
    d The nursing staff go on strike.

Section One

Discussion, questions and answers

These questions ask you to examine issues concerning the applications of the scientific method to various aspects of health sciences research. Unlike the multiple choice and true or false questions, these discussion questions do not necessarily have a single correct answer. Rather, they are aimed at promoting a critical, integrative view of conducting research.

Our first discussion question involves theories and examines the relationships between theories, models, hypotheses and empirical observations. Theories are conceptual frameworks (as we discussed in Ch. 1) integrating a range of related observations and explanatory hypotheses. We may deduce empirically testable hypotheses from our theories.

On the basis of observations, in particular when the observations are carried out under controlled conditions, we establish the probable truth of our hypotheses, and thereby support or falsify the theories which were originally the sources for the hypotheses.

Some theories include models which represent specific aspects of a theory. Models are used to explain real situations and predict novel empirical outcomes. Models can be as follows:

1. *Physical models*. These models are constructed from materials, for example a 'pump' model of the heart for showing how the circulatory system works, or a construction of the DNA molecule to show how different nucleotides are organized in order to replicate genetic information.

2. *Mathematical models*. These models contain a series of equations that represent our theoretical interpretations of real-life situations. For example, epidemiologists may employ mathematical models to predict how a given epidemic might spread in a population, or a physiologist may employ a mathematical model of neuronal membranes to predict the behaviour of action potentials in a neurone. When our theories and related models are sufficiently detailed and well formed, we may use these in simulation research. We now use computers, which are capable of carrying out the complex calculations necessary for the simulation of a real-life situation and predicting numerical outcomes.

3. *'Paper and pencil' models*. Often, our theories are not sufficiently detailed to allow precise numerical predictions. Here the models are 'sketches' of a particular system, defining the key elements of the model and showing how these elements interact to produce various outcomes. Such models enable us to make testable predictions concerning the effects of variables as shown by the following model (Fig. D1.1) of the 'gate control theory' of pain (Melzack & Wall 1965). (Note that for teaching purposes this model is an incomplete and modified representation of the original. If you are interested in understanding pain problems, you should consult Melzack & Wall's original work.)

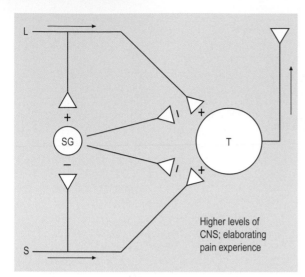

Figure D1.1 • Model of spinal gating of nociceptive input (adapted from Melzack & Wall 1965). See text for details.

Elements of the systems

(a) L: 'Large'-diameter axons of receptors, which convey information concerning mechanical stimuli, such as pressure and vibration.

(b) S: 'Small'-diameter axons of receptors, which convey information concerning noxious (tissue-damaging) stimuli.

(c) SG: Neurones within the substantia gelatinosa (SG) of the spinal cord. These receive converging information from L and S axons. The SG neurones control, or gate through pre-synaptic inhibition, the information flowing through to the T neurones.

(d) T: Transmission neurones in the spinal cord, which receive information from both L and S axons. The pattern of activity of T neurones is projected to higher levels of the central nervous system (CNS), where this information is elaborated into the experience of pain.

(e) Δ: Synapses, which may be either excitatory (+) or inhibitory (−). Excitatory synapses increase, while inhibitory synapses decrease the activity of the post-synaptic neurones.

(f) →: Arrows showing the direction of the information flow; in this case from the periphery towards the spinal cord and, subsequently, to higher levels of the CNS. The activity of large fibres (L) stimulates the gating mechanism (SG) which serves to inhibit nociceptive information conveyed by S axons to the T neurones.

The above model is an attempt to produce a representation of the events which take place in the mammalian nervous system when receiving and processing nociceptive input at a spinal cord level. The 'gate control' model integrates a broad range of research in the neurosciences and has been applied to explain aspects of pain control in clinical settings.

Questions

After this rather prolonged introduction to the model, we are ready to ask questions about how it may be applied to explaining and predicting observations about pain.

1. Use the above model to describe what happens in the nervous system during noxious (tissue-damaging) stimulation.

2. How would we use controlled observations to demonstrate that small (S), rather than large (L), neurones convey nociceptive information? (Assume that we have instrumentation for measuring the activity of single neurones in response to different kinds of stimuli.)

3. Explain how we would use evidence obtained by recording the activity of single neurones to demonstrate that T neurones are in fact involved in nociception.

4. Describe the effects of large (L) and small (S) axons on the activity of SG neurones.

5. Explain the mechanism by which SG neurones function as a 'pain-gating' system.

6. Propose a hypothesis for predicting the effects of selectively damaging T neurones on subsequent pain experience.

7. Propose a hypothesis for predicting the effects of damaging large axons (L) on subsequent pain experience.

8. A virus is identified which damages SG neurones. As a hypothetical case, imagine that people who have this virus report greatly reduced pain sensitivity. What would be the implication of this observation for the validity of the gate control theory of pain?

9. Would you discard the gate control theory on the bases of the hypothetical observations described in question 8? Explain.

10. A clinical technique called transcutaneous electrical nerve stimulation (TENS) for relieving pain involves the gentle peripheral electrical

stimulation of painful areas. Explain in terms of the model how TENS might work to reduce pain. (Hint: TENS does not directly reduce the activity of S axons.)

Answers

1. Small-diameter S axons convey nociceptive information towards spinal cord neurones, including the SG and the T neurones. The SG neurones are inhibited through nociceptive inputs while the T neurones are excited by the stimulation. Information concerning tissue damage is then conveyed by the axons of the T neurones to higher levels of the CNS. There it is elaborated into the experience of pain.

2. By showing that the activity of T neurones is correlated to the levels of peripheral noxious stimulation.

3. Mechanical stimuli – show that S axons are not responsive while L axons change rate of activity. Noxious stimuli – show that S axons change rate of activity while L remain unresponsive.

4. Large axons excite (increase the rate of activity of SG neurones) while small axons inhibit the rate of activity of the SG neurones.

5. The SG neurones inhibit the effect of the S axons on the T neurones. As L axons excite the SG neurones, the action of L fibres is to 'close' the pain gate. The S fibres 'open' the pain gate by inhibiting the SG neurones. In effect, the model is telling us that mechanical stimulation, such as gently scrubbing an injured area, will reduce nociceptive input. Conversely, noxious stimulation seems to maintain the effects of subsequent nociceptive inputs.

6. The T neurones are crucial for transmitting nociceptive information to higher levels of the CNS. Hypothesis: selectively damaging T neurones will reduce or eliminate pain experience following nociceptive stimulation.

7. Damage to L axons will result in reduced excitatory stimulation of the SG neurones, opening the spinal gate to noxious stimulation. Hypothesis: damaging L axons would increase the pain experienced following nociceptive stimulation.

8. As the model proposes that SG neurones are involved in the gating of noxious stimuli, we would predict that damage to the SG neurones would increase pain sensitivity. Reduced pain sensitivity is evidence which would falsify the gate control theory.

9. Probably not; as we discussed in the context of Lakatos' ideas. Theories have a 'protective belt' of assumptions, which means that a single empirical falsification need not result in the rejection of the theory. In this case, we may look for additional effects of the virus; say in destroying CNS tissue involved in elaborating pain experience. However, in the long run, such disconfirmations will lead to discarding the theory.

10. In terms of the model, TENS works by stimulating the L axons, and thereby 'closing' the pain gate, as outlined in questions 4 and 5.

Section **Two**

Research planning

SECTION CONTENTS

The first stage of research involves the detailed planning of the project. The plan for what is to occur in the project is written up in a document called the research protocol. Before the research project may proceed, the protocol is examined by ethics committees and funding bodies to ensure that it conforms with general methodological and ethical principles. The three chapters of Section 2 aim to outline the basic considerations for the successful preparation of a research protocol.

The primary reason for carrying out a research project is to obtain empirical evidence that will advance theory and practice in the health sciences. Before all else, we must be sure that we are asking the right questions, that is, raising issues and problems which are central to progress in contemporary health care. We must convince the critical reader that our aims or the hypotheses which we are attempting to resolve are of central importance. Asking the right research questions depends on being creative, for example identifying previously ignored patterns in the data, or the construction of novel theories that predict new, as yet unobserved phenomena. Of course, we are not suggesting that

researchers are geniuses, or that only brilliant, ground-breaking research is funded. Much important research is carried out by perfectly ordinary men and women who are interested in their patients and their problems, who have a good knowledge of their professional practices and who understand research methods.

To justify the research proposal it is necessary to write a 'literature review'. The literature review is a summary and critical evaluation of previous research and theory relevant to the problem we are intending to investigate. In this way the literature review provides both a conceptual background for our proposal and justifies the need for further empirical evidence by identifying 'gaps' in our knowledge.

The proposed research may be descriptive, for example collecting information concerning health needs of a community and/or the impact of illness or injury on a group of patients. In Chapter 3, non-experimental research strategies are described. Non-experimental research which includes both quantitative and qualitative surveys (Section 3) aims to provide a clear picture or description of the health of individuals, groups or whole communities. Experimental research strategies are appropriate when we are testing hypotheses about the causes of illness, and when we attempt to gain control over extraneous variables which may influence treatment outcomes. The notions of causality and control are central for health research and are explored in Chapter 4. Of course, when we write a research protocol, we must be sure that we select the appropriate research strategy.

No research can proceed unless it is judged to be ethical by an appropriate committee. A research proposal is judged ethical if it conforms with our rules and values concerning caregiving. These rules and values are made explicit in documents representing the standards of professional groups and of institutions (e.g. hospitals, universities and research councils). The research protocol must be described in sufficient detail so that a decision can be made as to whether any harm might occur to participants in the research project.

Economic considerations, or the availability of resources, also have a strong influence on research planning. For example, you may have designed a qualitative research project which involves 100 'in-depth' interviews with persons suffering from a disorder. Say you have only one year and a very limited amount of money to complete your project. You would be advised either to reduce your sample size or, if this is not possible, change your topic. Ethics or funding committees will only approve projects which can feasibly be completed with the available resources.

The way in which samples are selected is discussed in Chapter 3. Selection of an appropriate sample is crucial for the generalizability (or external validity) of your findings. Our aim is to select a representative sample of the population but this may not always be possible in health sciences research. We need a sample size which is sufficiently large to identify the phenomena in which we are interested, but not too large or we are simply wasting resources.

Thus, research planning is a process by which we transform our ideas into well-planned, ethical and economically feasible projects, as described in a research protocol.

Chapter Two

Research planning

CHAPTER CONTENTS

Introduction

Before the actual collection of information or data begins, researchers generally invest considerable time and effort in the planning of their investigations. The first step is to select and to justify the research problem. The second step is to transform the problem into clear researchable aims and research questions and, in the case of quantitative research, hypotheses are also usually specified. Research planning includes the selection of an appropriate research strategy for providing the required evidence to answer the research question. The selection of the appropriate research strategy may depend not only on the research questions being asked, but also on ethical issues and resource constraints that may define the scope and form of the investigation.

The specific aims of this chapter are to:

1. Discuss how research questions are selected and justified and derived from research aims.
2. Broadly outline research strategies available for specific types of investigations.
3. Discuss the ethical and economic constraints on the planning and implementation of research.

Sources of research questions

Advances in health research depend on the identification of questions and problems that promote the development of more powerful theories of health, illness and disability, and then devising more effective ways of assessing, treating and preventing health problems. This advancement depends very much on researchers asking the 'right' questions and identifying solvable problems and then applying sound investigation methods to these questions and problems.

The formulation of research questions depends on the expertise of researchers who have a combination of theoretical knowledge and practical experience for identifying problems and asking the right questions. The professional background of researchers is an important consideration, as one's educational background and practices will influence what are seen as theoretically and professionally interesting problems.

The formulation of even apparently simple research questions is often the culmination of intensive preliminary observations, spending long hours in the library reading through and critically analysing related research, discussing the issues and thinking through a range of issues.

The health care setting in which the researcher works may also have a strong influence on the formulation of research questions. For example, it is an important consideration if the researcher works in a laboratory, a hospital, a community clinic or in private practice. These settings will often influence how the patients' problems are perceived, and how researchers define professionally relevant solutions to these problems.

In many areas of health care, including areas such as rehabilitation, community health and neurosciences, researchers sharing similar interests may join together in multidisciplinary research teams. Because of the broad range of expertise and perspectives, such teams may be in a position to formulate interesting research questions that can be simultaneously addressed from these different perspectives.

The formulation of research questions

The formulation of research questions is a creative act. It draws upon consideration of previous relevant work in the area under study. This work may be reviewed and the review may give rise to questions that have not been answered by previous work. A literature review is the usual way in which knowledge gaps are identified. The purpose of the review is to answer the questions 'What do we know?' and 'What do we not know?'

Inspiration for research questions often stems from personal experience. Exposure to an issue or problems may raise questions suitable for a research study. Most health practitioners constantly pose questions like 'What is the best and most effective method of treating this condition?' and 'How can we ensure that patients or clients get what they want from this service?'

The justification of research questions

When researchers call on public funds to conduct their studies, they must explain in what way their intended study will contribute to scientific knowledge and/or clinical practice. In 'pure' or 'basic' scientific research, a proposed investigation is justified in terms of its potential contribution to existing knowledge. In the context of 'applied' health research, the investigator may be required to demonstrate that the research will in some way contribute to the improved practice of health care, and benefit patients.

Before embarking on the design and conduct of a research project, the investigator must review previous work and publications relevant to the aims of the intended project. This process is essential, both for providing the appropriate background and context for the investigation, and for justifying the investigation in contributing to existing knowledge. It is a waste of money to duplicate very similar research (although deliberate replication of previous studies may be a legitimate activity if there are uncertainties about the validity of a previous study).

Literature searching may be carried out at appropriate research centres or libraries where scientific and professional journals are stored and, of course, by using the Internet. There are powerful web-based search methods that can simplify the search.

The most widely used search tool for health research publications is probably PubMed, the web-based Public Medline (see http://www.ncbi.nlm.nih.gov/entrez/). Professional library staff can help you to locate the relevant literature. However, the critical evaluation of the literature depends on the application of research methods for the identification of controversies or 'gaps' in the available evidence.

Formulation of research aims

Hypotheses in quantitative research

Quantitative research is normally structured so as to test a research hypothesis. Hypotheses are propositions about relationships between variables or differences between groups that are to be tested. Hypotheses may be concerned with relationships between observations or variables (for example, 'Is there an association between level of exercise and annual health care expenditure?') or differences between groups (for example, 'Do patients treated under therapy x exhibit greater improvement than those treated under therapy y?'). A *variable* is a property that varies, for example the room temperature, the ages of the patients, or their improvement on a clinical measurement scale.

Some quantitative research projects do not have a hypothesis to be tested in any formal sense. For example, if you are assessing the health needs of a local community, there need not be any specific expectation or hypothesis to be tested. The purpose of the research may be simply to describe accurately the characteristics of the study sample and target population. The goal is not to test a specific hypothesis. This does not mean the research is deficient; it just means it has a different objective from other types of quantitative research projects. So hypothesis testing is a characteristic of many, but not all, quantitative projects.

Qualitative research does not usually test hypotheses. It is concerned with understanding the personal meanings and interpretations of people concerning specified issues. However, most qualitative researchers work with specified research aims and questions to guide their investigation.

The formulation of adequate research aims generally involves a process during which the researcher gradually refines a broadly based issue into more specific operationally defined statements. This process must take into account the logical requirements of designs for information and data collection and ethical standards for conducting health research. In addition, the research aims must inform a realistic data collection procedure which can be supported by the resources available for researchers. We will examine these issues in the rest of this chapter.

Research strategies

Research planning also involves the selection or formulation of research strategies. Research strategies are established procedures for designing and executing research. The research strategies that are outlined in this book include experimental and quasi-experimental strategies, single case research, surveys and qualitative research. Before detailed discussion of the differences between these strategies is undertaken in the following sections, it is instructive to compare the basic structures of survey research and experimental research. As we shall see in subsequent sections, these are fundamentally different ways of conducting research.

Survey research strategies

The three essential steps involved in survey research strategies are shown in Figure 2.1. You will note in Figure 2.1 that the researcher defines the population of interest, selects the cases to be studied and then observes or studies them, generating the data. There is no intended active intervention in the situation by the researcher. Indeed, intervention that would change the phenomenon being studied is discouraged and avoided. In this type of research strategy there is a constant tension between the requirements for close and detailed observation (proximity to the phenomenon under study) and the possibility that the behaviour of the research participants under study may change because they are being studied. There are techniques for dealing with this problem, such as the use of unobtrusive

Figure 2.1 • Structure of a survey research strategy.

Figure 2.2 • Experimental research strategies.

measures and participant observation, which will be discussed in subsequent chapters.

Experimental research strategies

Experimental research strategies involve a sequence of steps, as illustrated in Figure 2.2. As with the survey research strategy, cases are selected for study from a defined population. However, these cases are then assigned (generally by chance or random method) to a treatment (intervention) or non-treatment (non-intervention) group, and then given the intervention or, in clinical contexts, the treatment. The term 'treatment' is used here in the sense that the subject or event is being systematically influenced or manipulated by the investigator; that is, in a broader sense than with medical or physical treatment. For this reason the broader term 'intervention' is often used in place of the term 'treatment'. The intervention and non-intervention groups are then observed and compared. If everything went according to plan, any differences in the results for the intervention and non-intervention groups should be a result of the effects of the intervention. This type of design is often called a randomized controlled (sometimes clinical) trial or RCT. In some review systems such as the Cochrane Collaboration system, the RCT is considered to be the 'best' level of evidence to establish the effectiveness of an intervention.

Thus, there is quite a difference in the structure of experimental and survey (non-experimental) and qualitative research strategies. Cook & Campbell (1979) proposed a separate class of '*quasi-experimental*' strategies (which are really just tightly structured non-experimental strategies) that we will also cover later in this book.

The decision of the investigator to adopt specific research strategies depends on the phenomenon being studied and the specific question type of research (causal or descriptive) being investigated.

Research planning: ethical considerations

In health research, where the health and lives of people participating in the study may be at stake, ethical considerations play a key role in research planning and implementation. For instance, consider the question of whether cigarette smoking has negative impacts on health. One way of investigating this question would be through experiments, which are generally considered to be the design best suited to establishing causal relationships. However, it would be ethically unacceptable to have a number of people randomly assigned to a group involved in long-term, heavy cigarette smoking as this would very likely damage their health. Clearly, to meet ethical criteria, evidence must come from studies in which investigators observe the effects of smoking in persons who have themselves chosen to smoke.

A research process is judged to be *ethical* by the extent to which it conforms to or complies with the set of standards or conventions in the context in which the research is to be carried out. In different countries, the various medical research councils have developed detailed statements concerning these standards. In the United Kingdom the Medical Research Council has a series of statements and publications available at its web-site (http://www.mrc.ac.uk), as does the Australian National Health and Medical Research Council on its web-site at http://www.nhmrc.gov.au. Canada has the statements by the Interagency Advisory Panel on Research Ethics (http://www.pre.ethics.gc.ca). In the United States there is a proliferation of bodies with research ethics guidelines, mostly based upon the 1979 work by the Belmont group. All of these guidelines draw upon the pioneering 1964 Helsinki declaration from the World Medical Association.

Most health services and higher education institutions now have their own ethics committees to oversee health research involving humans and/or animals. Ethics committees, along with the researcher, are responsible for interpreting and enforcing ethical standards. It should be noted, however, that even when a given research proposal is judged to be ethical, it may not be seen as *moral* by specific individuals or groups in a community. A good example is animal experimentation when the research involves painful or stressful procedures such as surgery. According to the value systems of some persons and groups, such work may be considered to be intrinsically immoral. From this viewpoint, there may be no acceptable justification for inflicting suffering on animals, even when the results may be beneficial for humans. Others may argue that such procedures are morally justified, given that they are necessary for the advancement of the biological and medical sciences and provided that reasonable steps are taken to limit the suffering of the animals. There are no absolute solutions for such controversies as they involve human values, but discussing these issues in public may help to establish a degree of consensus in the community and guidance for the ethical decisions of researchers.

It is beyond the scope of this discussion to examine in full the ethics of health research, but the following issues are central to making decisions in these areas:

1. *Benefits.* Who is to benefit from the research? One likes to think that 'humanity', 'the participants', or 'health science' are going to be the beneficiaries of health research. A slightly more cynical analysis points to the investigators as having the most to gain, at least in the short term. After all, given a successful outcome for the research project, they stand to satisfy their curiosity, improve their career prospects or to raise their esteem before colleagues. In practice, benefits accruing to the investigator, the participants and health science have to be carefully weighed in relation to the conduct of any project. The protection of the rights and welfare of the participants is the primary consideration of research ethics.

2. *Informed consent.* Informed consent by the participants is a necessary condition for ethically acceptable research. This means that all the risks involved in the investigation must be explained to prospective participants, as well as the possible benefits, and they must decide about their participation or non-participation in an informed manner. Honest explanation of the procedures to the participant takes considerable skill, as disclosing the design of the study may influence the expectations and behaviour of the participants. Also, special care needs to be taken when the participants are in some way limited in their ability to understand the risks; for example, people who are intellectually disabled, or confused under the influence of drugs. Informed consent implies a freedom of choice: participants must feel confident that refusal to participate will not prejudice their subsequent clinical treatment.

3. *Protection of participants.* It is the investigator's responsibility to minimise the chances of long-term deleterious effects to subjects. Dangers can arise from administering new interventions or treatments with unknown side effects, denying interventions of known effectiveness or using invasive assessment techniques. The welfare of laboratory animals must not be ignored. There are nowadays legally enforceable constraints in most jurisdictions on the conditions for using animals in research.

4. *Minimizing discomfort.* The investigator must also minimize even short-term pain, anxiety, discomfort or embarrassment involved in an investigation, especially if it is not part of routine therapeutic practice. This is an important issue, as some therapists and researchers take a mistakenly 'proprietary' view of their patients, imagining that they should put up with some discomfort for the good of medical science. In the past, patients in public wards of hospitals and long-term prisoners have been most vulnerable to questionable ethical practices.

5. *Privacy.* Health care research may involve collecting information that can lead to the embarrassment

or stigmatization of the participants. The identity of participants must be protected; for instance, by 'coding' their real names so that they may not be identified even inadvertently. In qualitative research where the full text of comments may be reported, it is important that this text does not inadvertently identify people through the reporting of identifiable scenarios or names.

6. *Community values.* Some research, such as that involving the assessment of sexual function-ing or the investigation of human fetuses, calls for very sensitive planning. Anatomical research involving the use of human cadaver material must be planned to ensure respectful handling and disposal. Even if the investigator does not agree, the values and taboos of groups in the community must be taken into consideration when planning the investigation.

7. *Conservation of resources.* A fundamental value is that the time and effort of researchers and sub-jects and the resources of the community should not be wasted on a badly planned investigation. Of course, there can never be a guarantee that an investigation will produce clinically useful results. However, some poorly designed projects are doomed to failure even before the data collection begins, and lead to confusion and controversy in the professional literature. Therefore, the appro-priate use of high-quality and sound research methods is not only useful for solving problems, but constitutes an ethical necessity. Many ethics committees also vet projects for scientific merit before the project is approved.

A responsible investigator is required to take into consideration ethical principles and to plan research projects accordingly so that no, or the minimum possible, harm is caused. Therefore, the health researcher must use considerable ingenuity in designing valid investigations, while maintaining ethical values. One of the roles of ethics committees is to guide investigators on complex issues, and to ensure that research is conducted in accordance with accepted community principles.

Selection of research strategies: economic considerations

Selection of appropriate research strategies can also be influenced by the resources available to investigators. Some projects involving the evalu-ation of the safety and effectiveness of new drugs, or the identification of risk factors in cardiac disease, have taken tens of millions of dollars to finance. Research planning takes into account eco-nomic issues, such as:

1. *Availability of participants.* Here the investigator has to consider if enough people can participate in the project under the required conditions. Attention has to be paid to issues such as the frequency of the disorder in the community, problems in identifying participants and their level of voluntary participation. As will be shown in Chapter 3, selection of participants is crucial for the validity of a study.

2. *Availability of equipment.* Some equipment is costly to acquire or to operate (for example, CT (computed tomography) scanners, biochemical assays, experimental drugs). Research planning should take these expenses into account.

3. *Availability of expertise.* Specialized assessment techniques and the administration of clinical treat-ments require professional expertise. If these are beyond the investigator's competence or if the experimental design requires an unbiased, 'blind' therapist or assessor (see Ch. 5), there must be means for securing them.

4. *Availability of time.* Research projects have a tendency to take considerably longer than an inexperienced researcher might expect, due to the erratic and at times disastrous workings of Murphy's law: 'If anything can go wrong, it will'. Equipment breaks down and needs to be repaired, subjects 'disappear', collaborators might not deliver services promised. Research planning should take into account possible prob-lems and how these might affect the time scale of investigations. This is a particularly important issue for postgraduate students.

The availability of resources strongly influences the scope of the research programme and also the research strategy selected by the investigator. A research project must be shown to be feasible from a cost viewpoint before it is initiated. It is only after the ethical constraints and economic resources have been evaluated that the researchers' questions can be transformed into clearly defined hypotheses or aims.

It is important when conducting research that the identities of all supporting agencies and individuals are disclosed to the participants in order that their agreement to participate is fully informed.

Steps in research planning

The following steps should be considered in quantitative research before actual data collection begins. The term 'data' refers to the set of observations recorded during an investigation.

1. Identification of the research problem.
2. Retrieval and critical evaluation of relevant literature for justifying and giving the context of the research problem.
3. Formulation of precise research aims and questions in the light of:
   (a) the information to be collected
   (b) the appropriate research strategies
   (c) the ethical considerations required to protect participants and the community
   (d) the projected cost of the project.
4. In addition, as to be discussed in this book, research planning takes into account:
   (a) how the participants are to be selected
   (b) the design of the investigation
   (c) how the data are to be collected
   (d) how the data are to be analysed.

The above points are written up in the form of a *research protocol*. This protocol is submitted to supervisors, colleagues or ethical committees, for scrutiny of methodological and ethical problems. It is only when the protocol is acceptable to all these parties that the actual data collection begins. It is often desirable to carry out a small-scale preliminary study, called a 'pilot'. This is an economical way of identifying and eliminating potential problems in the large-scale investigation.

Summary

The planning of a research project requires the transformation of a vague question or problem into clearly stated aims or questions. To achieve this, the researcher should review the relevant literature and evaluate ethical considerations and economic constraints in conducting the investigation. Next, an appropriate research strategy needs

to be selected. On the basis of the above, the researcher is in a position to state precisely the aims or hypotheses being investigated.

Before data collection begins, a protocol for the complete investigation is scrutinized by colleagues to correct methodological problems, or to prevent unethical research.

Self-assessment

Explain the meaning of the following terms:

ethics
informed consent
literature review
Murphy's law
non-experimental study
pilot study
research strategy
variable

True or false

1. Scientific research always involves the testing of hypotheses.
2. A sample is a subset of the data.
3. The population being studied is defined after the sample has been selected.
4. A research protocol is a summary of the data obtained in an investigation.
5. A pilot is a small-scale research programme to demonstrate the feasibility of an investigation.
6. Human cadavers are not sentient beings, therefore their treatment falls outside the scope of medical ethics.
7. Planning quantitative research includes specifying the variables to be studied and how these are to be measured.
8. Abstract constructs, like 'intelligence' or 'motivation', cannot have empirical referents.
9. A literature review is necessary for providing the appropriate background and rationale for an investigation.
10. Well-established data collection techniques are called research findings.
11. A non-experimental design involves the assignment of subjects to treatment groups.
12. Both experimental and non-experimental designs involve the drawing of an appropriate sample from the population being studied.

13. An anthropologist studying how ethnic groups relate to illness would tend to adopt a quantitative research strategy.
14. The clear explanation of the risks involved in a research project is a necessary condition for obtaining informed consent from a subject.
15. The use of correct research methods does not constitute an ethical necessity.
16. A hypothesis is a proposition about the relationship existing between variables or prediction of differences between groups.
17. Some scientific research projects do not involve the testing of hypotheses.
18. Existing theories are the only appropriate sources for experimental hypotheses.
19. In a non-experimental study there is no need to pay attention to sampling.
20. Experimental designs involve the assignment of the sampled subjects into treatment groups.
21. Experimental designs are more appropriate than non-experimental designs for demonstrating causal relationships.
22. The subjects participating in medical research are generally the most likely beneficiaries of the project.
23. Informed consent of human subjects is necessary even when the investigation is not apparently embarrassing or dangerous.
24. It is unethical to study human sexual behaviour because people find it embarrassing to serve as subjects.
25. Medical researchers should expect that patients who receive free hospital treatment should participate in medical experiments.
26. The correct use of research methods in conducting an investigation is useful, but not an ethical necessity.
27. A well-designed, relevant research project will always be financed, regardless of the expense.
28. A variable is a property or attribute which varies from subject to subject.

Multiple choice

1. The aim of research planning is to:
   a generate appropriate aims or clear-cut research hypotheses
   b select an appropriate research strategy
   c identify possible ethical or economic limitations in conducting the investigation
   d a and b
   e all of the above.

2. A 'literature review':
   a is a list of research publications relevant to an investigation
   b should discredit research findings which are inconsistent with the hypothesis
   c should include only findings which directly support the hypothesis being investigated
   d should be a critical review of findings relevant to an investigation.

3. Which of the following is common to both experimental and non-experimental research strategies?
   a random assignment
   b selection of cases to be studied
   c experimental hypothesis
   d participant observation
   e field research.

4. Which of the following is unique to the experimental research strategy?
   a random assignment
   b selection of cases to be studied
   c definition of population
   d participant observation
   e field research.

5. The availability of resources to conduct an investigation:
   a is not the concern of a scientific researcher
   b has an influence on the scope and design of the investigation
   c is determined by Murphy's law
   d none of the above.

6. 32 degrees Centigrade is an example of:
   a a variable
   b the value of a variable
   c a ratio
   d a null hypothesis.

7. A variable is:
   a a property which can take different values across different individuals
   b a property which can take different values within an individual
   c both a and b
   d neither a nor b.

8. Which of the following ethical requirements is the *most* difficult to satisfy when conducting a placebo-controlled randomized clinical trial?
   a Ensuring the privacy of the research participants.
   b Obtaining informed consent from all research participants.

c Protecting research participants from unnecessary risks.

d Providing the best available treatment for all research participants.

9. Which of the following represents the most explicitly formulated research aim?

a The aim of the present project was to investigate if health care workers in Gotham City were satisfied with their pay and career prospects.

b The aim of the present project was to investigate if emotionally disturbed persons living in Gotham City received adequate medical care.

c The aim of the present project was to identify the reasons why health professionals in Gotham City leave their professions, and turn to other types of employment.

d The aim of the present project was to identify the proportion of teenagers in Gotham City smoking more than 10 cigarettes a day.

10. A research protocol should make explicit:

a the justification for undertaking the research project

b the way in which the data are to be collected

c the empirical evidence provided by the investigation

d a and b.

11. Which of the following represents a non-researchable problem (in the context of the scientific method)?

a Is aspirin preferable to steroids in reducing the symptoms of arthritis?

b Does the use of alcohol result in greater levels of brain damage than the use of marijuana?

c Are painful experiments involving animals justified if they lead to benefits to patients?

d Do people coming from a low socioeconomic class receive poorer health care than people from a higher class?

Chapter Three

3

Sampling methods and external validity

Introduction

Research in the health sciences usually involves the collection of information from a sample of participants, rather than on the entire population in which the investigator is interested. Studies that involve an entire population or group are called *census* studies but these are relatively rare and generally expensive to perform. A sample drawn from the target population is studied because it is usually impossible or too costly to study entire populations. For instance, when individuals who have conditions such as diabetes, cerebral palsy or emphysema are being studied, it is not possible to study everyone because of the large size of such populations. Also because many people do not seek treatment or may be wrongly diagnosed, we may not be able to identify all members of the entire population in order to study them. Therefore, in most research, the researcher studies a subset or sample of the target population, and then attempts to generalize the findings to the population from which the participants were drawn. This general principle applies to both qualitative and quantitative studies.

The aim of this chapter is to examine ways that samples can be drawn to permit the investigator to make valid generalizations from the study sample to the target population. We will also consider the question of generalizing the findings of an investigation to other samples and situations. This is referred to as 'external validity' or 'generalizability'.

The specific aims of this chapter are to:

1. Define what is meant by sampling and representative samples.
2. Outline the relative advantages and disadvantages of commonly used sampling methods.
3. Discuss the relationship between sampling error and sample size.
4. Examine the concept of external validity for generalizing research findings to other settings.

What is sampled in a study

While this chapter will focus on the selection of the research participants in a study, many other things are also selected or sampled. These include:

1. the information to be collected by the researcher
2. the procedures used for the collection of the information
3. where the research is conducted, e.g. in a field setting or in a structured research setting
4. the clinicians and researchers who are involved.

Many researchers focus on the selection of the research participants as the key or only issue in maximizing the generalizability of their research, and they do not pay enough attention to the other factors they are sampling or the context in which the research is being conducted. It is not at all unusual to see studies that employ large and sophisticated participant samples, yet with only one or two highly selected clinicians involved in the research in perhaps only one health setting. While the study sample may be highly representative, the context in which the research is conducted may not be and it may be that the researchers and clinicians involved in the study have a particularly unusual or idiosyncratic approach to their work that is not reflective of others. It is our contention that in many qualitative studies there is strong consideration of the research context and its impact upon the research findings. However, there is often less emphasis upon sampling of research participants. This impacts upon the ability to generalize the findings more broadly from the actual research participants to other groups.

Basic issues in sampling

As we have discussed, often, because of the numbers involved, it is not within the resources of the researcher to study the whole target population. In any event, in most situations it would be wasteful to study all of the population. If a sample is representative, one can generalize validly from the sample's results to the population without going to the expense of studying everyone.

The population is the target group of individuals or cases in which the researcher is interested. Examples of valid study populations include: all English women under 25; all children with diagnosed spina bifida in the state of Alberta; all the students at a particular Australian college. The researcher defines the population to which he/she wishes to generalize. Note that a population need not consist of human or animal subjects. Objects or events can also be sampled, as shown in Table 3.1.

As shown in Table 3.1, a population is an entire set of persons, objects or events which the researcher intends to study. A sample is a subset of the population. Sampling involves the selection of the sample from the population.

Representative samples

There is a variety of different ways by which one can select the sample from the population. These are called sampling methods.

The ultimate aim of all sampling methods is to draw a representative sample from the population. The advantage of a representative sample is clear: one can confidently generalize from a representative sample to the rest of the population without having to take the trouble of studying the rest of the population. If the sample is biased (not representative of the population) one can generalize less validly from the sample to the population. This might lead to quite incorrect conclusions or inferences about the population. This would mean that the results obtained in the study would not necessarily generalize to other studies using the same population. Figure 3.1 illustrates the concept of a representative sample.

Table 3.1 Examples of populations and samples

Population	Possible sample selection
All working podiatrists in a state	50 podiatrists selected for a study of job satisfaction
All working pathologists in a state	25 pathologists selected for detailed tax evaluation by an inspector
The temperature of a patient during a 24-hour period	Hourly measurements of the patient's temperature recorded by staff
Stuttering in a child's speech	Number of stutters made during 5 minutes of reading a standard piece of material
All patients in a state with frontal lobe damage	30 patients with frontal lobe damage selected for evaluating a rehabilitation programme
All surgical gauzes held by a given hospital	10 gauzes selected by a bacteriologist to test for sterility

Figure 3.1 • A simple representative sample.

Figure 3.1 illustrates a hypothetical population composed of three different types of study participants or categories of participants. A representative sample is a precise miniaturized representation of the population. An unrepresentative or biased sample does not adequately represent the key groups or characteristics in the population, and this may lead to mistaken conclusions about the state of the population.

The selection of the appropriate sampling method depends upon the aims and resources of the researchers. For instance, if someone is designing a very expensive health or social welfare programme on the basis of a survey of clients' needs, it is imperative that the researcher uses a good sampling method and obtains a representative sample of the clients, so that appropriate conclusions may be reached about the population. Good sampling methods are somewhat more expensive and more difficult to implement than poor methods but they are worth it. The main sampling methods used in health research are incidental and random sampling.

Incidental samples

Incidental sampling is the cheapest, easiest and most commonly used sampling method in clinical studies. It involves the selection of the most accessible and available members of the target population. For example, a researcher who stands in the middle of a city street and quizzes people about their health status is practising incidental sampling. However, it is quite likely that this sample would not be representative of the general voting population. There would probably be an over-representation of businessmen and white-collar workers, and an under-representation of factory workers and housewives. The sample is likely to be unrepresentative and biased.

A further example of incidental sampling might involve a researcher surveying the needs of a group of spina bifida children at a local community health centre. Their measured needs may be representative of those of other spina bifida children, but then again they may not if these children are not typical of the wider population of children with spina bifida.

Thus, incidental sampling is cheap and easy to implement but may give a biased sample that is not representative of the population.

Quota sampling

Sometimes it is known in advance that there are important subgroups within the population that

Table 3.2 Distribution of percentages of gender and occupational variables in the general population

	Blue collar	White collar	Not employed	Total
Male	19	21	9	49
Female	15	15	21	51
Total	34	36	30	100

need to be included in the sample. Two such important groups within the human population are males and females. Further, it is known that they occur in the ratio of approximately 49:51 in the general population. Our researcher might decide that it is very important that the sexes are proportionally represented in the sample. Thus, the researcher would set two quotas (of 49 male and 51 female respondents in a sample of 100) and sample accordingly in a city street. This is still a form of incidental sampling but has some significant advantages over simple incidental sampling because the study sample's composition on this key demographic variable is guaranteed to match that of the target population.

More sophisticated examples involving more than two groups can be accommodated as shown in Table 3.2. We can see from Table 3.2 that if our sample were to be representative regarding both sex and occupational status, in a sample of 100 people we would need 19 blue-collar males, 15 blue-collar females, and so on.

Quota sampling still has a number of shortcomings: before it can be used, one has to know which population groups are likely to be important to a particular question and the exact proportions of the various groups in the population. Sometimes we may not know these proportions. Also, the members of the sample within the quotas are still incidentally chosen. The blue-collar males, for example, selected in a city centre on a weekday may still be quite different from those working elsewhere. However, quota sampling is better than simple incidental sampling.

Random and systematic samples

Random sampling

This is one of the best but probably more expensive sampling methods to implement in drawing a study sample. A random sample is one in which all members of the population have an equal chance of selection. Thus a random sample is more likely to be representative of the relevant population than an incidental sample.

The procedure for drawing a random sample involves:

1. the construction of a list of all members of the population
2. using a method such as dice, coins, hat or random number tables to select randomly from the list the number of members required for the sample.

A simple example of a random sample is provided by a common raffle, where names on (preferably!) equal-size papers are put in a hat, shaken and selected 'blind'. Many national and state lotteries use numbered balls that are drawn randomly from a barrel. Another way to draw a random sample is to construct a list of all the members of the population and assign a number to each element. Then a table of random numbers, generated by a computer, could be used to select a random sample.

Cases that are selected from a list using a random selection method constitute a random sample. Sometimes, because of issues such as refusal to participate in the study, dropping out and failure to satisfy the sample inclusion criteria, it is necessary to select replacements for some cases that are unavailable for the study. This can introduce bias into the sample, as the people who refuse may differ consistently from those who accept or volunteer. This impact on sampling validity is sometimes called the volunteer effect.

However, random sampling methods have a number of important advantages over incidental or non-random methods:

- Because the exact sizes of the sample and population are known, it is possible to estimate exactly how representative the sample is; that is, the size of the sampling error. This cannot usually be done with non-random sampling methods.
- Because random samples are usually more representative than non-random samples, the

sample size needed for good representation of the population is smaller.

The major disadvantages of random sampling methods are:

- The researcher needs to be able to list every member of the population. Often this is impossible because the full extent of the population is not known. For example, it would be very difficult to sample randomly from the population of Canadians with coronary disease, because no such list exists. Even if it did exist it would be constantly changing.
- Cost. It is usually easier to use conveniently available groups. Random sampling usually involves considerable planning and expense, especially with large populations.

Stratified random sampling

This involves the same approach as quota sampling with set quotas from specific subgroups, except that each quota is filled by randomly sampling from each subgroup, rather than sampling incidentally. For example, if one was drawing a sample stratified with respect to sex, one would prepare a list of all females and all males in the target population and then sample randomly from these lists with the numbers of each group in the sample corresponding to the population proportions. These groups collectively are called the strata.

The advantages of stratified random sampling are:

- All the important groups are proportionally represented.
- The exact representativeness of the sample is known. This has important statistical ramifications.

The disadvantages are:

- A list of all members of the population, their characteristics and the proportions of the important groups within the population need to be known.
- Cost.
- The gain in sample accuracy is usually small in comparison to simple random sampling.

Area sampling

In area sampling, one samples on the basis of location of cases. For example, on the basis of census data the investigator may select several areas in a city or county with known characteristics, such as high or low unemployment rates. The areas could then be further divided into specific streets and the occupants of, say, every third house contacted for participation in the study. In other words, the locations are randomly selected and then one interviews the occupants of those locations. This can be a very effective, cheap method of sampling in social surveys. It does not require a list of the individual members of the population, merely the location where they live. Recent research has shown that where people live can be an important factor in their health status and their use of health services. The study of the impact of where people live upon health and social issues is sometimes called (geo-) spatial analysis.

Systematic sampling

This involves working through a list of the population and choosing, say, every 10th or 20th case for inclusion in the sample. It is not a truly random technique but it will usually give a representative sample. It is based on the (usually justified) supposition that cases are not added to the list in a systematic way which coincides with the sampling system. Provided a list of cases is available, systematic sampling is an easy and convenient sampling method. In clinical practice we are using systematic sampling when, for instance, we measure temperature and blood pressure every hour.

Sample size

One of the most poorly understood aspects of sampling is the number of cases that should be included in a study sample. The whole issue of sampling is conceptualized somewhat differently for qualitative and quantitative studies, although the issue of to what extent the results of a study are generalizable is the same whatever the study design.

It is obvious that in one sense the more cases selected the merrier (or the better the sample representativeness), but the costs associated with the sampling and data collection must be weighed up against the greater generalizability that is generally associated with larger samples. Also, some studies may involve discomfort, pain or even danger to patients or laboratory animals. Therefore, in this case it is ethically and logistically desirable to ensure that no more than the bare minimum of subjects is used to achieve the desired sample accuracy. Health researchers 'walk a tightrope' in deciding the optimum sample sizes for their studies. However, there are some principles available to guide the researcher.

First of all, let us say quite definitely that there is no magic number that we can point to as an 'optimum' sample size. Rather, the optimum sample size depends on the characteristics of an investigation in the context of which the sample is drawn. In general, the optimum sample size is one which is adequate for making correct generalizations from the sample to the target population. Let us discuss these issues by introducing the concept of sampling error.

Sampling error

In the quantitative research framework, sampling error is the discrepancy between the true population parameter and the sample statistic. For example, if I happen to know from census data that the actual average age of males in a district is 35 years and the average age of a sample of males I have surveyed from the district is 30 years, then I have a sampling error of 5 years. However, if we do not know the actual population parameters (which is commonly the case), we can only estimate the probable sampling error.

Sampling error is related to sample size by the following relationship:

$$\text{Sampling error} \propto \frac{1}{\sqrt{n}}$$

What the above equation claims is that the greater the sample size (n), the smaller the probability sampling error. In fact, the sampling error in a study sample is inversely proportional to the square root of the sample size.

From this relationship it can be seen that doubling the sample size would only result in a reduction of the error by a factor of the square root of 2 (1.414). Similarly, a ninefold increase in sample size would result in only a threefold reduction in

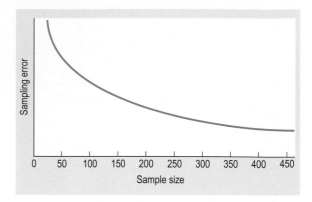

Figure 3.2 • The relationship between sample size and sampling error. The scaling but not the form of the curve will alter with the variability of the data.

the sampling error. Figure 3.2 illustrates this point by showing the graphical relationship between probable sampling error and sample size.

It can be seen from this graph that not much is gained from a sample size of over, say, n_1. Yet the cost of the sampling and data collection can be very high with large numbers (such as n_2), for relatively little gain in reducing sampling error. In some research situations, even large probable sampling errors have relatively little potential influence on our decisions. In such situations, we can live with a relatively small sample size. In other situations, we need large samples to justify our confidence in the truth of our decisions.

As an illustration, suppose that we are attempting to predict the outcome of an election fought between two political parties, A and B. A representative sample of 100 respondents is polled before the election. Say the outcome is as follows:

Intends to vote for A	Intends to vote for B	Estimated sampling error
25%	75%	10%

In this instance, the estimated sampling error is very small in relation to the size of the effect (that is, the difference between the percentage of intended votes for the two parties). We can predict confidently, assuming that the respondents were truthful and don't change their minds before the elections, that political party B will romp into government. Increasing sample size, say to 10 000, would enormously increase the cost of the survey. The corresponding reduction in sampling error would not justify this cost, as we would still come to the same conclusion. However, say the following sample statistics were obtained in the pre-election poll of $n = 100$ respondents:

Intends to vote for A	Intends to vote for B	Estimated sampling error
48%	58%	10%

Now the same level of estimated sampling error is too large, in relation to the apparent size of the effect, to make a decision concerning which party is likely to win the election. The poll would have to be repeated using a substantially increased sample size to reduce the sampling error.

The example illustrates the notion that the adequacy of the sample size is affected by the specific situation that we are trying to research. A sample size which is adequate in one situation may be inadequate in another. One benefit of a previous pilot study is that it allows the researcher to estimate the size of the phenomenon under study, and thereby make a more educated guess concerning the sample size required. The concept of statistical 'power' or the ability to detect real effects or differences is discussed later in this text.

Sampling issues in qualitative research

Qualitative research shares with quantitative research a concern with the extent to which findings from one study can be generalized to other settings and people. Therefore the representativeness of the information obtained from the sample is important in qualitative research. However, there are differences in the way in which a representative sample is conceptualized in qualitative research.

The key difference is the way in which the population is defined. In quantitative research we make the assumption that there is a true knowable state of the population. The true state of the population is represented by an actual parameter, such as '49% of the Australian population are females' or 'the average IQ of Canadian high school students is 104'. Qualitative research is not concerned with measuring quantities or counting frequencies but with the experiences and meanings of these experiences for individuals and communities. Sampling in qualitative research is referred to as purposive; the researchers deliberately select the participants who are best placed to provide the information for understanding the personal meanings of health-related events. For example, what is it like to survive a heart attack? What does it mean for patients to undergo transplantation surgery? Our sample provides the information which enables us to understand the emotional processes of coping with a heart attack or the psychological demands of being an organ recipient.

Let us consider an example of this approach. Say that you are intending to conduct qualitative research for clarifying issues relevant to the problem of family or 'domestic' violence. The first step would be to clarify the specific aspect of the problem you were studying and define the issues in which you were interested. For example, say that you wanted to collect data concerning the impact of physical violence on the lives of women. A key issue in defining the population is the cultural and historical setting in which it is enmeshed. The moral, legal and health-related problems involved in domestic violence are varied across cultures and change with time. In Western societies it is only relatively recently that violence in domestic settings has been recognized as a serious crime and this influences the experiences of the people involved in the events. Therefore, it is essential to define carefully the cultural characteristics of the group being studied and to keep in mind that we must be very cautious in generalizing the findings from one study to other settings and people.

Purposive sampling

Qualitative sampling is designed to be purposive, i.e. to select cases for inclusion in the research

Table 3.3 Nine of the commonly used purposive sampling methods

Sampling method	Brief description of sampling strategy
Extreme or deviant case sampling	The cases in these methods are chosen because of their deviance and the hope that this deviance may illustrate issues about more regular or mainstream cases
Maximum variation sampling	Purposefully picking a wide range of variation on dimensions of interest. Documents unique or diverse variations that have emerged in adapting to different conditions. Identifies important common patterns that cut across variations
Homogenous sampling	Focuses, reduces variation, simplifies analysis, facilitates group interviewing
Stratified purposeful sampling	Illustrates characteristics of particular subgroups previously found to be of interest. Facilitates comparisons of issues across groups
Snowball or chain sampling	Identifies cases of interest from contacts who know of suitable interview participants; that is, people who are likely to be good sources of information
Theory-based or operational construct sampling	Finding manifestations of theoretical construct of interest so as to elaborate and examine the construct
Opportunistic sampling	Following new leads during fieldwork, taking advantage of the unexpected, flexibility for discovering new issues
Random purposive sampling	(Still small sample size.) Adds credibility to sample when potential purposeful sample is larger than one can handle. Reduces judgment within a purposeful category. Unlike qualitative research, this strategy is not used for generalizations or representativeness
Convenience sampling	Similarly to quantitative sampling, this strategy saves time, money and effort. Poorest rationale, lowest credibility for findings. Yields information-poor cases

that are likely to be illustrative of particular issues or circumstances. Patton (1990) has proposed a typology of sampling that is widely used in qualitative research. Table 3.3 shows nine of the commonly used purposive sampling methods. Interested readers can follow up in Patton (1990) or Liamputtong Rice & Ezzy (1999) for more detailed information.

To illustrate qualitative sampling we have selected four strategies. Considering the example of physical violence against women in domestic settings, what would be the researcher's purpose for selecting the following strategies?

- *Extreme or deviant case sampling*. We would select respondents who experienced severe, even life-threatening, physical violence. Alternatively, we could select women who experienced minimal violence (such as verbal abuse). Both extremes would illustrate the consequences of violence from the victims' perspective and the understanding of

these issues could contribute to developing sensitive and effective interventions.

- *Maximum variation sampling*. Here we would select across all the categories and severities of domestic violence which have been previously identified. Our purpose here is to identify the common themes emerging from the victims' experiences. This approach would also help to understand how different types of violence might result in varying outcomes from the individual's perspective.

- *Snowball or chain sampling*. The assumption here is that people sharing similar important experiences might become aware of each other in a community. In particular, key informants who are sympathetic to the researcher's work might be helpful in identifying 'information-rich' cases. For example, people who are actively involved in victim support groups would be a good source for further contacts with possible participants. In addition, such key informants can act as 'gatekeepers', protecting participants from unsafe researchers. However, 'snowball' sampling can lead to the biased selection of participants and an inaccurate representation of the issues.

- *Theory-based sampling*. A researcher might hold the theory that the occurrence and experience of family violence might be shaped by patriarchal traditions. Here the researcher might purposely select couples who have more-or-less equal relationships and couples where there has been an imbalance of power. The theoretical construct of interest might be 'power' or 'oppression' and this construct might be manifested in the ways in which women experience and interpret violence.

To summarize, we want to make sure the people we are interviewing or the situations we are observing are representative of the targeted issues. We want to gain as complete a picture of the issues from the perspectives of our participants as possible. The usual approach to qualitative sampling is to interview or observe people in situations that fit our criteria until we have reached a point where little or no new observations are being made. This is called saturation.

External validity and sampling

The term *external validity* refers to the extent to which the results of an investigation can be generalized to other samples or situations. External validity can be classified into two types: population and ecological (Huck et al 1974).

Population validity

This refers to generalizing the findings from the sample to the population from which it was drawn. We have already examined the importance of having a representative sample in the generalizing of results from a sample to a population. However, an investigator in the health sciences might face another problem; that the accessible population from which the sample was taken might not be the same as the target population, that is, the one of general interest.

Let us illustrate this point with an example. A physiotherapist working in a large private maternity hospital intends to examine the effectiveness of a new antenatal exercise procedure for pregnant women for controlling levels of pain during delivery. A random sample of 50 pregnant women is chosen for the investigation from the population attending the hospital. The sample is then randomly assigned into two groups: one receiving the new antenatal exercise procedure, the other receiving the traditional programme. The researcher finds a statistically and clinically significant difference between the two procedures, such that the new programme is shown to be effective.

Strictly speaking, these findings can be generalized only to the population of women who attend the hospital. If the target population is *all* women who are having babies, then the generalization will lack external validity, because women attending different hospitals or having children at home had no chance of being included in the study sample. They might have different characteristics and these different characteristics may interact with the treatment in different ways to that of the sample. For instance, women who chose to deliver at home might respond better than those who chose to go to hospital but we would not know this from this study.

Ecological validity

There is another facet of external validity: the situation in which an investigation is carried out might not be generalizable to other situations. This is called ecological validity. Consider the following examples:

1. It has been shown that for clinical pain (due to disease or injury), morphine is an excellent analgesic. However, in laboratory studies of pain induced by electric shocks, morphine had little effect on subjects' reports of pain threshold. Clearly, generalizing from laboratory to clinical settings, or vice versa, has to be done with extreme caution (Beecher 1959).

2. Coronary arteriography involves the insertion of a small-gauge catheter into the coronary arteries, and injection of a dye for X-ray visualization. It was initially reported that the mortality rates for this rather dangerous-sounding practice were only 0.1% (1 per 1000) in a first-class medical institution. However, later reports from various other institutions showed mortality rates as high as 8% (80 per 1000) (Taylor 1979). Clearly, the effectiveness of treatments or the usefulness of clinical evaluations can well depend on who implements them.

The above examples illustrate the caution necessary in generalizing findings.

Summary

Appropriate sampling strategies ensure the external validity of studies and their findings. The aim of sampling strategies is to ensure the selection of a sample that is *representative* of the population of objects, persons or events the investigator aims to study. Incidental and quota samples are chosen for convenience, but these sampling strategies do not guarantee a representative sample. Random and stratified random sampling methods ensure that all important groups and characteristics in the population have the best chance to be selected and included in the study sample. Random sampling strategies are the most desirable to obtain a representative sample, although random sampling is not always feasible or desirable in health research. Area sampling and systematic sampling are also strategies that can be used to obtain representative samples.

An adequate sample size reduces the chance of large sampling errors. The probable sampling error is inversely proportional to the square root of the sample size. It was argued that optimum sample size is not the maximum number of obtainable subjects or a constant number or proportion. Rather, it has to be estimated for a specific investigation on the basis of the parameters of the phenomenon being studied and the study circumstances. Two types of external validity were discussed: population and ecological. External validity is related to inference, which involves using evidence from a limited set of elements to formulate general propositions.

Various approaches to purposive sampling in qualitative research were reviewed and an example of their application to a hypothetical study situation was presented.

Self-assessment

Explain the meaning of the following terms:

area sample
biased sample
ecological validity
external validity
incidental sample
population
population validity
random sample
random sampling
representative sample
sample
sampling error (probable)

True or false

1. The basic idea underlying sampling is to select a representative sample from which the investigator can make inferences to the population.
2. A sample is said to be random when it is not representative of the population.
3. If a population contains 50% males and 50% females, and our sample has 10% males and 90% females, then our sample is said to be biased.
4. When you take a patient's blood pressure daily, you are in fact sampling from a population of potential blood pressure readings.
5. If the patient's blood pressure fluctuates considerably during the day, then a single reading will be an inadequate sample.
6. Stratified random sampling involves the selection of the most accessible elements of the population.
7. Say that important subgroups of the population are known and subjects are sampled incidentally in proportion to these subgroups. This sampling method is known as area sampling.
8. A random sample is one in which 50% of the elements of a population have equal chances of being sampled.
9. Random sampling in health sciences is the least expensive and time-consuming strategy for selecting a sample.
10. When you take blood pressures hourly, you are in fact using a random sampling method.
11. The larger the sample size, the larger the sampling error.
12. The problem of internal validity might emerge when we generalize results obtained in one research setting to another.
13. An incidental sample cannot be, in principle, representative of the population.

14. If a sample is representative, it yields valid data for making generalizations about the population from which it was drawn.

15. The main difference between random and quota sampling is that in quota sampling particular subgroups of the population are represented proportionately.

16. Incidental sampling generates less bias than systematic sampling.

17. Area sampling involves selecting an area at random and assessing the inhabitants of that area.

18. A sample that is unbiased is a representative sample of the population from which it is drawn.

19. Sample error decreases as the sample size increases.

20. If the sample size is halved, the sampling error will be doubled.

21. If a sample is large (say $n > 500$) then the sample must be representative.

22. Generalizing findings from laboratory to clinical settings raises questions of ecological validity.

23. The problem of population validity refers to a population which contains invalid elements.

Multiple choice

1. As sample size increases:
   a the sampling error decreases
   b the ecological validity of the investigation increases
   c the population becomes more accessible
   d the sample becomes more biased.

2. A representative sample:
   a consists of at least 500 cases
   b must be a random sample
   c is defined as the inverse of the square root of the sample size
   d reflects precisely the crucial dimensions of a population.

3. An incidental sample is:
   a not necessarily biased
   b generally obtained through costly and difficult sampling procedures
   c used only in non-experimental investigations
   d none of the above.

An investigator wishes to study individuals suffering from agoraphobia (fear of open spaces). The investigator places an advertisement in the paper asking for subjects. One hundred replies are received, of which the investigator randomly selects 30. However, only 15 subjects actually turn up for their appointment. Questions 4–6 refer to the above information.

4. Which of the following statements is true?
   a The final 15 subjects are likely to be a representative sample of the subjects selected by the investigator.
   b The final 15 subjects are likely to be a representative sample of the population of agoraphobics.
   c The randomly selected 30 subjects are likely to be a representative sample of those agoraphobics who replied to the newspaper advertisement.
   d None of the above are true.

5. The problem with drawing a representative sample of subjects with clinical conditions such as agoraphobia is that:
   a the subjects who consent to participate may be unrepresentative of the target population
   b no sampling strategies are appropriate
   c no complete lists of sufferers' names are usually available
   d a and c.

6. The basic problem confronted by the investigator is that:
   a the accessible population might be different from the target population
   b the sample has been chosen using an unethical method
   c the sample size was too small
   d agoraphobics are impossible to study in a scientific way.

7. Say that it is known that coronary disease occurs twice as frequently among males as females and three times more commonly among over 50-year-olds than those under 50. Given a sample of 120 obtained by quota sampling, how many subjects would you expect to be female and under 50?
   a 60
   b 40
   c 30
   d 10.

8. Referring to the population in Question 7, and given a sample obtained by stratified random sampling, how many females over 50 would you expect in the sample?
   a 40
   b 30
   c 10
   d 5.

9. If a study is externally valid then:
   a its results can be generalized to other equivalent settings
   b it must have been an experiment
   c quota sampling must have been used
   d all the subjects in the sample must have been equivalent.

10. A random sample is one in which:
    a all the elements had an equal chance of selection
    b a chance method was used to select the elements included in the sample
    c both a and b
    d neither a nor b.

11. When we say that a study lacks ecological validity we are implying that:
    a the study was carried out in a laboratory
    b the results cannot be generalized to other settings
    c the target population is different to the accessible population
    d all of the above.

12. Pilot studies are useful for establishing:
    a the approximate sample size necessary for the investigation
    b the appropriateness of the sampling model being employed
    c both a and b
    d neither a nor b.

13. If a pilot study indicates that the effect is likely to be small in relation to the sampling error then the investigator should:
    a abandon the research project
    b use a relatively small sample
    c use a relatively large sample
    d use an incidental method of sampling.

Chapter Four

4

Causal research and internal validity

Introduction

Some types of research have purely descriptive goals: the aim of the investigator is to gather data, make observations and measure phenomena. For example, we may gather statistics on the incidence or prevalence of schizophrenia or neonate deaths within a community. However, in the health sciences there is often a need to identify the causes of illness and disabilities, not just to describe them. It is by understanding these causes that we can formulate and justify our assessments and interventions. Furthermore, we can justify the interventions we use in that we can point to evidence that demonstrates that the interventions are causing the beneficial changes in patients' symptoms. In health research the concept of internal validity is related to the design of research projects and the extent to which we can unambiguously identify causal relationships between interventions and outcomes.

The specific aims of this chapter are to:

1. Examine the concept of causality.
2. Examine how threats to internal validity generate plausible alternative explanations.
3. Discuss how the use of control groups can overcome extraneous variables.

Causality

For philosophers the notion of causality is difficult and controversial. In health research we need to take a more pragmatic approach and look for the following criteria for demonstrating causal relationships so that we can determine to what extent an intervention has caused the observed outcomes. The criteria for demonstrating causality are:

1. The cause must precede (occur before) the effect.
2. The cause and effect co-vary. If the cause occurs then so does the effect.
3. If the cause does not occur, then the effect does not occur.

The first criterion is quite simple. For example, if we say that injury to the person's arm is the cause of that person's reported pain, we assume that the injury was sustained prior to the onset of the pain. Clearly, if the pain had been already present, the injury would not be seen as the cause of the pain. Second, we assume that there will be concomitant variation between the injury and the pain. The worse the injury, the more severe the pain. As the injury recovers, a decrease in the level of pain can be expected. In general, we are establishing a lawful relationship between the cause and the effect.

However, observing a relationship between two events is not sufficient to demonstrate causality. For example, night follows day in a predictable, lawful fashion, but we do not say that day causes the night. We must attempt to eliminate plausible alternative explanations or hypotheses that offer rival causal explanations for the findings. For example, pain might persist even after the injury has healed. There might be other variables operating which maintain a person's experience of pain.

Threats to internal validity in intervention studies

Cook & Campbell (1979) defined a number of threats to the internal validity of intervention studies, including experiments and quasi-experiments. These threats to internal validity compromise the ability of the researcher to conclude that the different interventions administered to groups of subjects are in fact responsible for the differences or lack of differences that are observed. Threats to internal validity are sources of alternative explanations for the outcome of an investigation.

The main threats to internal validity include:

1. *History.* This refers to events that intervene between the pre-intervention test and post-intervention test that do not form part of the treatment or intervention being investigated by the researcher. For example, in a study of the effects of an exercise programme on hypertension, some of the patients might take up additional exercise, such as playing tennis. The effects occurring as a result of these unplanned activities are history effects.

2. *Maturation.* In a study over time, the patients may naturally mature or change. This is a particular issue with paediatric and geriatric populations and studies that are conducted over an extended time period (longitudinal studies). Maturation refers to any time-dependent internal changes in respondents or patients which might influence the outcome. For example, simple infection will resolve without interventions through the action of the immune system.

3. *Testing.* The patient may, as a result of familiarity with the testing procedures, appear to improve spontaneously. These are sometimes called practice effects. For instance, the re-administration of an IQ test might lead to better performance without an actual improvement in the subjects' intellects.

4. *Instrumentation.* During the time between measurements, the measuring instrument might change, for example start reading heavier or lighter, leading to apparent improvement or deterioration when no such change has occurred.

5. *Regression to the mean.* This is a special effect that originates from the unreliability of test measures. Often, clinical research involves the selection for study of patients who have achieved particularly low or high scores on one or more measures, for example the most depressed patients or those with the highest measured cholesterol levels. It is often found that such patient groups, when retested, will show apparent spontaneous improvement (or decline) known as regression towards the mean.

6. *Selection or assignment errors.* The groups being compared may be different at the outset prior to any intervention because of inadequate assignment or selection procedures. If the groups are different to start with, then this difference is likely

to persist after the intervention. Thus a post-intervention difference may not reflect the effects of the intervention when the groups were different at the start.

7. *Mortality*. You do not have to have anyone die in a study to have research study mortality! Mortality in a study refers to when a participant withdraws from the study before its completion. There may be more dropouts in one group than in others, making the groups different. For example, participants in a placebo group might reject an ineffectual treatment and refuse to participate to the conclusion of the study. Since the participants who drop out might be different from those who stay, the experimental and the control group no longer remain equivalent. Once again, if the groups are different, it is difficult to ascribe these differences to their different treatments.

The following investigation illustrates that some of the above threats to validity generate plausible alternative explanations for outcomes. A recent study attempted to demonstrate the effects of an exercise programme in patients with occlusions (blockages) of some of the major arteries in the leg. The 'effect' or the dependent variables measured included the distance walked by the patient to 'limits to the pain tolerance'. The independent variable or the 'cause' was the exercise programme, which included daily walking, with encouragement to increase the distance daily. In addition the patients were also strongly advised to stop smoking and were given a diet low in animal fats and carbohydrates. More than half the patients were smokers and reported that their smoking declined markedly by the end of the programme. The procedure for the study involved pre-tests on the dependent variables (including walking), the administration of the treatment, and then a re-test six weeks after the programme commenced. The results (Fig. 4.1) appeared to indicate an increase in the walking distance. The study was done under the guidance of a vascular surgeon, who also selected the patients.

Figure 4.1 shows that there was an increase in the patients' average walking distance. The question here is: 'Was this change in the dependent variable (effect) caused by the independent variable or by other uncontrolled extraneous variables?' Extraneous variables are variables other than the independent variables which plausibly influence the

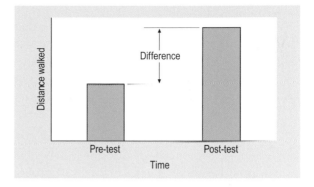

Figure 4.1 • Walking tolerance: before and after exercise programme.

dependent variable. As discussed earlier, uncontrolled extraneous variables are the sources of threats to internal validity.

1. *History*. The threat here is from simultaneous changes in walking, smoking pattern, and diet, any of which might have been responsible for some or all of the changes in the dependent variable reported in the study.

2. *Maturation*. The degree of this threat depends on the natural history of the illness. Natural improvements (or, for that matter, deterioration) in the condition might account for at least some of the difference in walking.

3. *Testing*. Both the pre-test and the exercise programme included walking. It is possible that the difference between pre-test and post-test is simply due to practice effects, the patients becoming more confident in walking to real tolerance limits.

4. *Instrumentation*. This threat is not relevant in this instance, in that no sophisticated or potentially inaccurate measuring devices were used to measure the dependent variable.

5. *Regression to the mean*. Possibly the vascular surgeon selected extreme cases for the study: those most in need of treatment. Their performances might have drifted back towards the mean on the post-test.

6–7. *Selection errors and mortality*. These threats are not relevant, as no control group was included in the hypothetical study.

We have not shown that the extraneous variables described above necessarily caused the reported difference. Rather, because of the lack of control, the investigator cannot claim that the differences found in the dependent variable necessarily reflect changes due to the independent variable, i.e. that the change observed in the outcome measure was caused by the treatment.

The need for control

We have seen how uncontrolled extraneous events and variables can result in plausible alternative explanations for the outcomes of an investigation. In causal research, the adoption of an appropriate design potentially enables us to remove the confounding influences of extraneous variables. If we can do this, i.e. correctly attribute any effects we observe to our interventions and eliminate the effects of other uncontrolled factors upon outcome, we can say that the experiment is internally valid or has internal validity.

In the context of laboratory research, an investigator can use several types of strategy to achieve control over extraneous variables. For example, a physicist studying electricity will make sure that the apparatus is insulated against extraneous electrical disturbances; a researcher studying biofeedback would make sure that the subjects were in a noise-insulated, temperature-controlled room. In 'field' research, in applied clinical settings, such tight control is not feasible. Other methods, such as the inclusion of control groups in the design, are used to maximize internal validity.

A control group consists of subjects that undergo exactly the same conditions as the group receiving the intervention under investigation. For example, in drug trials control group participants will often receive an injection of saline solution, if the experimental treatment is administered via injection, in order to control for the effects of actual injection. If the medication were administrated orally, similar-looking inert tablets would be used for control subjects. It has been found that if people receive any form of 'therapy', improvement may occur even when the 'treatment' or intervention is physiologically and chemically inert. This is referred to as a placebo effect. The control group allows the researcher to measure the size of the placebo effect, and to take it into account when interpreting the study results.

If we are to include a control group in our intervention studies, it is essential that at the outset the experimental and control groups are as similar as possible. We have to take the group of subjects participating in the study and split them up into the experimental and control groups as equally as possible. This process is called assignment. The assignment of subjects to their groups by the investigator is an essential feature of an intervention study.

The use of control groups in clinical research

Let us re-examine the investigation outlined on page 45 in terms of the impact upon internal validity when we use a control group in the study.

1. Assess the walking distances of the patients in a pre-treatment test.
2. Assign subjects into experimental or control groups by matching on the basis of pre-test performance, and random assignment within pairs.
3. Administer:
   (a) experimental intervention (total package of exercise plan, walking, diet and smoking reduction) and
   (b) control intervention (an alternative activity, walking, diet and smoking reduction). The *only* difference between the two groups is that one group receives the exercise programme, and the other some alternative activity.
4. Test both groups on walking distance, following the treatment.

The results of this fictional study are presented in Figure 4.2.

Let us examine how this new design stands up to threats of internal validity in contrast to the original investigation outlined on page 45.

1. *History*. Both groups had walking, smoking decrement and diet; it is unlikely that the difference between post-test results shown in Figure 4.2 is due to these variables.
2. *Maturation*. Both control and experimental groups had the same time to recover or deteriorate; it is unlikely that this factor explains the difference.

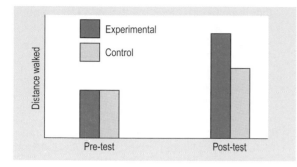

Figure 4.2 • Hypothetical results of a pre-test/post-test study.

3. *Testing*. Both groups had the pre-test and the walking; it is unlikely that this factor explains the difference.
4. *Instrumentation*. Not relevant to this study.
5. *Regression to the mean*. Both groups were similar on pre-test performance, given that they were matched.
6. *Selection error*. Random or matched assignment would have controlled for this, so initial differ ences between the two groups is minimized.
7. *Mortality*. This depends on the actual data; internal validity is preserved if drop-out rates are equivalent in the two groups.

We can see that using a design with a control group resulted in an improvement of the internal validity of the investigation. Note that the use of a control group has not removed the effects of history and other extraneous variables in this study. It is still possible, but much less likely, that the differences in the outcomes for the two groups were not a result of the different interventions they received. Now the investigator has a much sounder basis for deciding whether or not the exercise programme was effective.

It should be noted that there are ways, other than the use of control groups, to minimize the effects of uncontrolled extraneous variables. For example, if 'noise' is a possible extraneous variable in administering a test, we may 'insulate' from it by using a quiet setting. However, if noisy settings are the norm in real life, then the search for higher internal validity may be at the cost of external validity.

Summary

The demonstration of causality involves the discounting of plausible alternative explanations for the study outcomes. If there are uncontrolled extraneous variables, these may generate plausible alternative explanations to the research hypothesis that the intervention alone was responsible for the study outcomes. In this case the investigation is said to have low internal validity. When designing a study to investigate the causal effects of an intervention we aim to reduce the threats to internal validity. When the design includes an appropriate control group, the ability to attribute causal effects to the intervention and not to other extraneous events becomes more convincing.

However, in field research involving human subjects, complete control over the phenomena is not possible. To some extent, control might have to be sacrificed in order to ensure the external validity of the results. In the next chapter, we examine a variety of research strategies and the designs used within these strategies aimed at maximizing internal and external validity.

Self-assessment

Explain the meaning of the following terms:

assignment errors
causality
causal explanations
control
dependent variables
extraneous variables
history
independent variables
instrumentation
internal validity
maturation
mortality
regression to the mean
testing

True or false

1. It is possible to have an effect occur prior to its cause.

2. If a group of children were found to have improved their reading skills in a long-term treatment programme, it would be easy to eliminate maturation as a rival explanation to treatment for their improvement.

3. If two groups in a study start off on an unequal basis, this would probably be an example of assignment errors.

4. In a test of skill that is easily learned, testing effects are unlikely to be a problem.

5. Control groups will eliminate assignment errors.

6. If the researcher can attribute the outcomes in a study to the treatment programmes employed and not other factors, then the study is internally valid.

7. If a study is internally valid then it must be externally valid.

8. Mortality refers to the difficulty of patients dying while undergoing the treatment programme.

9. Regression to the mean occurs mainly in studies where groups have been selected to participate on the basis of some form of extreme score in a pre-test.

10. Control refers to the need to eliminate alternative conflicting explanations for the outcomes observed in a study.

Multiple choice

1. If a group of participants in a study are selected on the basis of a particularly poor pre-assessment, it is likely that they will appear to 'improve' when re-assessed soon after, without any treatment. This phenomenon is known as:
   a regression to the mean
   b maturation
   c history
   d assignment error.

2. If, after a 12-month programme, a group of children with reading problems had improved their reading ages by an average of 9 months, a viable alternative explanation for the results, other than the effectiveness of the programme, would be:
   a regression to the mean
   b maturation
   c history
   d assignment error.

3. If, after the evaluation of the effectiveness of two different rehabilitation programmes, it was found that the participants in the 'better' programme had all attended a disability workshop together, a viable alternative explanation for the results other than the programme would be:
   a regression to the mean
   b maturation
   c history
   d assignment error.

4. If, after the evaluation of the effectiveness of two different rehabilitation programmes, it was found that the participants in the 'better' programme were selected from a less-impaired group, then a viable alternative explanation for the results other than the programme would be:
   a regression to the mean
   b maturation
   c history
   d assignment error.

5. The advantage of including a control or comparison group in a study of treatment effectiveness is that:
   a effects such as maturation can be eliminated
   b effects such as maturation can be reduced
   c effects such as maturation can be measured
   d effects such as maturation can be ignored.

6. If a well-designed study demonstrates a convincing advantage of one therapeutic technique over another, but is based on a sample of five people in the two groups, then the study is likely to have:
   a high internal and low external validity
   b high external and low internal validity
   c low internal and external validity
   d high external and internal validity.

7. Those patients that receive inert treatment in a control comparison group yet respond as if they had received real treatment are demonstrating:
   a the placebo effect
   b external validity
   c internal validity
   d regression to the mean.

8. In a long-term treatment study with a single group with no comparison or control group, it is possible to attribute any improvements observed to:
   a the treatment
   b history effects
   c maturation
   d all of the above.

Section Two

Discussion, questions and answers

Our next discussion question takes us back over 50 years in time, to the setting of the closed psychiatric institutions where persons with serious mental illnesses were often confined under dismal and overcrowded conditions. Psychiatric researchers were desperately seeking new and effective treatments which could enable the residents to return to the community and thus to relieve the pressure on the institutions. A team of Italian researchers, led by the psychiatrist Cerletti, were working on a new technique which they hoped would provide a quick and effective treatment for schizophrenia.

Unfortunately, their research programme was guided by what was later shown to be a false hypothesis: that persons who suffered from epilepsy did not develop schizophrenia. On the basis of this false hypothesis it was predicted that inducing epileptic convulsions would help to reduce the signs and symptoms of schizophrenia. Thus, in the late 1930s thousands of mentally ill persons were administered convulsants, such as the drugs cardiazol and metrazol. The drugs induced convulsions that were difficult to control and proved to be very dangerous. Cerletti argued that the use of electrical shocks to induce epileptic convulsions would be a safer approach than the drugs.

In an article which outlines the historical development of electroshock, Krzyzowski (1989) reported what happened when Cerletti and his assistant Bini first presented these ideas to their colleagues.

Bini, at a conference in Munich in 1936, and Cerletti in the same year in Milan, mention the possible application of electric current to cause therapeutically desired epileptic attacks. The idea was almost unanimously rejected on the grounds of its barbarity and associated hazard. It should be noted that the electric chair had just been introduced in America.

(Krzyzowski 1989, p. 51)

Despite this hostile reaction, Cerletti and his team continued research into electric shock, experimenting with animals in Rome's slaughterhouses. According to Krzyzowski (1989, pp 51–52) the team was ready for their first human subject by 1938.

On April 15 1938, a patient manifesting distinct symptoms of mental illness was admitted into the clinic in Rome after having been arrested by the police for travelling on a train without a ticket. The condition of the patient was then as follows: fully normal orientation, expressed distinct introversion and persecution delusions often using neologisms. He considered himself to be under telepathic influence directing his behaviour. At the same time he exhibited hallucinations thematically related to the delusions. He was depressed and altered neurological conditions were found. Schizophrenia was diagnosed.

Having selected their first subject, the team administered the first electroconvulsive therapy (ECT) procedure.

Two electrodes were attached symmetrically in the vicinity of the crown and forehead and then a relatively low 80 V current was passed for 1.5 s. On switching the current on, the patient sat upright on the bed, his muscles contracted and he fell back onto the bed, not losing consciousness, however. He cried out for a while and then became quiet.

It appeared that the voltage applied was too low to induce the convulsion required for the therapeutic effectiveness of the ECT procedure. What happened next is discussed by Krzyzowski:

Continuation of the treatment was postponed until the next day. The patient, on hearing of such suggestions, roused himself and shouted normally: 'No more. It could kill me'. The words were spoken aloud normally, while previously he used only a specific and hardly understandable jargon, self-devised and full of neologisms. This normal utterance confirmed and assured Cerletti of the effectiveness of the method and, in spite of the strong reservations of his assistants, he decided to repeat the ECT without delay. This time a 110 V current with a pulse duration of 1.5 s was used. Once again a short lived, general contraction of all muscles was observed followed by a full classic epileptic type attack of convulsions. All those present uneasily watched the pallidness and cyanosis accompanying the attack, relaxing as the patient gradually recovered.

The story, you will be pleased to hear, had a happy ending.

After prolonged treatment consisting of 11 full and 3 incomplete shocks, the patient was discharged from the clinic in good health. At follow-up a year later, the mental state of the patient was seen to be good and stable. Subsequent years evidenced a widening application of ECT.

(Krzyzowski 1989, p. 52)

As a matter of interest, ECT is still used by contemporary psychiatrists, but in a greatly modified fashion:

- It is used with anaesthetized patients, with electrodes placed only on one side of the head.
- It is not used with persons with schizophrenia (for whom it was found to be ineffective) but rather with persons who are profoundly depressed.
- It is used as a 'last resort' when current pharmaceutical treatments are ineffective.

Questions

The following questions concerning research planning are related to the above narrative:

1. On the basis of the information given propose aims and/or hypotheses which might have guided the above study.
2. Given the state of psychiatric knowledge and practice of the late 1930s, do you think the above study was justified?
3. Give three or four reasons why a contemporary ethics committee might reject such a research project.
4. By present ethical standards, what should have been done after the patient shouted 'No more, it could kill me'?
5. Cerletti proceeded with a more severe shock on the grounds that the previous shock 'improved' the patient's condition. Comment on this logic, in the context of scientific methodology.
6. Do you think such dangerous experiments are ever justified in the context of health care? If yes, under what conditions?
7. Discuss two or three problems with the 'internal validity' (Ch. 4) of this study. Suggest simple changes in 'control' which may help to improve internal validity.
8. Comment on the 'external validity' of this study in the light of the fact that in subsequent studies ECT was shown to be ineffectual as a treatment for schizophrenia.
9. Do you think Cerletti and his colleagues were guided by a rather simplistic paradigm of schizophrenia? Explain, by comparing the biomedical and biopsychosocial approaches discussed in Section 1.

Answers

1. The research seems to have been guided by several interrelated aims and/or hypotheses.
   (a) The first aim was to find the electrical shock intensity that was sufficient to induce an epileptic seizure in a human.
   (b) The second aim was to demonstrate that the seizure did not result in death or disability; that is, that the treatment was 'safe'.
   (c) The hypothesis implicit in the research might be stated as: 'A course of ECT is effective for reducing the signs and symptoms of schizophrenia'.

   You may be able to suggest other aims and hypotheses. None of the outcomes was stated precisely in the paper quoted.

2. As you may have judged from this brief excerpt, the state of knowledge concerning the biological causes of mental illness was confused and had a weak empirical basis. Biological treatments, such as drug-induced epileptic seizures, were poorly theorized, dangerous and generally ineffective. In this context, in the late 1930s, it could be argued that experimenting with new and safer treatments was justified.

3. We outlined some relevant ethical guidelines in Chapter 2 in terms of which the present study would be judged as problematic, e.g. questionable benefits for patients, lack of informed consent, dangerous and painful intervention and lack of consultation with the relatives/guardians of a mentally ill person.

4. Obviously, discontinue the research. Even though the person was confused when admitted to the hospital, his request was rational and reasonable. There was no doubt whatsoever concerning the patient's desires, and by present ethical standards researchers must comply with such requests.

5. The first electrical shock did not induce the epileptic convulsion which was postulated as the factor 'causing' the therapeutic change. As the first shock simply hurt the man, there was no theoretical or empirical justification for his apparent improvement being due to this shock.

6. One could argue that risking people's health and lives in the context of 'heroic' medicine is never justified. Rather, we should look to prevention or gentler, more natural treatments. The other point of view is that aggressive medical treatment is justified if there are incapacitating and chronic problems, such as schizophrenia. According to this approach, painful and potentially harmful experimental treatments are justified provided that the study is well designed and the participants are well informed and have consented.

7. The issue is whether or not the apparent improvement in the patient's condition was due to the ECT or to other 'extraneous' factors or variables. There are several possibilities which provide plausible alternative explanations, such as:
   (a) *History*. The patient may have been frightened by the treatment and 'pretended' to be better to escape the situation.
   (b) *Maturation*. The patient may have recovered anyway: his condition may be cyclical.
   (c) *Testing or instrumentation*. There may have been inaccuracies and bias in the way in which the patient's condition was assessed.

   Control may be introduced by using groups of persons who have (a) no treatment and/or (b) another treatment for schizophrenia. The appropriate designs for showing causal effects are outlined in Section 3. However, because of the poorly designed research in the area, there were almost two decades of useless treatments before it became evident that ECT was not an effective treatment for schizophrenia

8. Clearly, there was no evidence that the improvement claimed in this study was caused by ECT. In addition, it is tricky to make inferences from unrepresentative samples to populations. In this study, the patient may have shown symptoms of depression, which perhaps responded to the treatment. But this may not be generalizable to persons who show other patterns of schizophrenia. External validity is ensured by appropriate sampling procedures (Ch. 3) and clear operational definition and assessment of the condition, as outlined in Chapter 12. Without appropriate sampling and assessment procedures, we may use inappropriate treatments, unsuitable for the specific needs of our patients.

9. The researchers were working in the context of a 'biomedical' model, assuming that schizophrenia was simply a biological disorder which could be suddenly cured by a heroic treatment such as ECT. A biopsychosocial approach takes a more complex view of chronic disorders, and research programmes include identifying and treating both psychological disabilities and social handicaps entailed in schizophrenia. Biopsychosocial research may involve both quantitative and qualitative methods.

Section **Three**

Research designs

SECTION CONTENTS

In the previous section, we identified broad categories of descriptive (non-experimental) and causal (experimental) strategies for conducting research. The aim of Section 3 is to discuss these issues in more detail by examining various research designs and outlining their applications for conducting health sciences research. As in other areas of creative human activity, such as architecture or the fashion industry, designs refer to explicit plans for completing an object or an activity.

The conceptual basis for experiments is the need for control, as outlined in Chapter 4. In experimental research (see Ch. 5) we manipulate one or more variables (independent variables), while controlling the extraneous variables, by using appropriate controls such as control groups. If the experiment is well designed and properly conducted we are in a position to demonstrate the causal effects of the independent variables on the outcome or dependent variables. The random assignment of subjects to experimental groups is a common way to achieve control. However, health and illness outcomes often have multiple and interacting causes requiring multivariate experimental designs.

Another issue we will address is reactivity of human beings to social situations, such as being involved in research. Appropriate experiments attempt to control for the biases of both the participants and the experimenters involved in a research project.

There are situations where for practical or ethical reasons we cannot randomly assign subjects to control or treatment groups. Here we use quasi-experimental methods which involve comparing pre-existing groups undergoing different treatments (see Ch. 6). There are other research designs discussed in Chapter 6, including naturalistic comparisons, correlational designs and surveys. Naturalistic comparisons and correlational designs enable us to describe and predict relationships among variables, but should be used only with extreme caution in attempting to understand causal effects. Surveys that include the use of questionnaires and interviews to study a person's knowledge, attitudes and beliefs concerning aspects of health and illness are essentially a tool for descriptive research. The accuracy of the information collected within the framework of non-experimental designs depends to a large extent on the use of appropriate sampling strategies for selecting the partipants.

An interesting and commonly used design in clinical settings is the $n = 1$ or 'single case' design. The advantage is that using $n = 1$ designs we may be able to demonstrate causal effects using only one or two subjects, without the need for separate control groups. The major limitation of $n = 1$ (and other types of clinical case studies) is that the findings may not be generalizable to other cases or situations.

Chapter 8 describes some of the elementary characteristics of qualitative field research designs. This chapter aims to compare and contrast quantitative and qualitative research, and describes the importance of qualitative research for understanding the personal experiences of our clients and/or patients. Qualitative data collection strategies (such as in-depth interviewing and participant observation) are outlined in Section 4 and quantitative data analysis in Section 6.

Chapter Five

5

Experimental designs and intervention studies

Introduction

Experiments are an important form of intervention studies. A well-designed experiment enables researchers to demonstrate how manipulating one set of variables (*independent* variables) produces systematic changes in another set of variables (outcome or *dependent* variables). Experimental designs attempt to ensure that all variables other than the independent variable(s) are controlled; that is, that there are no uncontrolled extraneous variables that might systematically influence or bias changes in the outcome variable(s). Control is most readily exercised in the sheltered environment of research laboratories and this is one of the reasons why these settings are the preferred habitats of experimentalists. Much of clinical experimentation, however, takes place in field settings (e.g. hospitals and clinics), where the phenomena of health, illness and treatment are naturally located. Even in these natural settings researchers can exercise control over extraneous variables. The randomized controlled trial (RCT) is an experimental research design aimed at assessing the effectiveness of a clinical intervention. The experimental approach has also been used more broadly in the 'hard' sciences.

The specific aims of this chapter are to:

1. Examine the basic structure of experimental research designs and RCTs.
2. Consider threats to the validity of the results obtained from experiments and RCTs.

Experimental research

Experimental studies and RCTs involve the following steps:

1. *Definition of the population.* Researchers define the population to which they wish to generalize. For example, this might be males over 55 years with coronary heart disease or the local community or a certain type of health care organization.
2. *Selection of the sample.* Using an appropriate sampling method, the study sample is selected from the population. It is desirable that the sample is representative of the population. It is important to note that steps 1 and 2 are common to all research designs.
3. *Assignment procedures.* Using a randomized assignment procedure the participants are allocated to the intervention groups. Random assignment means that each participant has equal chance of being assigned to any of the groups. In an RCT, one of the groups receives a control intervention with the active component of the intervention missing. For example, in an experimental study of the effectiveness of different types of weight-loss programmes, one group might receive an instruction manual, another might receive supervised dietary training and a third group may receive no intervention. The purpose of the randomized assignment procedure is to ensure that the groups are as similar as possible on all the relevant variables. If the groups are substantially different, it will be very difficult to attribute any differences in final outcome to the 'treatments' being administered.
4. *Administration of intervention (treatment).* The researcher then administers the intervention(s) to the various groups participating in the experiment. This is called the independent variable(s). It is important that the intervention is administered in an unbiased way, in order that a fair test of any differences in outcomes may be provided. As will be discussed later, awareness of the expected outcomes on the part of participants may lead to a spurious biasing of the outcomes for those participants. Therefore, the

true aims and expectations of the researcher are sometimes concealed from the participants in an attempt to control expectancy effects.

5. *Measurement of outcomes.* The researcher assesses the outcome of the experiment through measurement of the dependent or outcome variable(s). Sometimes, the dependent variable is measured both before and after the experimental intervention (this is called a pre-test/post-test design) and other times only afterwards (this is called a post-test only design).

Thus, in an experimental study the researcher actively manipulates the independent variable(s) and monitors outcomes through measurement of the outcome or dependent variable(s).

Assignment of participants into groups

Random assignment

The simplest approach is to assign the participants randomly to independent groups. Each intervention group represents a 'level' of the independent variable. Say, for instance, we were interested in the effects of a new drug (we will call this drug A) in helping to relieve the symptoms of depression. We also decide to have a placebo control group, which involves giving patients a capsule identical to A, but not containing the active ingredient.

Given a sample size of 20, we would assign each participant randomly to either the experimental (drug A) or the control (placebo control) group. Random assignment could involve encoding all the 20 names into a computer program and using random numbers to generate two groups of 10. In this case, we would end up with the two equivalent groups:

	Levels of the independent variables	
	Control group (Placebo)	Experimental group (Drug A)
Number of participants	$n_c = 10$	$n_e = 10$

Here n_c and n_e refer to the number of participants in each of the groups, given that the total sample size (n) was 20. We can have more than two groups if we want. For example, if we also included another drug 'B', the independent variables would have three levels. We would require a total of 30 participants if the group sizes remained at 10.

Matched groups

Random assignment does not guarantee that the two groups will be equivalent. Rather, the argument is that there is no reason that the groups should be different. While this is true in the long run, with small sample sizes chance differences among the groups may distort the results of an experiment or RCT. Matched assignment of the participants into groups minimizes group differences caused by chance variation.

Using the hypothetical example discussed previously, say that the researcher required that the two groups should be equivalent at the start of the study on the measure of depression used in the experiment. Using a matched groups design the participants would be assessed for level of depression before the treatment and paired for scores from highest to lowest. Subsequently, the two participants in each pair would be randomly assigned to either the experimental group or the placebo control group. In this way, it would be likely that the two groups would have similar average pre-test depression scores.

Different experimental designs

Four types of experimental design will be discussed. These are the post-test only, pre-test/post-test, repeated measures and factorial designs.

Post-test only design

At first it may appear that this would make measurement of change impossible. At an individual level this is certainly true. However, if we assume that the control and experimental groups were initially identical and that no change had occurred in the controls, direct comparison of the post-test scores will indicate the extent of the change. This type of design is fraught with danger in clinical research and should only be used in special circumstances, such as when pre-test measures are impossible or unethical to carry out. The assumptions of initial equivalence and of no change in the control group often may not be supported and, in such cases, interpretation of group differences is difficult and ambiguous.

Pre-test/post-test design

In this design, measurements of the outcome or dependent variables are taken both before and after intervention. This allows the measurement of actual changes for individual cases. However, the measurement process itself may produce change, thereby introducing difficulties in the clear attribution of change to the intervention on its own. For example, in an experimental study of weight loss, simply administering a questionnaire concerning dietary habits may lead to changes in those habits by encouraging people to scrutinize their own behaviour and hence modify it. Alternatively, in measures of skill, there may be a practice effect such that, without any intervention, the performance on a second test will improve. In order to overcome these difficulties, many researchers turn to the post-test only design.

Repeated measures

In order to economize with the number of participants required in an experimental design, the researchers will sometimes re-use participants in the design. Thus, at different times the participants may receive, say, drug A or drug B. If it were the case that every subject encountered more than one level of the drug variable or factor, then 'drug' would be termed a repeated measures factor. An important consideration is using a 'counterbalanced' design to avoid series effects. For example, half the participants should receive drug A first, and half drug B. If all the participants received drug A first and then drug B, the study would not be counterbalanced and we would not be able to determine whether the order of administration of the drugs was important. Time is a common

Table 5.1 Examples of a factorial design		
	Drug A	**No drug**
Rogerian therapy	1	2
No psychological therapy	3	4

repeated measures factor in many studies. A pretest/post-test design involves the measurement of the same participants twice. If 'time' is included in the analysis of the study, then this is a repeated measures factor. In statistical analysis, repeated measures factors are treated differently from factors where each level is represented by a separate, independent group. This is true both for matched groups, discussed earlier, as well as for repeated measures, discussed above.

Factorial designs

A researcher will often not be content with the manipulation of one intervention factor or variable in isolation. For example, a clinical psychologist may wish to investigate the effectiveness of both the type of psychological therapy and the use of drug therapy for a group of patients. Let us assume that the psychologist was interested in the effects of therapy versus no psychological treatment, and of drug A versus no treatment. These two variables lead to four possible combinations of treatment (see Table 5.1).

This design enables us to investigate the separate and combined effects of both independent variables upon the outcome measure(s). In other words, we are looking for interactions among the two (or more) factors. If all possible combinations of the values or levels of the independent variables are included in the study, the design is said to be fully crossed. If one or more is left out, it is said to be incomplete. With an incomplete factorial design, there are some difficulties in determining the complete joint and separate effects of the independent variables.

In order that the terminology in experimental designs is clear, it is instructive to consider the way in which research methodologists would typically

describe the example design in Table 5.1. This is a study with two independent variables (sometimes called factors), namely, type of psychological therapy and drug treatment. Each independent variable or factor has two levels or values. In the case of psychological therapy, the two levels are Rogerian therapy and no psychological therapy. This would commonly be described as a 2 by 2 design (each factor having two levels). There are four groups (2 × 2) in the design.

If a third level, drug B, was added to the drug factor, then it would become a 2 by 3 design with six groups required. Two groups, drug B with Rogerian therapy and drug B with no psychological therapy, would be added. It is possible to overdo the number of factors and levels in experimental studies. A 4 × 4 × 4 design would require 64 groups: that is a lot of research participants to find for a study. It is relevant to note that when we evaluate two or more groups over a period of time we are also using a factorial design.

Multiple dependent variables

Just as it is possible to have multiple independent variables in an experimental study, it is also sometimes appropriate to have multiple outcome or dependent measures. For example, in order to assess the effectiveness of an intervention such as icing of an injury, factors such as extent of oedema and area of bruising are both important outcome measures. In this instance, there would be two outcome measures. The use of multiple dependent variables is very common in health research. The outcomes measured are usually evaluated individually, although there are more complex statistical techniques which enable the simultaneous analysis of multiple dependent variables.

External validity of experiments and RCTs

We have already discussed external validity in Chapter 3. There are further criteria for ensuring the generalizability of an investigation, depending on the procedures used and the interaction between the patients and the therapist.

The Rosenthal effect

A series of classic experiments by Rosenthal (1976) and other researchers have shown the importance of expectancy effects, where the expectations of the experimenter are conveyed to the experimental subject. This type of expectancy effect has been termed the *Rosenthal effect* and is best explained by consideration of some of the original literature in this area.

Rosenthal and his colleagues performed an experiment involving the training of two groups of rats in a maze-learning task. A bright strain and a dull strain of rats, specially bred for the purpose, were trained by undergraduate student experimenters to negotiate the maze. After a suitable training interval, the relative performances of the two groups were compared. Not surprisingly, the 'bright' strain significantly outperformed the 'dull' strain.

What was surprising is that the two groups of rats were actually genetically identical. The researchers had deceived the student experimenters for the purposes of the study. The students' expectations of the rats likely had resulted in different handling and recording which had apparently affected the rats' measured learning outcomes. Rosenthal's results have been confirmed time and time again in a variety of experimental settings, and with a variety of participants.

If the Rosenthal effect is so pervasive, how can we control for its effects? One method of control is to ensure that the 'experimenters' do not know the true purpose of the study; that is, the experimental hypothesis. This can be done by withholding information – just not telling people what you are doing – or by deception.

Deception is riskier and less ethically acceptable. Most organizations engaged in research activity have ethics committees that carefully monitor and limit the use of deception in research. If the people carrying out the data collection are unaware of the research aims being tested we say that they were 'blind' to the research aims.

The Hawthorne effect

As well as the impact of the expectations of participants in experimental studies, there is also the issue of whether attention paid to participants in the experimental setting alters the results.

In the late 1920s, a group of researchers at the Western Electric Hawthorne Works in Chicago investigated the effects of lighting, heating and other physical conditions upon the productivity of production workers. Much to the surprise of the researchers, the productivity of the workers kept improving independently of the actual physical conditions. Even with dim lighting, productivity reached new highs. It was obvious that the improvements observed were not due to the manipulations of the independent variables themselves, but some other aspect of the research situation. The researchers concluded that there was a facilitation effect caused by the presence of the researchers. This type of effect has been labelled the *Hawthorne effect* and has been found to be prevalent in many settings. Of particular interest to us is the Hawthorne effect in clinical research settings. It must be considered that even 'inert' or useless treatments might result in significant improvements in the patients' condition under certain circumstances. The existence of the placebo effect reinforces the importance of having adequate controls in applied clinical research. Although we cannot eliminate it, we can at least measure the size of it through observation of the control group, and evaluate the experimental results accordingly.

Controlled research involving human participants

Investigations involving human participants require that researchers should consider both psychological and ethical issues when designing experiments. Human beings respond actively to being studied. When recruited as a research participant, a person might formulate a set of beliefs about the aims of the study and will have expectations about the outcomes. In health research, placebo effects are positive changes in signs and symptoms in people who believe that they are being offered effective treatment by health professionals. These improvements in signs and symptoms are in fact elicited by inert treatments probably mediated by the patients' expectations. Health professionals who hold strong beliefs about the effectiveness of their treatments communicate this attitude to their patients and possibly increase the placebo effects.

Placebo responses as such are not a problem in everyday health care. Skilled therapists utilize this effect to the patients' benefit. Of course, charlatans exploit this phenomenon, masking the poor efficacy of their interventions. In health research, however, we need to demonstrate that an intervention has therapeutic effects greater than a placebo, hence the need for a placebo control group. The ideal standard for an experiment is a *double-blind* design, in which neither the research participants nor the health providers/experimenters know which participants are receiving the active form of the treatment.

It is not always possible, however, to form placebo control groups. In the area of drug research and some other physical treatments it can be possible; but with certain behaviourally-based interventions, in areas such as psychotherapy, physiotherapy or occupational therapy, double-blind placebo interventions may be impossible to implement. For instance, how could a physiotherapist offering a complex and intensive exercise programme be 'blind' to the treatment programme being offered? In these situations researchers employ no treatment or traditional intervention control groups when evaluating the safety and effectiveness of a novel intervention.

Also, there are ethical issues that need to be taken into account when using placebo or non-intervention control groups. Where people are suffering from acute or life-threatening conditions, assignment into a placebo or no-treatment control group could have serious consequences. This is particularly true for illnesses where prolonged participation in a placebo control group could have irreversible consequences for the sufferers. Under such circumstances, placebo or no-treatment controls might well be unethical and the selection of a traditional treatment group would be preferred.

Summary

The experimental (RCT) approach to research design involves the active manipulation of the independent variable(s) through the administration of an intervention often with a non-intervention control group and the measurement of outcome through the dependent variable(s). Good experimental design requires careful sampling, assignment and measurement procedures to maximize both internal and external validity.

The Hawthorne and Rosenthal effects are important factors affecting the validity of experimental studies, and we attempt to control for these by 'blinding' when ethically possible.

Common experimental designs include the pre-test/post-test, post-test only, repeated measures and factorial approaches. These designs ensure that investigations can show causal effects. More recent approaches to evidence-based health care have emphasized the importance of employing experimental trials wherever possible.

Self-assessment

Explain the meaning of the following terms:

control group
double blind
factorial design
Hawthorne effect
history
independent variable
instrumentation
internal validity
matching
mathematical model
maturation
mortality
physical model
placebo effects
post-test only design
pre-test/post-test design
random assignment
Rosenthal effect
selection error

True or false

1. The dependent variable is the variable measured by the investigator.

2. Selection or assignment errors arise when, after the assignment of the participants, the groups are not equivalent.
3. If in a clinical investigation more people die in the control group than the experimental group, the investigation lacks internal validity.
4. Ideally, the control group and the experimental group should receive exactly the same treatments.
5. Given that a placebo is an inert substance, its administration has no effects on the participants' behaviours.
6. The random assignment of participants is always preferable to assignment by matching.
7. Persons can serve as their own controls.
8. We reduce the effects of subject and experimenter expectancies by blindfolding.
9. Dependent variables are manipulated by the researcher.
10. Control can be exercised by keeping the values of extraneous variables constant.
11. Confounding extraneous variables generate explanations other than the independent variable.
12. Placebo effects can be seen as confounding extraneous variables.
13. If A antecedes B, then A must be the cause of B.
14. 'Double-blind' experiments are impossible for evaluating some health interventions.
15. 'Maturation', that is natural recovery, can be an extraneous variable.
16. The use of placebo control groups is always unethical.

Multiple choice

1. The aim of controlled observation is to:
   a remove the effects of confounding influences
   b identify the effects of the independent variable on the dependent variable
   c establish causal relationships
   d all of the above.
2. To say that an investigation lacks internal validity means that:
   a the independent variable had no effect
   b the dependent variable was not measured
   c uncontrolled variables may have affected the outcome
   d there were several dependent variables.

3. Which of the following is most representative of a placebo effect?
   a Headache is reduced when an antidepressant is administered.
   b Headache is reduced one second after swallowing an analgesic, well before it is absorbed by the body.
   c Headache is increased after a fierce argument with a 'significant other'.
   d Headache is decreased after the use of biofeedback.

A researcher is studying the effect of a new drug on healing of ulcers. Patients are assigned randomly, by the physician who treats them, to receive either the standard treatment or the new drug. Patients are informed that they are being studied, but they do not know which treatment they are getting. The measure of rate of healing is the number of days until the ulcer is completely healed.

4. The independent variable in the above study was:
   a ulcers
   b the new drug
   c type of treatment
   d rate of healing.
5. The dependent variable in the above study was:
   a ulcers
   b the new drug
   c type of treatment
   d rate of healing.
6. This study is:
   a double blind because the patients do not know what treatment they are getting or which is expected to be more effective
   b double blind because neither the researcher nor the patients know what treatment each person is getting
   c single blind because the patients do not know what treatment they are getting but the physician who treats them does
   d not blind at all as the patients know they are being studied.
7. Which of the following threats to internal validity is not controlled for in this study?
   a maturation
   b regression to the mean
   c repeated testing
   d history
   e none of the above.

8. This investigation is an example of:
   a an experiment, because patients are assigned randomly
   b a study, because the treating doctor did the assigning
   c an experiment, because two treatments are compared
   d a study, because there is no control group.
9. If an experiment is internally valid, this means that:
   a the study's results cannot be generalized to other equivalent settings
   b the sampling method is appropriate
   c the study is not really an experiment
   d the independent variable is responsible for any trends observed
   e the dependent variable has face validity.

A researcher wishes to study the effectiveness of a new drug for treating arthritis. Participants are selected randomly from patients attending a clinic and are assigned randomly to treatment with the new drug (A) or with the current standard treatment (B). A pre-test/post-test design is used. A number of arthritic symptoms are assessed using a checklist of seven items.

10. The dependent variable in this study is:
    a the number of arthritic symptoms
    b the new drug
    c the method of assignment
    d the type of treatment.
11. The independent variable in this study is:
    a the number of arthritic symptoms
    b the new drug
    c the method of assessment
    d the type of treatment.
12. The actual outcome of the study is illustrated by the following graph. Even though the participants were assigned randomly, the graph indicates possible threat(s) to internal validity due to:
    a maturation
    b regression to the mean
    c assignment
    d b and c
    e all of the above.
13. A factorial design involves:
    a more than one independent variable
    b more than one dependent variable

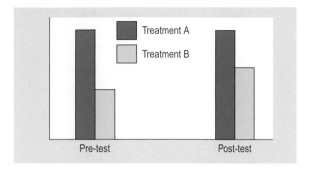

c only one independent variable, but with more than one level
d no control group
e none of the above.
14. Simulation research means:
    a using computers to analyse data
    b studying differences between different artificial limbs
    c studying a model of a situation to reach conclusions about a situation
    d pretending to research one behaviour while actually studying another.
15. An appropriate design for an investigation will be one which:
    a minimizes all possible sources of error
    b is experimental
    c gives you the answer you expect
    d none of the above.
16. If a study is externally valid, then:
    a it must have been an experiment
    b the dependent variable has face validity
    c it cannot be internally valid
    d its results can be generalized to other equivalent settings.
17. The placebo effect:
    a happens only in drug studies
    b occurs in experimental as well as control groups
    c is another name for relaxing participants
    d occurs only if you do not have double blinding.
18. Random selection of participants in a study is typically employed to:
    a maximize generality of the results
    b minimize random measurement error
    c control assignment errors
    d minimize the Rosenthal effect
    e minimize the Hawthorne effect.

19. Random assignment of participants in an experiment is typically employed to:
    a minimize random measurement error
    b minimize the Rosenthal effect
    c minimize the Hawthorne effect
    d ensure that the experimental and control groups are similar at the outset
    e maximize generality of the results.

20. The principal advantage of a factorial design is that:
    a all important factors are taken into account
    b only one factor is considered
    c the dependent variable is more reliable
    d the joint effects of two or more independent variables may be assessed
    e the independent variable has more levels.

Chapter Six

6

Surveys and quasi-experimental designs

Introduction

In the previous chapter, the basic features of the experiment were presented. Experiments or randomized controlled trials (RCTs), when properly designed and implemented, allow the study of causal relationships between variables. However, there are many other legitimate research designs. Although the RCT is held up by some commentators, such as those using the Cochrane Collaboration framework, as producing the highest level of research evidence, most health sciences research does not use an experimental design. For example, Bloch (1987) reported that of the 757 articles on back pain interventions published in 1985, only eight employed RCT or experimental designs. In this chapter we will examine a variety of approaches used for investigation of research questions that do not lend themselves to an experimental approach.

The specific aims of this chapter are to:

1. Examine the uses of naturalistic non-experimental designs.
2. Discuss the use of surveys in health sciences research.
3. Outline the characteristics of designs involving naturalistic comparisons, correlations and quasi-experiments.
4. Identify some of the limitations of these designs.

Naturalistic non-experimental research designs

If experimental designs are supposed to provide the tightest possible control of extraneous factors, why should we resort to alternative non-experimental research methods? There are a number of reasons why non-experimental research designs ought to be employed instead of experimental designs.

1. Many variables are not amenable to experimental manipulation, i.e. they are static. For example, if the research question is concerned with sex differences in responses to heart surgery, then sex cannot be manipulated by the researcher. Similarly, if the researcher is interested in age differences, the ages of the participants cannot be altered by the researcher.

2. Often, it is ethically inappropriate to investigate research questions using an experimental design. For example, if a researcher wished to perform a study on the effects of smoking upon health, studying this in an experimental design would require the experimenter to allocate participants randomly to the smoking or non-smoking group. Clearly, it is unethical to force some participants to smoke and others not to smoke. In experimental designs using a non-treatment control group, valuable and effective treatment might be withheld from participants. This situation involves serious ethical concerns that might lead to an experiment not being approved.

3. Experiments are best used to study simple causal relationships between variables, i.e. does the intervention cause positive therapeutic effects? However, many human diseases and illnesses are not determined by a single cause but rather by a number of causes interacting in a complex fashion. For example, heart disease may be caused by factors such as smoking, excessive stress, inappropriate diet or genetic factors. To identify such possible causal (or risk) factors, we need to study systems as they function in nature. That is, we should investigate patients in their natural setting, even with the difficulties this entails.

Naturalistic non-experimental designs are appropriate alternatives to experimental methods. In the health sciences, experimental methods are focused on a rather narrow band of research questions that relate to the effectiveness of interventions. There are many other interesting research questions that do not relate to intervention effectiveness and, even when the questions do relate to interventions, there are circumstances in which non-experimental methods are more appropriate.

Surveys

Surveys are investigations aimed at describing accurately the characteristics of populations for specific variables (see Fig. 2.1). Surveys are commonly used in health research for the following purposes:

1. To establish the attitudes, opinions or beliefs of persons concerning health-related issues. The data collection techniques often include questionnaires or interviews.

2. To study characteristics of populations on health-related variables, such as utilization of health care, blood pressure, emotional problems or drug use patterns.

3. To collect information about the demographic characteristics (age, sex, income, etc.) of populations. A government census can be an important source of knowledge concerning population characteristics.

The statistics obtained from surveys can present us with an overview of the patterns of states of health, illness and the use of health services in a given community. In this way, we can gain insights into issues such as the prevalent causes of death or the health-related requirements of the population. The outcomes of the surveys can be the bases for hypotheses and theories concerning the causes of illness in a community. The area of health science concerned with such matters is called *epidemiology*.

Epidemiology

Epidemiology is the field of study that is concerned with the distribution and determinants of health and illnesses in groups of people. Last (1988) defined epidemiology as:

The study of the distribution and determinants of health related states or events in specified populations and the application of this study to control of health problems.

Epidemiology is a frequently used approach in public health as it is concerned with the study of the health of populations. It differs from much clinical research in that it is oriented to the population or group rather than individual level.

Epidemiology goes back to the time of Hippocrates who was concerned with the effects of environments upon the health of populations. The work of John Snow in the 19th century concerning the epidemiology of cholera is also considered to be a major landmark in the development of the discipline. Snow mapped the distribution of cholera cases in London and demonstrated that the water supply to different houses supplied by different water companies was involved with the transmission of the disease. The existence of the cholera organism was inferred from these observational data.

Epidemiology focuses on specific target populations and compares the occurrence of different health or disease states within these populations. Thus the numbers of cases, new cases and the relative risk of having the target condition are key components of the epidemiological approach. Two key terms in epidemiology are incidence and prevalence. The *incidence* of a disease is the rate at which new cases occur in a specified population during a specified period. The *prevalence* of a disease is the proportion of a specified population that have the target condition at a specified point in time.

These basic definitions are often used to construct indicators of population health that can be compared across different countries. The World Health Organization (WHO) maintains statistics concerning rates such as the birth rate, the infant mortality rate and perinatal mortality rate. The WHO web-sites provide a wealth of comparative epidemiological data (http://www.who.int/en/).

Epidemiology is also concerned with how diseases are transmitted or spread within populations. The classic epidemiological approach conceptualizes disease within the framework of host, agent, vector and environment. The host is the human, the agent is the infection or health problem, the vector is the means by which the disease is carried, e.g. in the case of malaria this may be a mosquito, and the environment is the setting or mechanism that promotes the exposure. Disease can be transmitted directly (from person to person) or indirectly (via water, such as was demonstrated in Snow's classic study of London water supplies). Although this framework was developed initially within the context of infectious diseases, it is actually much more broadly applicable.

The pattern of outbreaks of disease within populations is also an area of interest to epidemiologists. Common patterns of occurrence of diseases include endemic, epidemic and pandemic patterns. A disease is said to be endemic to a particular area if it habitually occurs within the area. An epidemic is the occurrence of a disease that is over and beyond the usually expected rate. We often talk of flu epidemics, meaning an unexpectedly high rate of the occurrence of influenza. A pandemic is a worldwide epidemic. We have become acutely aware of pandemics such as human immunodeficiency virus/acquired immuno-deficiency syndrome (HIV/AIDS) and other feared pandemics such as severe acute respiratory syndrome (SARS), and, more recently, avian flu.

Epidemiology uses both experimental and non-experimental designs for collecting evidence. Beaglehole et al (2000) provide a useful discussion of equivalences of epidemiological and other research terminology.

Naturalistic comparison studies

Essentially, this type of study involves the comparison of naturally occurring groups or populations. For example, a researcher may be interested in the relative performances of males and females on a test of spatial abilities. The researcher might take a sample of each sex studying at a university and then compare the relative performances of the males and females on the test. Alternatively, a researcher might be interested in whether people growing up in different cultures have different pain reactions. Here, the researcher would select a sample of volunteers from the cultural groups of interest and compare their pain responses to standard pain stimuli.

There are extraneous variables which can be controlled in this type of investigation. In these studies, the researcher can control variables such as the ages or educational backgrounds of the participants by selecting similar groups. However, the researchers have not actually changed or manipulated the variables being studied. All that has been done is the measure of differences between naturally occurring groups.

To relate this to our first example, if our researcher determines that there is indeed a statistically significant difference in the performance of males and females on the measure(s) chosen, well and good. If our researcher then claims that biological factors are solely responsible for the differences, this is another matter altogether. This inference is only one of a number of alternative explanations that could be advanced to account for the differences observed. It is possible, for instance, that males and females in a sample have been exposed to different types of toys and games during their development, so that males might perform better or worse on some tasks. In the second example, any significant results in the pain responses might not be due to 'culture', but rather to systematic biological differences among the groups or a complicated interaction between these factors.

The simple fact of the matter is that it is difficult to demonstrate causation in natural comparison studies. However, if consistent evidence emerges from a logical sequence of studies, the investigators will gain crucial information about the differences between groups on clinically relevant measures. Natural comparison studies are vital components of the researcher's methodological tools.

Correlational studies

The aim of correlational studies in the health sciences is to identify interrelationships among variables. In epidemiology these studies are referred to as 'ecological' designs. A correlation is a statistic that expresses numerically the strength of association that exists between two or more variables.

Let us look at a simple illustration of correlational or epidemiological studies. Say that clinical observations indicate that people who suffer from coronary heart disease tend to be overweight. Such observations might generate the hypothesis: 'There is a positive correlation between being overweight and the probability of coronary heart disease'. Here, the investigator will need to draw a representative sample of the population of interest (let's say 500 men and 500 women randomly selected from a population of healthy men and women aged 40 living in a specified district). The next step would be to measure the participants' weights and heights. These measures might be monitored over a period of time to check for drastic changes in weight. The second variable would be measured by the criterion of whether or not the participant suffered from heart disease during a specified period (e.g. ten years), representing the length of the study. The incidence of coronary disease can then be converted into a probability for a particular category of weight (see Table 6.1).

It can be seen from Table 6.1 that the higher an individual scores on one variable (percentage overweight), the higher the scores on the other variable (probability of coronary heart disease). In this way, the fictional data presented in Table 6.1 are consistent with the predictions of the hypothesis stated above.

Two points should be considered at this stage. First, no evidence has been presented that one variable is causally related to another. This type of investigation does not, by itself, allow us to conclude that, for instance, 'being overweight causes coronary heart disease'. There are several alternative hypotheses, such as 'stress causes both being overweight and heart disease', which can also account for the findings. Second, it is clear that, at least for the period of the investigation, the variable 'percentage overweight' does not account for all of the other variable 'probability of coronary heart disease'. That is, according to the data presented in Table 6.1, there are normal or underweight individuals who suffer from coronary heart disease and very overweight people who do not. Clearly, there must be other variables which influence the incidence of coronary heart disease. There are many other variables such as smoking, blood cholesterol level, personality type, stress and family history of heart disease that also correlate with the probability of coronary heart disease.

Some diseases, for example lung cancer and chronic back pain, have complex, interacting causes. Natural comparison, correlational and

Table 6.1 Fictional data representing the relationship between variables 'percentage overweight' and 'probability of coronary heart disease' (for a 10-year period)

Percentage overweight	Number of participants	Number suffering coronary heart disease	Probability of coronary heart disease
Underweight or normal	600	30	30/600 = 0.05
10–19% overweight	200	20	20/200 = 0.10
20–29% overweight	100	15	15/100 = 0.15
30–39% overweight	75	20	20/75 = 0.27
40% or more overweight	25	10	10/25 = 0.40

ecological designs can help us to identify risk factors; that is, factors that might elevate the risk of the onset or progress of these illnesses.

Quasi-experimental designs

If preventive interventions are to be undertaken to reduce the risk factors associated with a disease, then we require reasonable evidence that these factors are, in fact, causally related to the disease. *Quasi-experimental* designs are often used for this purpose.

Quasi-experimental designs can resemble experiments, with the important difference that there is no random assignment into treatment groups. However, the investigator can control the time at which a treatment is introduced or withdrawn. One such method is a time-series design. This type of design is used by both clinical and epidemiological researchers.

Time-series designs

Time-series designs involve repeated observations before and after a given treatment. In this way, changes in the sequence of observations following the introduction of a treatment may represent the effects of the treatment on the observed variable. Let us look at an example illustrating the use of time-series designs in health sciences research.

Returning to the risk factor of 'being overweight' we discussed previously, the following

investigation using a time-series design could provide evidence for a causal relationship between this variable and cardiac disease.

1. Select an appropriate population to study.
2. Specify the dependent variable; that is, some clear-cut measure of 'coronary heart disease'. A commonly used measure may be the incidence of the disease. By 'incidence' we mean the number of new cases of the disease reported in relation to the population within a specified period of time (for example, 50 per 100 000 per year).
3. Introduce an appropriate treatment which reduces the magnitude of the risk factor. In our example, a health promotion package could be introduced, emphasizing exercise and good eating habits. Let us assume that this intervention is adequately financed and a significant proportion of the population adheres to the programme. It could then be hypothesized that introduction of the health promotion package will result in a decrease in the incidence of coronary heart disease in the community.
4. Monitor the dependent variable over a period of time. It is essential to have readings of the variable both before and after the introduction of treatment. In this instance, the incidence of coronary illness would be determined from the medical records of hospitals, clinics and physicians. Public health authorities often gather and make available such statistics.

Epidemiologists are involved in the monitoring and surveillance of the health of human populations to track the occurrence of existing and possibly new health problems. The existence of HIV/AIDS was established very early by epidemiologists at the

US Centers for Disease Control using sophisticated monitoring and surveillance systems. At the heart of such systems are sophisticated data-gathering procedures.

While the language and concepts of epidemiology are different from the classical clinical disciplines, the approaches to data collection are quite similar to those disciplines. Epidemiologists rely upon the collection of (especially longitudinal) survey data as the basis for their analyses of the distribution and transmission of diseases, are involved in the analysis of RCTs and, like clinicians, attempt to build causal and statistical models of disease occurrence.

Figure 6.1A and B represents two of the many possible empirical outcomes using time-series designs. We will assume that the incidence of the illness was monitored for six years before and after the introduction of the treatment.

There are, of course, other possible outcomes. However, in this case, Figure 6.1A would be consistent with the predictions of our hypothesis, while the outcome shown in Figure 6.1B would

be inconsistent with our hypothesis. Discussion of the way in which data generated by time-series designs are analysed is beyond the scope of the present text. Briefly, it involves the analysis of trends (increase or decrease) found in the dependent or outcome variable.

Time-series designs may have problems with internal validity. What assurance have we that the decrease in the incidence of coronary heart disease, shown in Figure 6.1A, was caused by the introduction of the health promotion programme? Perhaps there was another cause, such as the introduction of drugs to control high blood pressure.

Multiple-group time-series designs

The introduction of multiple-group time-series designs involves the comparison of two or more naturally occurring groups. Let us examine a simple illustration of such designs by a fictional further investigation of the coronary heart disease problem.

Using a multiple-group time-series design, the investigator would select a community which is as similar as possible on demographic variables (socio-economic classes, age, size of the community, etc.) to the community being studied. In this way we would have:

- *Community A*. Control. Do not introduce health promotion programme.
- *Community B*. Introduce health promotion programme.

Figure 6.2 shows two of the several possible outcomes for such an investigation. Some researchers would call this type of design a prospective cohort design; prospective refers to the fact that the data are collected after the commencement of the intervention and cohort refers to the fact that we have multiple intervention/non-intervention groups in the study.

Where the two communities show different trends, the outcome shown in Figure 6.2A is consistent with our previously stated hypothesis. However, in Figure 6.2B there is a trend for decrease in both communities A and B, therefore the evidence is not consistent with the prediction of the hypothesis.

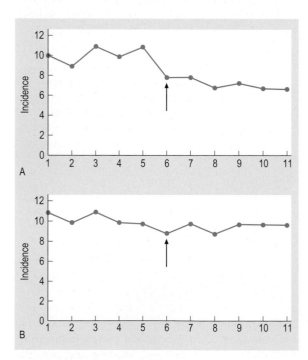

Figure 6.1 A,B • Possible outcomes of time-series designs.

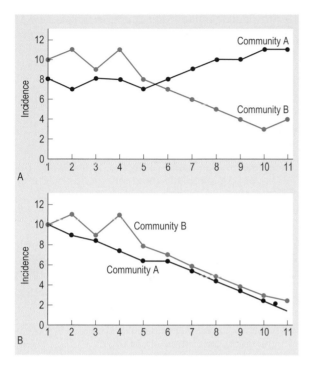

Figure 6.2 A,B • Possible outcomes of multiple-group time-series designs.

Even with multiple-group time-series (prospective cohort) designs, some threats to internal validity remain. There are no guarantees that the communities A and B were equivalent on all relevant factors, or that there were no important changes during the study in the communities which might have influenced the incidence of coronary heart disease. The best that researchers can do is to identify and try to estimate the effect of such extraneous factors on the dependent variable. There are problems such as insulating the two groups: when people in community B learn about the programme being carried out in community A they, by themselves, might initiate aspects of the programme.

The internal and external validity of naturalistic designs

We have noted several types of problems concerning the internal validity of investigations using natural comparison, correlational and time-series designs. These are similar to the problems of internal validity found in experimental RCT investigations. However, because researchers have generally less control over the phenomena being investigated, the use of natural comparison designs makes it more difficult to evaluate causal hypotheses. That is, given uncontrolled extraneous variables, a variety of plausible alternative hypotheses might be offered to account for the findings. Therefore, in areas such as epidemiology, researchers use evidence arising from a variety of investigations using different types of designs to evaluate their theories and models of the causes of human diseases.

When evaluating evidence from natural comparison designs, the external validity of the findings must be considered. In Chapters 3 and 5, we stated that external validity refers to the generalizability of the results of an investigation. Strictly speaking, the results of an investigation should be generalized only to the population from which the sample was selected. For instance, consider the example discussed previously, where a sample of male and female students were compared on a test of spatial ability. Any differences between these two groups can be generalized validly only to the population of students from which the samples were drawn. Investigators sometimes forget this obvious point, and try to make inferences about males and females in general. Such sweeping generalizations are invalid. For instance, other cultures with alternative child-rearing practices might well have males and females with completely different relative spatial abilities. Just because a variable is found to be a risk factor in one community does not guarantee that it will have the same influence on diseases in another community. Clearly, the finding that cigarette smoking is a serious risk factor for coronary heart disease in Western societies does not necessarily mean that cigarette smoking is a risk factor for coronary heart disease among other cultural groups and settings. Given the complex, interacting causes of coronary heart disease, there may be different risk factors in communities which follow different lifestyles or have different physical constitutions. It is not surprising, therefore, that advances in knowledge concerning systematic differences between culturally, racially or sexually different groups have been slow and controversial.

Summary

Descriptive surveys were shown to be important ways of studying the attitudes, behaviours and health problems of a community. Evidence of this kind can be used to propose theories or test hypotheses of the nature and causes of illness. We examined several types of non-experimental research designs including epidemiological approaches, naturalistic comparisons, correlational and ecological designs, and time-series and pro-spective cohort designs. It was argued that these designs are appropriate alternatives to experimen-tal designs, especially in field settings. However, as with experimental RCT designs, investigations using these designs must confront the same prob-lems of internal and external validity.

Self-assessment

Explain the meaning of the following terms:

cohort studies
correlational studies
ecological designs
epidemiology
incidence
multiple-group time-series
naturalistic comparisons
prevalence
quasi-experimental designs
risk factors
surveys
time-series

True or false

1. If it is impracticable to manipulate an independ-ent variable, the investigator might adopt a non-experimental design.
2. The finding that the incidence of birth abnor-mality has increased in a community since the fluoridation of the water supply is sufficient evi-dence that fluoridation caused the birth defects.
3. If there is a high correlation between levels of stress and heart disease, we can say that stress is a risk factor in heart disease.
4. Time-series designs involve the repeated observation of participants before and after treatment.
5. An important difference between experimen-tal and quasi-experimental designs is that in a quasi-experimental study the participants are not assigned into treatment groups by the investigator.
6. A quasi-experimental design affords greater control over extraneous variables than an experiment.
7. It might be invalid to infer that there are general differences between males and females on the basis of findings involving a sample.
8. An investigator compares the IQs of two ethnic groups, but does not control for systematic differences in socioeconomic status. Therefore, the study lacks internal validity.
9. When we speak of the 'insulation' of one group from another, we mean attempting to prevent participants in a control group learning about and adopting the treatment given to an experi-mental group.
10. If a risk factor is, in fact, a cause for a disorder, we can predict that reducing the risk factor should lead to a reduction in the incidence of the disorder.
11. Surveys are utilized in the social, but not in the medical, sciences.
12. 'Naturalistic' designs are useful when it is physic-ally or ethically impossible to manipulate the independent variable.
13. The advantage of naturalistic designs over experimental designs is that they enable the investigator to exercise more control over the independent variable.
14. Naturalistic designs should not be employed to investigate conditions which have complex, interacting causes.
15. Naturalistic comparisons yield data which unequivocally establish the causal effects of the independent variable.
16. A risk factor is a possible cause of a disease.
17. Quasi-experimental designs can involve the production of 'time-series'.
18. Time-series designs involve the calculation of correlation between time and space.

19. A multiple-group time-series design involves the comparison of two or more naturally occurring groups over a period of time.
20. A multiple-group time-series design can be employed only if the participants can be randomly assigned into treatment groups.
21. For a factor to be recognized as a 'risk factor' it must be shown that it correlates with aspects of a disorder across cultures.
22. Epidemiologists are interested in the frequency and causes of diseases.

Multiple choice

1. Naturalistic designs are appropriate when:
   a it is ethically inappropriate to manipulate the independent variable
   b only a small sample of participants is available
   c the independent variable is extremely difficult or impossible to manipulate
   d a and c
   e all of the above.
2. Naturalistic comparisons differ from experimental designs in that:
   a random selection of participants is not possible with naturalistic comparisons
   b random assignment of participants is not necessary with naturalistic comparisons
   c naturalistic comparisons lack external validity
   d all of the above.
3. A risk factor is:
   a a sufficient cause for a complex disorder
   b a necessary cause for a complex disorder
   c both a and b
   d neither a nor b.

We compare a representative sample of Kamchatkans and Patagonians currently resident in Australia on a test of visual acuity.
   Questions 4 and 5 refer to the above.

4. The design employed in the above investigation is:
   a a naturalistic comparison
   b a true experiment
   c a factorial design
   d a time-series design.
5. Given that the sample of Kamchatkans are found to have higher visual acuity than the sample of Patagonians, we can conclude that:
   a Patagonians have poor eyesight
   b Kamchatkans have higher visual acuity than Patagonians

c living in Kamchatka improves one's visual acuity
d Kamchatkans living in Australia probably have higher visual acuity than Patagonians living in Australia
e both a and d.

6. We employ correlational designs in order to:
   a establish the magnitude and direction of association between variables
   b establish unequivocally causal effects
   c identify the possible causes of disease entities
   d both a and c.
7. We intend to investigate if the use of ice is more effective than an exercise programme in treating a particular type of physical injury. The design most appropriate for investigating this problem is:
   a an experimental design
   b a correlational design
   c a model
   d a time-series design.
8. An investigator intends to establish if there is a relationship between levels of atmospheric lead and learning deficits in children. The design most appropriate for investigating this problem is:
   a an experimental design
   b a correlational design
   c a model
   d a time-series design.

The graph below summarizes changes in infant mortality rates over a period of years in two communities, A and B. In community A, a programme of intensive fetal monitoring was introduced at the time indicated by the arrow. No such programme was introduced in community B.
   Questions 9 and 10 refer to the above information.

9. The investigation should be described as:
   a a correlational study
   b an experiment
   c a time-series design
   d a multiple-group time-series design.

10. The findings summarized in the above graph appear to be consistent with the conclusion that:
    a the introduction of fetal monitoring had no effect on infant mortality rate
    b the introduction of fetal monitoring decreased mortality rate
    c the introduction of fetal monitoring increased infant mortality rate
    d none of the above conclusions is consistent with the data.

11. Risk factors of diseases:
    a can be identified by correlational designs
    b are not necessarily the sole causes of diseases
    c are not necessarily the same across cultures
    d all of the above.

A multiple-group time-series design is introduced to study the effects of an insecticide on the number of spontaneous abortions. The insecticide was introduced (not by the investigator) in community A, but not in a similar community B. The graph below represents the hypothetical data.

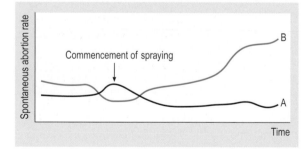

12. On the basis of the graph above, one can conclude that:
    a there is evidence that the introduction of the insecticide increased spontaneous abortions in community A
    b there is no evidence that the introduction of the insecticide increased spontaneous abortions in community A
    c there appears to be a contamination of community B by the insecticide
    d a and c.

13. An investigator distributes a questionnaire to a sample of ex-nurses in an attempt to discover their reasons for leaving the profession. This is best described as:
    a a quasi-experiment
    b an experiment
    c a survey
    d a social model.

14. In an attempt to demonstrate the causal relationship between intake of animal fat and heart disease, an investigator studies the eating habits and heart disease rates of demographically defined groups. Which of the following (hypothetical) findings is most inconsistent with the hypothesis that 'The intake of high levels of animal fats causes heart disease'.
    a Vegetarians have a lower rate of heart disease than meat eaters.
    b Canadian males have a lower rate of heart disease than Canadian females.
    c The increase of protein and fat intake in China has correlated with an increased incidence of heart disease.
    d Eskimos, whose diet consists mainly of animal fats, have lower incidence of heart disease than Egyptians who eat mainly grains.

Chapter Seven

7

Single case (*n* = 1) designs

Introduction

We have discussed research designs involving the comparison of groups of participants selected from a population. These designs provide evidence concerning the general causes of diseases, or the overall effectiveness of interventions. However, health professionals often work with individual patients and need to understand the specific causes of their problems and the effectiveness of treatments as applied to them as individuals. *n* − 1 designs illustrate the close relationship between the principles for conducting research and everyday clinical practice.

The aim of the present chapter is to examine single subject (*n* = 1) designs, as applied by a variety of health professionals in natural clinical settings. You will be able to recognize close similarities between these designs and the quasi-experimental designs discussed in the previous chapter.

The aims of this chapter are to:

1. Identify methodological similarities between clinical problem solving and designing *n* = 1 studies.
2. Examine the use and comparative advantages of AB, ABAB, and multiple-baseline designs.
3. Comment on the validity of *n* = 1 designs.
4. Demonstrate how the interpretation of single case studies is related to generally applied methodological principles.

AB designs

Let us consider a simple example to illustrate the basic procedures involved in using *n* = 1 designs. Imagine that a patient is admitted to your ward suffering from a condition that involves having a high temperature. Before an appropriate intervention is devised, the patient's temperature is recorded every 15 minutes, for 2 hours. Following this time interval, the patient is given medication to reduce temperature. The question here is: 'How do we show that the medication was effective for reducing the patient's temperature?' Obviously, we need to show that the patient's temperature had fallen following the administration of the medication. Figure 7.1 illustrates a possible outcome.

Let us assume that the drug is known to act quickly, say in 20 minutes. The evidence shown in Figure 7.1 would be clearly consistent with the hypothesis that the medication caused a decrease in the patient's temperature. Let us generalize this example to *n* = 1 designs used in various settings. Figure 7.2 illustrates the general conventions used in *n* = 1 designs.

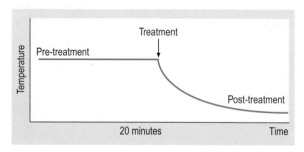

Figure 7.1 • Possible outcome of an AB design.

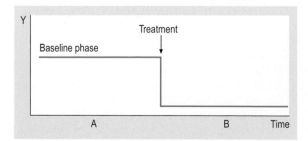

Figure 7.2 • General structure of *n* = 1 designs.

1. We can see that the y-axis (Y) represents the outcome or *dependent variable* (DV): observations made of specific physical characteristics or behaviours.
2. The x-axis represents the time over which the observations were carried out.
3. The period A represents the sessions during which no intervention was administered. This is the 'control' level of the *independent variable* (IV). The observations recorded during A form the baseline.
4. Period B represents the sessions during which intervention was administered, that is, the active stage.
5. The observations taken during A are compared with those taken during B. Systematic changes in the DV between A and B phases (increases or decreases) are assumed to reflect the influence of the intervention.

Therefore, an AB design involves taking observations during phase A, introducing an appropriate intervention, and then taking observations during B. It might have occurred to you that several of the threats to validity can be identified in AB designs. An obvious threat to validity is maturation, that is, recovery or deterioration occurring in the patient that might influence the readings on the outcome variable. Another possible threat is history, that is, influences on the patient other than the actual intervention. In the example we just looked at, one could also argue that perhaps the patient's temperature would have gone down even without the drug, because of the condition improving by itself or the environment of the ward (maturation), or perhaps the ward was air-conditioned and the patient would have cooled down anyway, drugs or not (history).

Next, we look at ABAB designs, which provide stronger control for extraneous variables than AB designs.

ABAB designs

The basic feature of ABAB designs is the alternation of intervention with no-intervention or baseline phases. That is, the researcher introduces the intervention following a baseline or no-intervention phase, then the intervention is withdrawn and then later re-introduced. Observations are recorded during each phase and this approach permits control for the previously discussed threats to validity.

Figure 7.3 illustrates the outcomes for a hypothetical drug study using an ABAB design. When the drug is withdrawn (second A) the patient's temperature returns to previous levels. When the drug is re-introduced (second B), the patient's temperature declines. Clearly, such an outcome is consistent with a causal relationship between the independent variable (intervention) and the outcome or dependent variable (observations of temperature). Figure 7.4 demonstrates the idealized results expected using ABAB designs with a highly effective rapid-onset intervention.

Although the above design is useful for demonstrating causal effects in a single individual, there are situations where it is inappropriate. ABAB designs are not particularly useful when there is a good reason to expect that the effects for an intervention are known to be irreversible following the intervention. For example, if the medication used in the previous example involved antibiotics, then the discontinuation of such drugs after a period might not result in the re-emergence of the symptoms since the antibiotics might well cure

the underlying problem. Even when reversal is possible, it might not be ethical. Clearly, if we have succeeded in establishing desirable effects in our client during the first B period, we might well be reluctant to reverse this for the sake of demonstrating causal relationships.

Multiple baseline designs

Multiple baseline designs involve the use of concurrent observations to generate two or more baselines. Given two or more baselines, the investigator has the opportunity to introduce intervention affecting only one set of observations, while using the other(s) as a control. We will examine a hypothetical clinical problem to illustrate these designs.

Imagine that we have a brain-damaged client showing aggressive behaviours that disrupt therapy. Therapy is offered in two situations, say occupational therapy (Situation 1) and speech therapy (Situation 2). A behavioural programme is devised, aimed at reducing the frequency of the aggressive outbursts. A multiple baseline design involves the observation of the frequency of the target behaviour in both Situations 1 and 2. After establishing a baseline, the intervention is introduced first in one of the situations and then in the other. Evidence demonstrating the effectiveness of the behavioural intervention is shown in Figure 7.5.

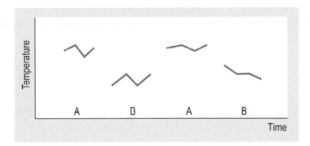

Figure 7.3 • Graph of patient's temperature under different treatment conditions.

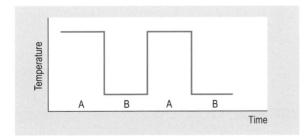

Figure 7.4 • General structure of ABAB designs.

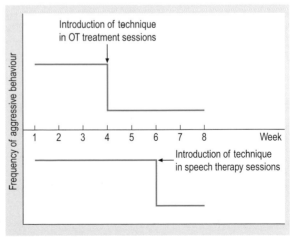

Figure 7.5 • Aggressive behaviour of a brain-damaged patient in two situations.

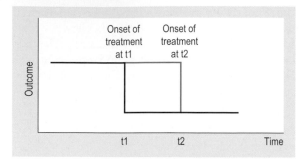

Figure 7.6 • General structure of multiple baseline designs.

The hypothetical data presented in Figure 7.5 indicates that the frequency of the target behaviour (aggression) declined in Situation 1 when the intervention was introduced, while it remained stable in Situation 2. The subsequent introduction of the intervention in Situation 2 resulted in a decrease of the behaviour.

Multiple baseline designs can also be introduced by generating baselines for two or more behaviours, or for two or more individuals. Just as in the example involving the different situations, the interventions would be introduced first for one of the behaviours or individuals and, subsequently, for the others. Figure 7.6 illustrates a general example for multiple baseline designs.

Clearly, by introducing the intervention at different times, we are controlling for the effects of extraneous variables that might have influenced our dependent variable. Both ABAB and multiple baseline designs are appropriate for demonstrating the benefits of therapeutic procedures in individual patients.

The interpretation of the results for *n* = 1 designs

The principles for conducting and interpreting health research are also relevant for evaluating the effectiveness of everyday health practices. The need for control and accurate measurement arises when we intend to demonstrate that particular interventions or preventive interventions are causally related to beneficial outcomes.

As we have seen previously we can exercise control by systematically introducing and withdrawing interventions and measuring concomitant changes in the signs and symptoms of a disorder.

Hypothetical example

Let us examine a hypothetical example for illustrating four different methodological principles relevant to the interpretation of *n* = 1 studies. Imagine that you are caring for a young man called John who had suffered a severe fracture of the femur following a motorbike accident. He is gradually recovering with intensive rehabilitation but he is still in severe pain when narcotic analgesics are not provided.

Previous research has shown that transcutaneous electrical nerve stimulation (TENS) was a safe and effective modality for managing acute pain. However the intervention is not equally effective for all patients so that there are no absolute guarantees that TENS will control pain in this particular patient. Also, even biologically inert pain control techniques can reduce pain through placebo effects. In this case you decide to investigate two clinically relevant research questions:

1. TENS is effective in reducing John's pain.
2. The pain reduction is causally related to the action of TENS.

Having obtained your patient's informed consent you decide to conduct an ABAB, *n* = 1 design for obtaining evidence to answer the above research questions. The variables here can be defined as follows:

1. *IV*. The independent variable is the pain control strategy using the TENS machine. The electrical stimulation produced by the TENS machine can be regulated such that you are in a position to vary the output of the machine. Two settings are selected:
   (a) A represents a TENS output which is known to be physiologically *ineffective* for activating the 'pain-gating' mechanisms (see Section 1). A represents the 'placebo control' level of the IV.
   (b) B represents a TENS output which is known to be physiologically *effective* in activating 'pain-gating' mechanisms. B represents the 'intervention' level of the IV.

2. *DV*. The outcome or dependent variable is an explicit measure of aspects of the signs and symptoms of the patent's condition. In this case we can select 'pain intensity' as a relevant dependent variable, measured on a 10-point scale (on this scale 0 represents 'no pain at all' and 10 'excruciating pain').

3. *EV*. Extraneous variables are variables other than the IV which can influence the DV and may 'confound' the demonstration of causal effects (Ch. 4). In the present $n = 1$ study we are controlling for extraneous variables by:

   (a) using a placebo control condition

   (b) introducing and withdrawing the active intervention over time (ABAB).

The therapeutic effectiveness of the TENS for pain control will be represented by the changes in the pain intensity or the differences between the A and B phases of the intervention. Table 7.1 provides the procedure for conducting the data collection.

The 'A' phase gives us the baseline against which we can compare the effectiveness of the active TENS intervention for reducing pain intensity. The outcome indicates a large and consistent difference between the A and B levels of the independent variable, and the large difference between A and B indicates a clinically useful reduction in the pain intensity experienced by John, your patient. You are now justified in continuing the intervention until he is sufficiently recovered to be painfree.

We hope you will agree that this was an inspiring little story, the problem with it being that things just do not normally happen this way in the real world. The data we hypothesized above

clearly illustrate an ideal, easily interpreted outcome appropriate for educational purposes. However, there may be some factors in the real world that impact upon these idealized findings. These include:

1. *Variability*. The above results are idealized, as opposed to 'variable'; that is to say, appearing to be all over the place. We will look at the concept of variability in Chapters 14 and 15. At this stage it suffices to say that the more variable the findings, the more difficult it is to identify the trends and differences in results of $n = 1$ studies.

2. *Effect size*. The effect size is indicated by the difference between the baseline (A) and the intervention (B) phases. If the effect size is large in relation to the variability of the data, changes in pain intensity will be easy to see. However, if the effect size is small in relation to the variability of the data, then changes in pain intensity will be hard to see. Thus, the ability to detect the effects of interventions is affected by natural variability in the measured variable.

The validity of $n = 1$ designs

We examined three (AB, ABAB, multiple baseline) designs in the previous subsections. However, more complicated, 'mixed' designs are available for $n = 1$ investigations. The mixed designs include elements of both reversal and multiple baseline strategies. We will not discuss these in detail in this text; interested readers are referred to Barlow & Hersen (1984).

A basic requirement for the valid interpretation of all $n = 1$ designs is the production of a stable baseline. Unless this requirement is met, the interpretation of the results is extremely difficult. In some clinical situations, the production of a stable baseline might be unethical as it could involve withholding treatment. The intervention phase must also be long enough for the effectiveness of the treatment to emerge. Some interventions, such as those involving physical rehabilitation or psychotherapy, might need to be administered for months before their effectiveness, or lack of it, becomes apparent. Clearly, we cannot assume that the baseline and intervention phases are of equal duration.

Table 7.1 Data collection procedure for hypothetical example

Time period	Independent variable level	Dependent variable
Week 1	A phase (placebo)	Daily assessment of pain intensity (at 0800 hours)
Week 2	B phase (treatment)	
Week 3	A phase (placebo)	
Week 4	B phase (treatment)	

It is essential that the observations should be valid and reliable. Some observations are straightforward, such as those based on taking temperatures. However, given a more complex variable such as 'aggression' we need to establish with clarity that different observers agree on the type of behaviours we are going to observe; behaviours that might seem 'aggressive' to one observer might not be classified as such by another.

We have already discussed how $n = 1$ designs attempt to control for the influence of extraneous variables. Although the $n = 1$ designs can be conceptually adequate to demonstrate causality, the patients, being in their natural setting, can be influenced by all sorts of uncontrolled events. After all, it is not possible to insulate individuals from their environment. Therefore, sources of invalidity must be evaluated with respect to each $n = 1$ investigation. It must also be remembered that no matter how sophisticated the $n = 1$ design, the observed outcomes for any given case may not generalize to other cases.

Summary

In this chapter, we examined three (AB, ABAB and multiple baseline) of the designs available for studying single individuals in their natural settings. It was argued that ABAB and multiple baseline studies provide a valid means for evaluating the causal effects of variables on therapeutic outcomes. These $n = 1$ designs are particularly useful for establishing the usefulness of interventions for individual patients. Although some limitations and ethical constraints might emerge in conducting $n = 1$ studies, they provide a useful tool for practising health professionals interested in evaluating the effectiveness of their interventions.

Although the statistical analysis of $n = 1$ studies is beyond the scope of this introductory text, it should be noted that graphing our observations, as discussed in this chapter, provides evidence for possible causal relationships. A precondition for interpreting the results of $n = 1$ studies is having an adequate number of stable observations across the various conditions.

The $n = 1$ designs are quite similar to quasi-experimental designs, in that the investigator has control over the type and timing of the interventions.

Self-assessment

Explain the meaning of the following terms:

AB design
ABAB design
baseline
designs reversal
multiple baseline

True or false

1. $n = 1$ designs are most appropriate for conducting epidemiological investigations.
2. The graphing of $n = 1$ findings involves graphing the magnitude of the dependent variable along the y-axis and time or sessions along the x-axis.
3. With an AB design, the time period A represents the time period during which the intervention is introduced.
4. A baseline is a series of observations recorded during a period when the intervention is administered.
5. With an AB design an intervention is introduced, withdrawn and then re-introduced.
6. A limitation in using ABAB designs in clinical investigations is that it might be possible, but unethical, to withdraw a treatment.
7. Using multiple baselines across two situations involves establishing baselines, then administering treatments simultaneously in both situations.
8. An advantage of using multiple baseline designs over AB designs is the increased control over threats to internal validity.
9. AB designs involve a period of initial treatment followed by the withdrawal of the treatment.
10. For $n = 1$ designs, the 'B' period is when the treatment is administered.
11. $n = 1$ designs cannot, in principle, indicate causal effects.
12. The major advantage of $n = 1$ designs is that no ethical issues need to be taken into account in planning such research.

13. An ABAB design involves introducing the treatment twice.
14. An ABAB design provides a more powerful control over possible extraneous variables than an AB design.
15. ABAB designs are particularly useful when changes in the symptoms following treatment are irreversible.
16. The production of a stable baseline might be unethical in some clinical situations.

Multiple choice

1. Quasi-experimental and $n = 1$ designs are similar in that:
   a they can both involve time-dependent sets of observations
   b both can involve control over the time at which a treatment is introduced
   c both a and b
   d neither a nor b.
2. An ABAB design:
   a involves the use of two individuals, A and B
   b has two baseline periods
   c depends on manipulating A and measuring B
   d involves correlating AA with BBC.

Consider the following outcome for an $n = 1$ type investigation.

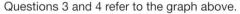

Questions 3 and 4 refer to the graph above.
3. This is a(n):
   a AB design
   b ABA design
   c ABAB design
   d 'mixed' design.
4. The above graph indicates that:
   a the treatment appears effective in reducing the symptom

b the treatment appears to exacerbate the symptom
c the treatment appears to have no effect on the symptom
d no conclusion can be reached on the basis of the obtained data.

A child with a serious behavioural problem at home is institutionalized. After a 1-week period of observation, a behavioural treatment is introduced. The graph below represents the fictitious results.

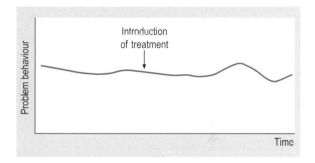

Questions 5 and 6 refer to the above data.

5. This is a(n):
   a AB design
   b ABA design
   c ABAB design
   d multiple baseline design.
6. The above graph indicates that:
   a the treatment appears to have improved the child's problem behaviour
   b the treatment appears to have exacerbated the child's problem behaviour
   c the treatment appears to have had no effect on the child's behaviour
   d a factorial design should have been used.
7. Treatment is undertaken to attempt to reduce anxiety in an individual. An ABAB design is used to evaluate treatment effectiveness. Because of different shifts at a hospital, six different observers are used to record the anxiety-related behaviours. Problem(s) with this investigation is (are) that:
   a the observers might not record exactly the same behaviours as reflecting 'anxiety'
   b the presence of the different observers might influence the behaviours in different ways
   c both a and b
   d neither a nor b.

A new technique to improve running speed in athletes is evaluated. The graph below represents fictional results for two athletes.

Questions 8 and 9 refer to the above data.

8. This design is:
    a AB
    b ABAB
    c multiple baseline
    d factorial.

9. The above graph indicates that:
    a the new technique appears to improve running speed
    b the new technique appears to reduce running speed
    c the new technique appears to have no effect on running speed
    d further investigations on the effects of the technique are necessary.

10. The use of an ABAB design is most useful for reducing threats due to:
    a placebo effects
    b experimenter expectancy
    c maturation
    d assignment.

Chapter Eight

8

Qualitative research

Introduction

The research strategies discussed in previous chapters can be called 'quantitative' in that the data obtained consist of measurements which can be statistically analysed. Quantitative research provides a particular perspective on health and illness. However, there are alternatives. Qualitative or interpretive research involves the investigation of individuals and groups in their social settings. The investigator seeks to understand the thoughts, feelings and experiences of the research participants as people coping with their conditions and treatments in a given social setting. The use of evidence from qualitative studies has traditionally been a fundamental source of knowledge in the clinical and social sciences.

The aims of this chapter are to:

1. Outline different conceptual approaches to qualitative research.
2. Compare and contrast specific dimensions of qualitative and quantitative approaches to research.
3. Emphasize the importance of using evidence from both qualitative and quantitative research.
4. Discuss basic strategies used for ensuring the validity of qualitative research.
5. Examine the scope and limitations of qualitative research in the health sciences.

What is qualitative research?

Qualitative research is disciplined enquiry examining the personal meanings of individuals' experiences and actions in the context of their social environments. 'Qualitative' refers to the nature of the data or evidence collected. Qualitative data consist of detailed descriptions based on language or pictures recorded by the investigator. By 'disciplined' we mean that the enquiry is guided by explicit methodological principles for defining problems, collecting and analysing the evidence, and formulating and evaluating theories.

'Personal meaning' refers to the way in which individuals subjectively perceive and explain their experiences, actions and social environments. Qualitative research provides systematic evidence for gaining insights into other persons' views of the world, 'putting ourselves into someone else's shoes'.

There are a variety of approaches to qualitative research and these take different positions concerning how data should be collected and analysed. There are also several diverse schools of thought that have contributed to the historical development of qualitative field research (see, for example, Denzin & Lincoln 1994, Liamputtong Rice & Ezzy 1999).

1. *Phenomenology*. Phenomenology, which is both a system of philosophy and an approach to psychology, emphasizes the direct study of personal experience and the understanding of the nature of human consciousness. Research in this area involves 'bracketing' or putting aside the usual preconceptions and prejudices that influence everyday perception so that we can uncover the pure constituents of conscious experience. Within this framework, conscious experience is seen as the basis for personal meaning as we reflect on our experiences in the context of our goals and purposes. An important concept adopted from phenomenology is the notion of 'multiple realities', that is, different people may consciously experience the world in quite diverse ways. This suggests that in order to understand the meanings of a person's actions, we must become adept, through empathy, at seeing things from their point of view.

2. *Symbolic interactionism*. Symbolic interactionists emphasize that a social situation has meaning only in the way people define and interpret what is happening. That is, people do not react to 'objective' aspects of their environments, but rather their actions are guided by their personal interpretations of the situation. It follows that different people, on the basis of their past experiences and their particular social positions, may come to interpret a specific situation in quite divergent ways, and act in conflicting fashions. For example, a male obstetrician might view childbirth in quite a different way from a female midwife, and in turn their views might be quite discordant with that of a woman giving birth. In social and health care settings, it is useful to explore different perceptions of events, as it is clear from the work of symbolic interactionists that 'shared perspectives' among people cannot be taken for granted.

3. *Ethnomethodology*. Ethnomethodologists study the processes associated with the way in which people perceive, describe and explain the world. Ethnomethodologists argue that the meanings of specific actions and events are not necessarily obvious, but are in fact rather ambiguous and problematic. People select and apply specific rules and principles in order to define and give meaning to situations in which they find themselves and in order to justify their actions in a given situation. Ethnomethodologists assert that we take an enormous amount of cultural context, such as norms and rules, for granted in our everyday communications and social interactions, and we tend to 'bracket' this as obvious or common sense. It must be remembered, however, that when the cultural backgrounds of individuals diverge, the understanding of personal meaning becomes less obvious or commonsense.

Although taking somewhat different views of personal meanings, the above three approaches have common themes and have all contributed to the development of qualitative field research. Table 8.1 shows key aspects of qualitative field research, in contrast to quantitative approaches.

Data collection and interpretation in qualitative field research

The fundamental aim of planning and designing qualitative field research is to position the investigator close to the participants, so as to gain access

Table 8.1 Contrast between quantitative and qualitative methods

	Quantitative	Qualitative
Perception of subject matter	Reductionistic: identification and operational definition of specific variables	Holistic: persons in the context of their social environments
Positioning of researcher	Objective: detached observation and precise measurement of variables	Subjective: close personal interaction with subjects
Database	Quantitative: interrelationships among specific variables	Qualitative: descriptions of actions and related personal meanings in context
Theories	Normative: general propositions explaining causal relationships among variables	Interpretive: providing insights into the nature and social contexts of personal meanings
Theory testing	Controlled: empirically supporting or falsifying hypotheses deduced from theories	Consensual: matching researcher's interpretations with those of subjects and other observers
Applications	Prediction and control of health-related factors in applied settings	Interacting with persons in a consensual, value-consonant fashion in health care settings

Adapted from McGartland & Polgar (1994). Copyright (1994) The Australian Psychological Society Ltd. Reproduced by permission

to and describe personal experiences, and to interpret their meanings in specific social settings. The following subsection develops in more detail the corresponding points presented in Table 8.1.

Perception of subject matter

Qualitative research is preferably carried out in a natural setting and there is no attempt made by the investigator to control for extraneous influences. Furthermore, there are no operational definitions provided for the study variables, but rather the health-related experiences being studied are perceived and described as a whole, in their social contexts.

Strong preconceptions or fixed hypotheses are not advantageous for qualitative field research. This is a different situation from that in quantitative research, where there are precisely defined hypotheses or aims for guiding the research. Qualitative researchers do have general aims and theoretical notions pertaining to the phenomena being studied but these are tentative and are open to modification as the data collection proceeds.

Qualitative field research focuses on the in-depth understanding of specific individuals and groups, rather than studying the general characteristics of a large population of individuals across specific variables. It should be kept in mind, however, that some quantitative designs may address single cases rather than large study populations. For example, we have reviewed $n = 1$ designs. The difference is that $n = 1$ designs address specific variables representing aspects of the individual's behaviour or clinical symptoms, rather than attempting to describe and understand individuals holistically in the context of their natural social settings. Such an approach is called 'idiographic' (describing a specific individual) as opposed to the 'nomothetic' (describing general phenomena) view of research in quantitative research.

Positioning of researcher

Accurate and replicable measurements are valued in quantitative research. The fundamental positioning of the researcher is 'objective', that is, aiming to perceive and record events without any personal bias or distortion. Within this quantitative framework we assume an objective reality that can be disclosed through accurate reproducible measurement or observation. The situation in qualitative field research is far more complex, as the researcher is more a part of the phenomenon being investigated than the detached observer in quantitative research. To understand personal meanings and subjective experiences one has to become involved with the lives of the subjects being studied. That is, some degree of empathy must develop between the researcher and the subject. By empathy we mean the ability to 'put ourselves in the other person's shoes' or to see things from their perspective(s). Reality is said to be constructed by the individual.

A particular reason for the advancement of quantitative research has been the development of valid and reliable measurement instruments. However, when standardized tests and measures are used to study a person, they become 'enframed' within the limitations of the instrument, and their possible unique self-expression may remain outside the scope of the enquiry. The qualitative researcher may find instruments intrusive, restricting the possibilities for understanding the ideas and emotions of the respondent.

There are advantages to a 'human measuring instrument' which is used in qualitative research. After all, we are more adaptable and multi-purpose than even very sophisticated machinery and we may be able to observe subtle behavioural changes and verbal and non-verbal cues in our participants. In addition, as the investigation progresses, the human 'instrument' becomes more aware of what is happening and as we tune in with each other's points of view the data collection becomes more accurate.

Database

The data obtained in quantitative research consist of sets of measurements of objective descriptions of physical and behavioural events. These are summarized and analysed in accordance with statistical principles outlined at an introductory level in Sections 4 and 5 of this book. The data in qualitative research are descriptive, a 'thick' or thorough description of what people said, their actions and activities, non-verbal behaviours and interactions with other people: 'The reality of the place should be conveyed through representation of its mundane aspects in a straightforward manner' (Lofland 1971, p. 4). An important aspect of field research is keeping thorough, up-to-date field notes. These should be recorded as closely as possible to the time of occurrence of the phenomena under study. The field notes should contain direct quotations from the participants and the settings in which the statements and actions were recorded. Where possible (where it is appropriate and not overly intrusive), the researcher may use audio and video recordings. This helps to record interviews, and improves accuracy in conveying what was said and done in a given setting, since it is possible to review the obtained information.

Although 'objectivity' does not mean remaining detached from the situation, it is essential in qualitative research that the reports of events should be truthful. The investigators should not allow ideological biases to distort or censor their observations, or deliberately lie to place their subjects in a good or bad light. This is a particularly important point as, given the close personal interaction with the subjects, one may be predisposed to report favourably.

By 'database', we mean the overall evidence that forms the basis for theory formation and specific applications for health care. In quantitative research, the database will consist of the statistically treated data which will enable us to see how specific variables are interrelated. In terms of qualitative field research, the database is essentially a narrative (or a story, if you like) that reports what has happened to people, what they did or said in specific situations. This narrative should be adequately detailed so as to illuminate for the reader the personal meanings that the health-related events had for the informants.

Theories

Theories represent our current state of knowledge about the state of the world. Theories are abstract, coherent explanatory systems which integrate a broad range of research findings. Theories may be constituted of premises stated in everyday language, with particular attention paid to the appropriate use of concepts and the logical development of the premises.

Theories based on quantitative evidence integrate patterns of findings concerning the interrelationships among variables. Such theories often contain 'models', which may be mathematical and/or systems representations of the patterns of findings. Models of anatomical and physiological processes, such as those of the circulatory or nervous systems, are good examples of successful quantitative models. Conversely, theories integrating evidence from qualitative research do not address facts about how objects are constituted and interact, but rather are the overall interpretations of personal meanings emerging in specific social settings.

Some commentators (Guba & Lincoln 1983) argued that data collection and theory formation should be intrinsically integrated rather than being different stages of the research process. In addition, it is suggested that personal meanings should be seen as unique and idiosyncratic, and thus no attempt should be made to integrate systematically such diverse personal positions. Theory, from an idiographic position, is seen essentially as the accurate presentation of the situation from a particular person's perspective.

Other qualitative researchers approach theory formation by attempting to identify common 'themes' or categories of meanings emerging from the data. The important point here is that the theoretical categories are developed from evidence expressing personal meanings, rather than 'facts' derived from the statistical treatment of objective measurements concerning variables. In this way, theory is said to be 'grounded' in the narratives of particular individuals.

Some researchers stress the broad, culture-interpreting aspects of qualitative field research. The formation of critical theory explains how personal meanings and actions emerge and are influenced by the person's social and cultural milieu. Critical theories identify the extent to which individuals' self-perception and freedom for action may become distorted and limited by the operation of power and coercion within a culture (e.g. Grundy 1987, pp 15–19, 106–114). As a general illustration, critical theories of the lives and experiences of Western women in the 1960s were crucial to the development of feminist movements.

Theory testing

Theories based on quantitative evidence lead to clear-cut, empirically testable predictions or hypotheses logically deduced from the theories. Theories are supported or falsified by a body of evidence collected under controlled conditions. Testing qualitative theories is somewhat different, as no causal mechanisms are included in the theoretical framework. The simplest verification of qualitative interpretations is to go to the subjects themselves, in order to establish if the researcher's interpretations make sense to them. The extent to which a consensus develops between researchers and their subjects is one of the important indications of the truth of qualitative theories.

Applications in health care delivery

The applications of quantitative evidence and theories are essentially technical, providing mechanisms in terms of which we can predict and control specific health-related variables. That is, we apply quantitative approaches for discovering the causes and progress of diseases and disabilities, for developing and validating assessment procedures and for evaluating the effectiveness of interventions.

In contrast, qualitative field research provides evidence and theories that enable us to understand our clients better as human beings. This research discloses how illnesses, disability and health care delivery affect people's lives interpreted from their points of view. In the following subsection, we will examine some of the applications of qualitative field research for improving health care delivery.

Qualitative field research

When there are significant differences in the cultural backgrounds and experiences of persons, the understanding of personal meanings becomes problematic. For example, an anthropologist might need to spend decades immersed in, and systematically studying, a different culture to be in a position to interpret accurately the actions and traditions of the participants.

There are numerous areas of health research where involving the interpretation of personal meanings is essential to ensure effective practices. The following three examples illustrate areas where qualitative field research can make strong contributions for clarifying personal meanings.

1. Understanding cultural differences between health workers and clients. In countries such as the US, Australia, Canada or the UK we live in multicultural societies. There is persuasive evidence that the way people experience their bodies, or events such as childbirth, pain or illness depends to a large extent on their cultural backgrounds. When health practitioners misconceive their clients' view concerning their illness or injury, the outcome may be erroneous diagnoses and useless interventions. A particularly important area of qualitative field research is to clarify personal meanings of clients and therapists with regard to health care problems, in an attempt to improve communications and enhance treatment outcomes.

2. Evaluating the effects of health care environments. Health care institutions, such as general and mental hospitals, can be seen as 'subcultures' having strong influences on the lives of both staff and clients. Persons with chronic illnesses and disabilities requiring long-term care might come to view themselves and their life situations from an 'institutionalized' perspective. The development of critical theories in these areas is particularly relevant for understanding the influences of health care environments. Research findings in this area have been applied to devise strategies to empower people such as those with intellectual disabilities to live and participate in the community.

3. Relating to people with neurological or psychiatric problems. People diagnosed as suffering from problems such as schizophrenia, intellectual disability or brain disorders may, to some extent, experience themselves and the world in ways different from 'ordinary' people. How such persons experience aspects of their world is by no means obvious, as these clients may demonstrate severe information-processing impairments such as delusions, hallucinations or memory problems, which may make it extremely

difficult to establish empathic relationships. However, in order to ensure that persons with such severe impairments or disabilities are treated appropriately and with understanding, health professionals must learn to see things from their perspectives. Qualitative field research has provided evidence which has helped to clarify the personal perspectives of people with severe disabilities.

The above are some obvious examples where qualitative research is appropriate for clarifying personal meanings, and enhancing understanding and communication in health care settings. However, personal meanings are relevant to all health care situations, not only in the obvious areas discussed above. The following exemplify questions which are appropriately approached through field research strategies:

- What is it like to have a speech disorder? In what ways does it disrupt the person's life, from their points of view?
- How do caregivers interact with terminally ill patients? How do health professionals experience the death of a patient?
- How do health professionals break the news of unfavourable diagnoses, such as heart disease, to their patients? How are such situations seen from the perspectives of the health professional or the patients?

The integration of quantitative and qualitative methodologies

When used jointly, quantitative research tools can be particularly powerful. One of the authors has conducted a study of how people evaluate primary health services (Thomas et al 1993). The first step in this process was to conduct focus group interviews with 20 groups of 8 participants specifically selected from a wide range of ethnic backgrounds, ages and sexes. The groups were conducted by a facilitator who presented questions concerned with knowledge and opinions of, and satisfaction with, health services. The discussions were recorded and transcribed.

One set of analyses of the transcripts involved consideration of everything that had been said about the health services with regard to satisfaction or dissatisfaction. This resulted in a range of separate categories or themes. These themes, therefore, were directly derived from the participants' own words and interpretations of their experiences.

The themes were then framed in the form of questions that sought information from people about their satisfaction and dissatisfaction with health services. The questions were then incorporated into a questionnaire (see Ch. 9). When the questionnaire was piloted with a sample of 500 people who attended several doctors' surgeries over a period of three weeks, it was found that none of the participants nominated new factors that affected their satisfaction and dissatisfaction. Thus, the procedure used in developing the questionnaire had very effectively captured how people decided whether they were satisfied or dissatisfied with their health services. This study is an example of where qualitative and quantitative research methodologies can combine powerfully. There are many productive ways for combining quantitative and qualitative approaches to health research. Interested readers are advised to consult Tashakkori & Teddlie (1998).

The validity of qualitative field research

It should be noted that the unstructured and descriptive nature of the data collection process in field research often sits uneasily with those favouring 'quantitative' research strategies. The major problem with the unstructured data collection techniques is that observer bias may cloud or distort the data being collected. As previously discussed, there are well-known observer effects such as the Rosenthal effect and the Hawthorne effect. Structured data collection methods are most likely to control for these effects, although there are no guarantees that they will be eliminated.

Furthermore, the sampling processes involved in qualitative field research are complex. Most social phenomena are profoundly affected by their participants. 'Real' situations may not reflect these biases. An important issue in understanding qualitative research is the specific culture dependence of the findings; what is true in one social setting

may not be true in another. Also cultures change with time. For example, the experiences of psychiatric patients who lived in large closed mental hospitals up to the 1970s might not be generalizable to mentally ill people who nowadays live in the community.

Therefore, as in other types of research, qualitative field studies also have to confront problems of external and internal validity. Guba & Lincoln (1983) recommended a variety of strategies to ensure the validity and reliability of field studies. These strategies included:

- asking subjects if the observations about them are credible (believable)
- prolonged engagement by the observers to minimize distortions caused by their presence
- triangulations, which involved pitting against each other different data and theoretical interpretations to provide cross-checks of observations and interpretations.

There are many other ways for ensuring the validity or rigour of qualitative research. These more advanced issues can be explored in books dedicated to qualitative research in health care (e.g. Liamputtong Rice & Ezzy 1999).

Therefore, despite controversies in the area, qualitative researchers pay considerable attention to methodological issues to ensure the adequacy (that is, validity and reliability) of their investigations. The situation is essentially no different from quantitative research, although qualitative researchers take somewhat different steps to ensure the accuracy and generalizability of their findings.

Summary

Qualitative research strategies include data collection which is aimed at understanding persons in their social environments. Rather than generating numerical data supporting or refuting clear-cut hypotheses, field research aims to produce accurate descriptions based on face-to-face knowledge of individuals and social groups in their natural settings. The role of the observer in this context is crucial and usually involves physical and social closeness between the subject and the observer. Data collection involves objective and accurate reporting of the activities and appearances of persons in their natural environments. As with other strategies of research, investigators must pay considerable attention to the external and internal validity of field research. We briefly looked at some ways in which field researchers can cross-check their descriptions in an attempt to ensure the validity of their reports and interpretations.

Different research designs may be used to generate evidence of the same processes, although from different perspectives. For instance, any complex clinical phenomenon, such as schizophrenia, may be studied using any of the research strategies outlined in Chapters 4–8. To understand the scope of the problems and the effectiveness of the appropriate treatments, it is desirable to use a variety of research strategies. Conversely, a comprehensive theory of a clinical problem should generate any number of hypotheses within the realm of the research strategies discussed in this book. We will look at the analysis of qualitative data in Chapter 21.

Self-assessment

Explain the meaning of the following terms:

critical theory
empathy
ethnomethodology
personal meaning
phenomenology
qualitative field research
quantitative research

True or false

1. Qualitative researchers focus on individuals behaving in their natural environments.
2. According to Lofland (1971), the field researcher should maintain a 'distance' from subjects in a physical and social sense.
3. A problem with unstructured data collection techniques is the possible distortion of the evidence through observer bias.
4. The basic aim of qualitative research is to test clearly defined hypotheses.

5. It is essential in qualitative research to place disadvantaged or oppressed people in a 'good light', to further their needs or causes.
6. Qualitative researchers need not concern themselves with issues of validity.
7. Qualitative research generally involves the use of precision instruments to measure specific subject variables.
8. Qualitative research generally produces intimate, face-to-face knowledge of other individuals.
9. Phenomenologists are concerned with the understanding of the nature of human conscious experience.
10. Quantitative research produces data well suited to the formulation of causal models.
11. Quantitative research is most appropriate for interpreting personal meanings in social settings.
12. Quantitative research is best suited to discovering how biological systems work.

Multiple choice

1. Qualitative research involves:
   a the testing of clear-cut hypotheses by employing sophisticated measuring instruments.
   b empathy with subjects' points of view
   c structured data collection
   d carrying out research in the open air.
2. Which of the following is not an example of qualitative research?
   a A researcher studying nursing conditions in major hospitals spends a week working as a nurse aide at Prince Henry's Hospital.
   b An anthropologist goes to live with a New Guinea tribe to find out about their religious practices.
   c A psychologist studying therapeutic processes attends group therapy as a client.
   d A speech pathologist compares two rival methods of treatment for stuttering.
   e A physiotherapy student spends a day in a wheelchair and uses this experience to write a report on some of the problems of the physically handicapped.
3. Which of the following disciplines would most likely employ qualitative designs?
   a nuclear physics
   b anatomy

  c genetics

  d sociology.

4. The medical model, as discussed in Chapter 1, is best supported by:

   a qualitative field research

   b quantitative research

   c philosophical speculation

   d all of the above.

5. Which of the following is not a characteristic of quantitative research?

   a A holistic approach to persons.

   b Precise definition of variables being studied.

   c Prediction and control of phenomena.

   d Theories including causal models.

6. An important basis of qualitative field research is:

   a phenomenology

   b numerology

   c measurement theory

   d the medical model.

7. A psychiatrist is interested in research to identify the relationship between brain dopamine levels and the occurrence of specific well-defined abnormal behaviours. This research would be:

   a based on phenomenological principles

   b a project in an ethnomethodological framework

   c a quantitative project

   d best described as qualitative field research.

Section Three

Discussion, questions and answers

The health sciences clinical researcher has a rich variety of research designs from which he or she may choose, including the experimental survey, single case and qualitative field approaches. Each approach has its unique strengths.

The experimental and single case designs are particularly suited to studies of the effects of health interventions. These are studies that are concerned with the clinical impact of administering different types of interventions (or non-interventions) upon people. In the classical two-group experimental study, similar groups of people are administered with either an intervention or a non-intervention condition and their outcomes are compared. The use of non-intervention with people who are ill has moral and ethical implications. So, often the experimental method is used to study the relative effects of two or more different types of intervention. There has been an affinity between the professions where health interventions are the norm and a form of enquiry which also involves intervention (i.e. the experimental and single case types of research design). However, much high-quality health sciences research involves other types of research design.

Sample surveys are frequently employed to study the opinions of large groups of people concerning health services and their experiences of health and illness. Epidemiological research, which is aimed at studying the distribution of health and illness and associated risk factors in populations, generally involves large-scale sample surveys. These surveys often draw upon hospital and other health agency records.

Qualitative field research involves the disciplined examination of the personal meanings of individuals' experiences and actions in the context of their social environment. The emphasis in such research is upon depth of interpretation rather than extent of sampling. Therefore such studies typically employ much smaller samples of participants than, for example, sample surveys.

It is useful to consider examples of the application of the various techniques to the same type of research questions.

Let us consider the situation of people with back injuries associated with manual labour. The major problem associated with back injuries is disability arising from pain. In countries such as the US and Australia older workers who come from non-English-speaking backgrounds are over-represented among people with these injuries. This is probably because such people are over-represented in jobs that have a greater risk of back injury and the effects are cumulative over a long period.

Experimental example

Let us consider an example of where a clinical researcher is interested in comparing the effectiveness of two alternate interventions for the treatment of back injury. There are two common approaches: a conservative approach such as physiotherapy, and surgery. So, if we took 20 workers with back injuries and, after random allocation, 10 of them were treated with a conservative intervention such as physiotherapy, and 10 were treated with surgery, we could compare their outcomes.

To achieve a true experimental design, the people need to be randomly allocated to surgery or physiotherapy. Incidentally, to implement this procedure in real life would require a lot of talking to the relevant ethics committees. All the participants would have to volunteer.

As far as the measurement of the outcome is concerned, most experimental studies would employ a quantitative measure of outcome. For example, the workers could fill in a pain questionnaire, perhaps on several occasions after the interventions, in order to compare the outcomes for the two groups. The use of a written questionnaire, especially if it is provided in English only to people from a non-English-speaking background, makes assumptions about the literacy of the participants which may not be valid.

Natural comparison example

If the clinical staff had chosen the interventions for the patients on a non-random basis, the study as described above would be a natural comparison study. Simply comparing groups does not mean we have an experimental design. Otherwise, the study could be structured in an identical fashion to the experimental example described above.

Single case example

A single case design involves the administration and withdrawal of interventions in a systematic fashion in order to observe their impact upon the phenomenon under study. The person in the single case trial is usually challenged with varied interventions to compare the effects of each. This type of design closely approximates the natural clinical history of interventions with many patients, particularly those with chronic illnesses.

However, the interventions in a single case study are structured much more rigorously.

In the present context, while it would be possible to administer and withdraw physiotherapy and to have baseline phases of no treatment, the surgical intervention cannot be withdrawn. Once the surgery is done, it permanently and drastically changes the person's body. Therefore a single case example could involve the alteration of baseline (no treatment) and physiotherapy and then, as the last link in the chain of event, the surgery. This is not a methodologically strong design, as there could be carry-over effects from the previous interventions that interact with the surgery, and the order of the administration of the surgery could not be readily altered.

Survey example

An alternative way of conducting the study of workers with back injuries would be to select a large group of such people and survey them for the different types of interventions they have had for their injury. The outcomes for different groups could then be compared because, as in a natural comparison study, we can compare men and women respondents. We could even give them the same pain questionnaire as in the types of study previously discussed.

Surveys do not, of course, necessarily involve the use of questionnaires. One could bypass the patients and survey their medical records (with necessary approvals) using a coding schedule. Alternatively, the information could be collected in the form of a structured survey interview.

Qualitative field research example

An additional way of studying this issue would be to conduct in-depth interviews with a small number of injured workers to study their interpretations of their situation. Workers who had surgery, as well as those who had physiotherapy, could be interviewed. The interviews would normally be recorded verbatim, transcribed and then exhaustively analysed for the theoretical constructs needed to describe the experiences of the participants. The use of checklists, survey inventories, etc. is normally avoided, although it is usual to have a list of issues to be introduced by the interviewer. The respondents typically describe their experiences and perceptions in their own natural discourse.

In studies which use questionnaires, there is limited interaction between the researcher and the respondent. As suggested by their name, the respondents respond to the questions framed solely by the researcher. Such an approach can be useful in eliciting factual information in an economical manner. However, it places the respondent in a relatively passive role. If the researcher and the respondent do not share the same constructs, ideas, feelings and motives, the 'wrong' questions may be asked. Schatzman & Strauss (1973, p. 57) note that the researcher 'harbours, wittingly or not, many expectations, conjectures and hypotheses which provide him with thought and directives on what to look for and what to ask about.' The respondent in most questionnaire studies has very little opportunity to contribute to the research agenda. Generally, a token 'any other comments' section is the extent of the invitation for the respondents to contribute to this agenda.

Questions

1. What would be the 'best' design to study the impact of physiotherapy and surgery upon the pain of workers with back injuries?
2. If the participant has been measured frequently over an extended time period, what type of data analysis is required?
3. What type of research design does an epidemiologist typically employ?
4. What special arrangements should be made for participants in research studies with low literacy in English?
5. Is it possible to use an experimental design with in-depth interviewing techniques?

Answers

1. No doubt this question will generate much lively debate. The authors' view is that there is no single best method to conduct such investigations. Each of the methods listed has legitimate insights to offer, each providing a perspective different from that of the others, provided the study is conducted well.
2. This type of design requires an analysis method that can handle repeated measures data, i.e. this is a repeated measures design.
3. Although they may use a variety of different designs, the epidemiologist is likely to use large-scale surveys, often of clinical records. The goal of epidemiologists is to determine the patterns of distribution of illnesses and their relationship with risk factors. Although the modelling may be complex, the research design is simple. Do a large survey.
4. Clinical researchers who are often fluent in English frequently do not make appropriate arrangements for participants with levels of literacy in English lower than their own. Such arrangements could include the provision of interpreters, translated instructions and questionnaires, and interviewers to read the questions to the participants.
5. Yes, it is possible to do so; however, it is very unusual. Experimenters typically employ quantitative outcome measures and researchers who use in-depth interviews tend to be disinclined to use experimental research designs. Perhaps both could learn from each other?

Section **Four**

Data collection

There are numerous methods available for data collection. The appropriate methods are chosen depending on the aims, design and resources of the research project.

Questionnaires are commonly used with survey designs. In Chapter 9, we examine a number of ways in which we can draw up and validate questionnaires. There are different types of questionnaires, ranging from highly structured, standardized scales to unstructured open-ended formats.

An interview (see Ch. 10) is, in a sense, a conversation between the interviewer and the person being interviewed. As they require the presence of an interviewer, this increases the cost and effort needed to obtain data. The presence of an interviewer may also influence the respondent's answers. Qualitative research studies often employ in-depth interviewing techniques which are preferably carried out in the 'natural' settings (homes, hospital, etc.) in which the respondents are living or receiving treatment.

Observational methods are also commonly used strategies for data collection. They may range from highly structured observational protocols, indicating precisely which behaviours or clinical signs should be recorded, to unstructured records of the experiences of participant observers, as used in qualitative research.

Depending on how the data are recorded and analysed, interviews and observations may be used for both quantitative and qualitative research. However, the use of instrumentation to produce numerical data is most appropriate for quantitative research. A variety of standardized measurement instruments are now available for measuring biological and psychological functions (see Ch. 10).

Whatever data collection strategy is being used, we must ensure that it is reliable (replicable) and valid (accurate). Otherwise, as discussed in Chapter 12, the measurement error due to unreliable and invalid data collection strategies may prevent the researchers from achieving their goals.

Chapter Nine

9

Questionnaire design

Introduction

In research investigations, information can be collected through the application of a variety of techniques such as interviews, questionnaires, observation, direct physical measurement and the use of standardized tests. This chapter focuses on questionnaires and questionnaire design, since they are frequently used to collect data in health sciences research.

The specific aims of this chapter are to:

1. Introduce basic concepts in questionnaire design.
2. Discuss the construction and administration of questionnaires.

Questionnaire construction

A questionnaire is a document designed with the purpose of seeking specific information from the respondents. Questionnaires are best used with literate people. The design of the questionnaire is crucial to its success. The process of design and implementation is usually termed *questionnaire construction*.

Questionnaire construction usually involves the following steps:

1. *The researcher specifies the information that is being sought*. This may involve considerable

thinking and discussion. Inspiration for selection of the required information comes from the investigator's research objectives, discussions with others, reading and other sources. At this stage, the document is typically a list of information yet to be translated into specific question form.

2. *Drafting of the questionnaire*. The researcher next takes the list of information he or she wishes to obtain from the respondent and attempts to devise draft questions. As is discussed later in this chapter, the phrasing and design of the questions and the overall design of the questionnaire are important for the validity of the obtained information. If the questionnaire is badly designed, then the responses obtained may not accurately reflect the real situation for the respondents.

3. *Questionnaire pilot*. It is wise to pilot or trial a new questionnaire with a small group of the intended respondents and with clinical or research colleagues, in order to improve its clarity and remove any problems before the main survey. The pilot respondents may be asked whether the questions were clear.

4. *Redrafting of the questionnaire*. If the pilot phase uncovers problems with the questionnaire, it will need to be redrafted in order to address these problems. If they are of a major nature, it is usual to repeat the pilot phase. If they are minor, the researcher may make the necessary changes and then proceed to administration of the revised questionnaire to the full sample of respondents.

5. *Administration of the questionnaire*. After the questionnaire has been developed, it is administered to the full sample of respondents. The responses are then analysed in terms of the researcher's aims and objectives.

As with all research, the ethics of conducting surveys and designing questionnaires must be considered. For example, respondents should not be misled concerning the aims of a survey. A blatant example of unethical conduct is if one is asked to respond to a general 'market survey' and then finds a high-pressure salesperson on the doorstep. If the survey is said to be anonymous, then it is questionable practice by the investigator to code the forms secretly. The follow-up of non-responders can cause a dilemma; people choosing not to participate in a survey should not be pestered. However, forms are sometimes mislaid or forgotten and it is necessary to follow these up to ensure that a representative sample is obtained.

In clinical research, the ethical issues relating to the possible effect of the contents of the questionnaire on the respondent must be taken into account. As an example, one of the present authors was once involved in a survey aimed at establishing levels of knowledge of Huntington's disease and certain attitudes of people at risk for the condition (Teltscher & Polgar 1981). Before the survey was undertaken, a pilot study was carried out to establish whether or not the questions were upsetting to the subjects. The actual subjects were randomly selected from a 'pedigree chart'. However, the questionnaires could not be sent out before it was clearly established that each of the prospective subjects already knew that they were at risk of developing the condition. It would have been appalling if people learned from receiving this questionnaire that they were at risk of a severe genetic disorder.

Questions and questionnaire formats

Questions and questionnaires come in a variety of formats. The researcher must decide which format is the most appropriate for the purpose of the study. Let us first consider the issue of the questionnaire format.

In some instances, researchers will not prepare a formal questionnaire to be filled in by the respondent, but will design an interview schedule to guide the interviewer who asks the questions. (Interviews are discussed in more detail in Ch. 10.) There are costs and benefits in both approaches, as shown in Table 9.1.

The interview schedule approach requires expert interviewers to administer the questions and this is expensive and time-consuming. Further, interviewer bias has been shown to influence responses, as some respondents may modify their responses to fit in with what they perceive to be the opinions of the interviewer. It is important to note that the structure and content of a questionnaire convey a lot of information about the researcher's agenda to the respondent. The respondent generally has little opportunity to influence the agenda. A questionnaire is not really a conversation or dialogue but

Table 9.1 Costs and benefits of interviews and questionnaires

	Costs	Benefits
Interview schedule administered by interviewer	Expensive to administer; requires expert help Responses much more susceptible to interviewer bias	Lower rejection rate More detailed responses can be elicited Greater control over filling out of response form
Self-administered questionnaire	Higher rejection rate Difficult to elicit detailed responses Less control over how response form is filled out	Cheap to administer Less susceptible to interviewer bias Can be administrated by mail

is essentially a monologue from the researcher to which the potential respondent may or may not respond.

However, the self-administered questionnaire approach is cheap, is less susceptible to interviewer bias and can be administered by post. The disadvantages of this approach include higher rejection or refusal rates and much less control over how the response forms are filled out. Anyone involved in self-administered questionnaire analysis will attest to the sometimes remarkable talents of respondents in returning incomplete questionnaire response forms.

Having decided whether the questionnaire will be self-administered or administered by interviewers, the researcher must then decide upon the format for the individual questions.

Open-ended and closed-response formats

There are two major question formats, the open-ended and closed-response types. The distinction between the two is best illustrated by example (see Table 9.2).

In Table 9.2 the first question is an open-ended question whereas the second question is a closed-response question. In an open-ended question, there is no predetermined response schedule into which the respondent must fit a response. In a closed-response question, the respondent is

Table 9.2 Open-ended and closed-response formats

Open-ended	Q1. How do you feel about the standard of the treatment you received while you were a patient at this hospital?
Closed-response	Q2. How would you rate the standard of the treatment you received while you were a patient at this hospital? (circle one number) excellent 1 good 2 moderately good 3 fair 4 poor 5

supplied with a predetermined list of response options. The advantages and disadvantages of both question types are represented in Table 9.3.

Although open-ended questions elicit more detailed responses, there are some possible disadvantages associated with this type of question. The responses generated by such questions require a large amount of effort to encode for data analysis and, when they are coded, tend to give rise to categorical scales. These scales necessitate the use of less powerful statistical methods. Further, some respondents may take a long time to answer this type of question.

Of course, to a researcher employing a qualitative orientation, these 'disadvantages' may not be seen as such. The opportunity to study

Table 9.3 Costs and benefits of open-ended and closed-response formats

	Costs	Benefits
Open-ended	Less structured Responses difficult to encode and analyse using powerful statistical methods Greater time taken by respondent to answer Respondent may find writing an essay more difficult than circling a number	More detailed answers elicited
Closed-response	Less 'depth' in answers May frustrate respondents	Tightly structured Responses easily encoded and analysed Less time taken to collect responses

respondents' interpretations expressed in their own words might lead a qualitative researcher to advocate extensive use of open-ended questions. It is more likely that interview techniques rather than a written questionnaire would be employed. Questionnaires, particularly of the self-administered variety, are generally used for convenience and speed, not for depth of analysis.

It is important that the lists of options for closed-response questions are carefully designed by the questionnaire designer. It is very easy to bias responses by restricting the range of answers in this type of question.

This brings to mind a short questionnaire distributed by an insurance company to one of the authors (see Table 9.4). Two features are remarkable about this question. First, it does not allow for any answers other than the ones listed. Second, the range of available answers is very limited. What we wanted to say was that the insurers were cheap and reliable, i.e. were likely to pay up in the event of a claim. Clearly, the survey designer was a marketing person who had not satisfactorily trialled the questions with a non-marketing audience. While the designers may well have obtained the answers they wanted, the answers may not have been the ones the respondents wished to give. In the health sciences, there are often large differences in the ways in which health professionals and consumers

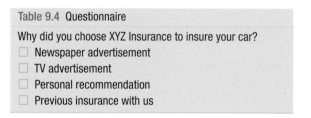

Table 9.4 Questionnaire

Why did you choose XYZ Insurance to insure your car?
- [ ] Newspaper advertisement
- [ ] TV advertisement
- [ ] Personal recommendation
- [ ] Previous insurance with us

approach the same problems. In questionnaire design, it is vital that the researchers do not impose their own conceptualizations of the situations under investigation to the extent that validity is compromised.

A further example of this danger is provided by the results of a survey conducted at a major teaching children's hospital in Australia (Thomas et al 1989). The survey was designed to study why many parents chose to stay with their children in the hospital, in order to plan better facilities and services. One of the questions asked of the respondents was 'Why did your child come to hospital today?' The investigators deliberately chose an open-ended response format for this question in order to tap into the parents' interpretations of the situation in their own words. What a treasure trove of answers! The answers provided considerable insight into the issues of importance to the parents, most of which we could not have

Table 9.5 Likert and forced-choice response formats

Q7. My medical practitioner always explains the chosen treatment to me (circle one number).

strongly agree	1
agree	2
undecided	3
disagree	4
strongly disagree	5

Q8. My medical practitioner always explains the chosen treatment to me (circle one number).

strongly agree	1
agree	2
disagree	3
strongly disagree	4

Table 9.6 Advantages and disadvantages of response formats

Response format	Advantages	Disadvantages
Likert-type	Allows middle 'undecided' response	Acquiescent response mode
Forced-choice	Respondent forced to give either a positive or a negative response	'Undecided' response not allowed

predicted. Thus, the ways in which the questions are asked and the answers sought can have a major impact on the value of the information collected.

Likert and forced-choice response formats

In attitudinal questions, two possible response formats may be chosen: the traditional five- or seven-point Likert-type format, or the four-point forced-choice format. These are best illustrated by examples, as shown in Table 9.5. The first example is a conventional five-point Likert-type scale. The second is a four-point forced-choice type. The advantages and disadvantages are summarized in Table 9.6.

The forced-choice format does not allow respondents to give a 'middle of the road' or undecided answer. This is to guard against respondents using an *acquiescent response mode*. Acquiescent response mode refers to the phenomenon that occurs when respondents give middle responses all the time. *Extreme response mode* occurs when a respondent never selects an intermediate point on the rating scale.

The wording and design of questions

The writing of good questions is an art, and a time-consuming art at that. In order to obtain valid and reliable responses one needs well-worded questions. There are a number of pitfalls to be avoided:

1. *Double-barrelled questions*. This is where two questions are included in one, for example 'Do you like maths or science?' These questions should be separated so that it is perfectly clear to the respondent (and the researcher) which component of the question is being answered.

2. *Ambiguous questions*. It is important to avoid vacuous words and terms that may mean different things to different people. For example, 'old people' may mean everyone above 30 years old to a teenager, but everyone above 60 to a 50-year-old.

3. *Level of wording*. It is important to tailor the level of wording of questions to accord with the intended respondents. Jargon is to be avoided, and it should be established in the pilot study that the respondents will understand the concepts. For instance, asking questions about 'Trisomy 21' might be inappropriate whereas 'Down syndrome' could be intelligible. Using double negatives should be avoided. In general, questions should be simple and concise.

4. *Bias and leading questions*. The wording of the question should not lead the respondent to feel committed to respond in a certain way. For example, the question 'How often do you go to church?' may lead respondents to respond in a way that is not entirely truthful if they in fact never go to church. Not only can the wording of a question be leading but the response format may also be leading. For example, if a 'never' response was excluded from the available answers to the above question, the respondent would be led to respond in an inaccurate way. Bias might also arise from possible carry-over effects from answering a pattern of questions. For example, a questionnaire on health workers' attitudes to abortion might

include the question 'Do you value human life?' followed by 'Do you think unborn babies should be murdered in their mothers' wombs?' In this case, the respondent is being led both by the context in which the second question is asked and the bias involved in the emotional wording of the questions. Surely one would have to be a monster to answer yes to the second question, given the way it was asked.

Finally, it should be kept in mind that even a good questionnaire might be invalidly completed. For example, a survey on 'attitudes to migration' might be answered less than honestly by respondents if the interviewer is obviously of immigrant background.

The overall structure of questionnaires

Questionnaires may be structured in different ways, but typically the following components are included.

1. *Introductory statement*. The introductory statement describes the purpose of the questionnaire, the information sought and how it is to be used. It also introduces the researchers and explains whether the information is confidential and/or anonymous.
2. *Demographic questions*. It is usual to collect information about respondents, including details such as age, sex, education history and so on. It is best to position these questions first as they are easily answered and serve as a 'warm-up' to what follows.
3. *Factual questions*. It is generally easier for respondents to answer direct factual questions, for example 'Do you have a driver's licence?' than to answer opinion questions. Often, this type of question is also positioned early on in the questionnaire to serve as a warm-up.
4. *Opinion questions*. Questions that require reflection on the part of the respondent are usually positioned after the demographic and factual questions.
5. *Closing statements and return instructions*. The closing statements in a questionnaire usually thank respondents for their participation, invite respondents to take up any issues they feel have not been satisfactorily addressed in the

questionnaire and provide information on how to return the questionnaire.

It is best to avoid complicated structures involving, for example, many conditional questions such as 'If you answered yes to Question 6 and no to Question 9, please answer Question 10'. Conditional questions usually confuse respondents and ought be avoided where possible.

Summary

Questionnaires are frequently used for data collection in health sciences research. This chapter has reviewed the principles of questionnaire design, including issues arising from the selection of appropriate questions and response formats.

Self-assessment

Explain the meaning of the following terms:

acquiescent response mode
bias
closed-response format
extreme response mode
forced-choice response format
Likert-type scale
open-ended format
piloting
questionnaire

True or false

1. The aim of survey research is to manipulate the attitudes or beliefs of the respondents.
2. A questionnaire is a measuring instrument which can be employed across a variety of research strategies.
3. If the draft questionnaire is well constructed, there is no need for 'piloting'.
4. As a questionnaire can cause no illness or pain, there is no need to worry about ethical issues when using this instrument.
5. The advantage of an interview schedule over a self-administered questionnaire is that interviews are generally cheaper and less time-consuming to administer.

6. Open-ended questions are easier to analyse and interpret than closed-response questions.
7. If we send out 100 copies of a well-constructed self-administered questionnaire we can expect that at least 95 correctly filled-in forms will be returned.
8. A forced-choice response format does not allow for 'undecided' responses.
9. 'Acquiescent response mode' refers to the phenomenon where respondents agree with only extreme points on a scale.
10. Survey research is more closely related to naturalistic designs than to true experimental designs.

Multiple choice

1. In which of the following ways is survey research similar to an experimental research design?
   a the selection of a representative sample from the population
   b the assignment of subjects into treatment groups
   c the manipulation of the independent variable by the investigator
   d a and c.
2. When a survey is employed as a research strategy:
   a the making of causal inferences from the data may be problematic
   b we must use a questionnaire for data collection
   c the respondents must be anonymous
   d the external validity of the investigation will be automatically assured.
3. Questionnaires:
   a might have ethical problems associated with their design and administration
   b are instruments for data collection
   c can be employed in experimental research
   d all of the above.
4. Redrafting a questionnaire involves:
   a eliminating questions which are not answered in the predicted direction
   b asking the 'pilot' subjects to write the questionnaire
   c rewriting the questionnaire on the basis of feedback from the 'pilot' administration
   d rewriting the questionnaire in such a way that 'pilot' subjects will select responses that are consistent with the investigator's predictions.

5. The question 'Do you attend gay parties?' is:
   a double-barrelled
   b leading
   c ambiguous
   d an acquiescent response.
6. The question 'Are you presently taking β-blockers?' is:
   a double-barrelled
   b ambiguous
   c biased
   d too technical.
7. The advantage of an interview schedule approach over a self-administered questionnaire is that:
   a it is cheaper to administer
   b there is greater control over administration
   c observer bias is minimized
   d people who look a little odd need not be interviewed
   e all of the above.

Do you think it is important for undergraduate students in the health sciences to study statistics (circle one)?

Strongly agree
Agree
Undecided
Disagree
Strongly disagree

8. The above is an example of:
   a an open-ended question
   b a Likert scale
   c a double-barrelled question
   d a leading question
   e none of the above.
9. The advantage of a closed-response format over an open-ended response format is that:
   a more 'in-depth' responses can be elicited
   b there is a lower response rate
   c the responses are easily encoded and analysed
   d it is more likely that the actual attitudes or feelings of the respondents will be revealed.

Chapter Ten

Interview techniques and the analysis of interview data

CHAPTER CONTENTS

Introduction

An interview can be thought of as a dialogue or conversation between interviewers and research participants with the purpose of eliciting information from the participants. Interviews are a key tool for the clinician and the health researcher as a means of collecting information. Interviews may vary substantially in their structure, content and the way in which they are conducted. This chapter is concerned with interviews and the analysis of interview data.

The aims of this chapter are to:

1. Distinguish between structured and unstructured interviews.
2. Outline commonly used strategies for conducting interviews.
3. Compare and contrast quantitative and qualitative strategies for conducting interviews.

Structured and unstructured interviews

Many researchers distinguish between structured and unstructured interviews. Sometimes the terms 'formal' and 'informal' or 'guided' and 'open-ended' are also used (see, for example, Morse & Field 2003).

Denzin & Lincoln (1994) distinguished between three forms of the interview: the schedule standardized interview in which the wording and order of all questions are exactly the same for every respondent; the non-schedule standardized interview where certain types of information are desired from all respondents but the particular phrasing of questions and their order are redefined; and the non-standardized interview in which no prescribed set of questions is employed.

If one defines an interview as a conversation, then a schedule standardized interview is a very rigid form of conversation, almost like a play with a fixed script. In its most structured form, a structured interview may involve the reading of a prepared questionnaire to respondents and then filling in an answer form or response sheet for them on the basis of their answers. The questions are provided in a systematic order, with minimal or no deviation from the prepared script. In a structured interview, the role of the interviewer is to ask the questions and the role of the respondent is to provide the answers with minimal extraneous information. Conversely, an unstructured interview may involve the interviewer in asking no direct questions, but simply prompting respondents to reflect on their current interests and concerns. Clearly, between these extremes lies a variety of different types of interview strategies and degrees of structure. The extent of 'structure' or 'formality' is determined by a number of factors, including the following:

1. *Whether there is a fixed set of questions or schedule*. In a structured interview, the interviewer has a preplanned set of questions or schedule. These questions may or may not be presented in a fixed order. In an unstructured interview, there may be particular 'themes' to be explored without a specific order required or specific question wordings.

2. *The way in which the information is recorded*. There are a number of ways in which interview information may be recorded. Structured interviews tend to employ preplanned answer sheets or response schedules. Unstructured interviews have less expectations and restrictions on the answer formats of the respondents. The interviewer may record the interview or take free-form notes.

3. *The types of questions*. Structured interviews tend to employ more closed-response questions in which the valid answers have been preplanned, rather than open-ended questions. With open-ended questions the respondents provide their answers in their own words, whereas closed-response questions involve a choice of answers provided by the interviewer.

4. *The extent of control by the interviewer*. In a structured interview, the interviewer explicitly guides or directs the conversation (e.g. 'Now Mr. Smith, let's discuss how your family feels about your problem') rather than the respondent setting the agenda. In an unstructured interview, the respondent may assume a more active role in the conversation.

It is useful to consider some of the advantages and disadvantages of the different types of interview approaches. These are summarized in Table 10.1.

The appropriateness of the different interview approaches is determined by the objectives of the researcher. If the researcher simply wished to collect some basic symptom data, an unstructured interview would be inefficient. However, if the researcher wished to study people's conceptualization and interpretation of their illness, an unstructured interview may be quite suitable.

Some clinical interviews, such as history taking, are highly structured whereas other clinical interviews, such as those involving management of a long-term problem, may be less so.

Methods of conducting interviews

Since an interview is a conversation, there exist several possible methods for conducting it. The interview may be conducted in person ('face to face') or by remote means such as by telephone. There are a number of advantages associated with face-to-face interviews. (These are also discussed in Ch. 9.) Face-to-face interviews permit the non-verbal reactions of the respondent to be observed and perhaps the development of a closer rapport arising from the more 'natural' setting. Interviewers may use their observations of non-verbal cues to supplement the verbal information being provided and use their own non-verbal cues in a similar fashion. However, the face-to-face interview may require a substantial amount of participant travel

Table 10.1 Advantages and disadvantages of structured and unstructured interviews

	Advantages	Disadvantages
Structured interviews	May be less time-consuming The same information is collected for all respondents	Responses may not be recorded in the respondents' own words
Unstructured interviews	Responses may be recorded in the 'own words' of the respondents, hence less bias through interpretation The respondent has some input into the research agenda	May be time-consuming Not all the same information is collected for all respondents

time and hence higher costs than for a telephone interview. With certain interview objectives, however, telephone interviews may not be suitable. If the interviewer and his or her credentials are not well known to the interviewee, it is unlikely that participants in a telephone interview would provide valid and reliable personal information about personal topics. Some people find disclosure of sensitive information to be easier by telephone or by the use of anonymous self-completion questionnaires. The face-to-face interview may be too confrontational or embarrassing for them.

The interview process

1. *Selection of interviewees*. One of the interviewer's first tasks is to select those to be interviewed. In qualitative research, techniques such as random sampling are used infrequently. Rather, the interviewer selects those who are most likely to provide the required insights into the situation or issue under study, i.e. the 'key informants'.

2. *Recruitment of research participants*. The interviewer must then enlist the participation of the research participants. Typically, the interviewer will contact the prospective participant, explain the purposes of the interview and make a number of assurances. These assurances may include protection of privacy, the ability to vet materials based on the interview and the extent of time involvement of the research participant. Often, the interviewer might write to participants first and then contact them via telephone to be less 'confronting'.

3. *The interview*. The process of the interview varies substantially according to the methodology to be

employed by the interviewer. The process of a structured interview is quite different from that of an unstructured interview. However, some basic goals are shared. The desirability of tapping the participant's views rather than reflecting those of the interviewer (i.e. maximization of validity) is paramount. To achieve this, interviewers need to be sensitive, non-evaluative, alert and skilled at delivering and sequencing their questions. In in-depth interviewing, multiple interviews may be required. In this type of approach, the emphasis is on depth of analysis with a smaller number of interviewees rather than the breadth of coverage of interviewees offered by a sample survey. Substantial practice and good interpersonal skills are required to achieve competence in interviewing. Both video and audio recording of interviews have one large advantage over other methods of recording interview information. This is that the interviewer's interpretation of the interviewee's answers is open to independent scrutiny, because the primary research materials are available for study by others (with appropriate ethical clearance).

4. *Use of response schedules/answer checklists*. When conducting an interview, the interviewer may record the information provided by the interviewee on a pre-designed response schedule/answer checklist. For example, the schedule may contain information such as the sex and age of respondents and areas for recording their answers to particular questions. Typically, the response sheet is completed during the interview, although it can be completed at some time following the interview. Immediate recording is probably more valid and reliable although, once again, the mere presence of a recording device may be of concern to the respondent. Unless the response sheet is well designed, there is a major

problem of handling novel or unexpected turns in the interview. The interviewer is interpreting, on the fly, the answers and information provided by the interviewee. If those do not conform to the assumptions designed into the response sheet, these interpretations may not be satisfactory or well considered. Telephone interviews may involve the use of computer assistance where the interviewer is prompted by, and records the responses on, a computerized schedule.

5. *Free-form (unstructured) notes*. This method of recording involves interviewers making free-form notes to record information they believe to be salient, either during or following the interview. This method of recording is used extensively by clinicians in case notes. There are a number of advantages and problems with such recording; these result from the process whereby the interview is distilled into the notes. This process involves substantial judgment and interpretation on the part of the interviewer. Such distillations result in highly refined (or biased) and reduced data, the validity of which, at least in terms of the interview, is inaccessible to scrutiny. Further, free-form note-taking may not result in the recording of the same type of data across interviewees. Often, when case audits from records are being performed, it is not possible to derive the required data from clinical notes because of this problem.

6. *Follow-up*. Having completed the interviews, the interviewer may wish to follow up the participants. Some interviewers undertake to give the interviewees copies of their findings and may offer the right of vetting the materials based on the interview.

Methods of recording interview information

Interviewers may use a number of different means of recording interview information, ranging from written summary notes of the interview to an actual video- or audiotaping of the live interview. These recording methods have a number of advantages and disadvantages, as discussed below.

1. *Video recording*. Video technology has reduced in cost and improved to such an extent that high-quality video recordings of interviews are well within the budgets of many organizations and individuals. Video recordings provide a wealth of information about the interview. It is possible to observe non-verbal communication channels as well as to construct audio transcripts of the interaction between the participants. However, some interviewees find the presence of the camera to be threatening. This may have a number of effects: one may be to refuse to participate, another may be to alter the normal flow of the interview. Some respondents may be unwilling to commit personal information and/or controversial views to tape, if they believe there is a risk that the interviewer might disclose the interview to others. Interviewees would find it difficult to deny their views when they have been videotaped expressing them. This is why the police in some countries videotape their interviews with suspects.

2. *Audio taping*. Many interviewers use audio recording of interviews in order to be able to prepare transcripts for later study. Many of the same issues that pertain to video recording are also relevant to audio recording. The use of audio recording may result in greater refusal rates and the 'sanitization' of the views expressed by participants for fear of reprisals arising from disclosure of the interview to others. Qualitative research methodologists have developed systematic methods in note-taking and coding of interview information. For an excellent treatment of these issues, the reader is referred to Kvale (1996).

Advantages and disadvantages of interview-recording methods

The advantages and disadvantages of the various recording methods are summarized in Table 10.2. Thus, video recording is intrusive, requires substantial post-interview analysis and may result in less disclosure, yet provides very rich information that can be independently analysed. The use of a recording method such as a response sheet requires great trust in the judgment and recording abilities of the interviewer. There is a potential for bias arising from the interviewer 'adjusting' the information provided by the interviewee to fit the recording method and/or expectations of the interviewer. Further, there is no opportunity for re-analysis.

So which information-recording method for interviews is the most appropriate? The appropriateness of the method of recording interview information is determined by the needs of the person using the information. For example, if the information user simply wants some basic data such

Table 10.2 Advantages and disadvantages of different ways of recording interview information

	Advantages	Disadvantages
Video recording	Full transcripts of interview possible Non-verbal data available Accessible to independent analysis	Intrusive Less disclosure Necessity for substantial, and costly, post-interview analysis Potentially greater rates of refusal to participate
Audio recording	Full transcripts of interview possible Accessible to independent analysis	Intrusive (but probably less than video) Reduced disclosure Necessity for substantial, and costly, post-interview analysis Potentially greater rates of refusal to participate
Response sheets	Same data recorded for all interviews Little post-interview analysis required, reducing costs	Unexpected answers may not be well handled Interviewers may bias data in their recording Inaccessible to independent analysis
Unstructured notes	Cheap and simple	Interviewers may bias data in their recording Some data may be omitted Inaccessible to independent analysis Necessity for some post-interview analysis

as the age, sex and symptom profile of a patient, it would be absurd to use video recording. This would be very time-consuming. Each tape would have to be made, then viewed again for analysis. In this instance, a simple response sheet or checklist would suffice. However, if the interviewer was interested in exploring reactions of interviewees to the death of a close relative, perhaps the use of audio or video recording would provide a richness of data suitable for that interest.

Although most interviews are conducted with one interviewer and one interviewee present, sometimes group interviews with many participants are conducted. The focus group, which is a form of group interview, involves a discussion among a small group of people, including a moderator or facilitator (Thomas et al 1992). The facilitator's role is to introduce the topics or questions for discussion and to facilitate the contributions of the group participants. As a matter of historical interest, Merton (1946) originally proposed the focused interview, which was the forerunner for the focus group.

Focus groups differ fundamentally from the individual interview in that the researcher is outnumbered and the participants may interact with each other, modify each other's responses and ask questions of each other. The researcher is less in control of the process than in other types of interview approaches. Focus groups often bring to the surface matters that would not have been raised in conventional interviews. Focus groups are now widely used in health research because they provide rich sources of insights and interpretations from the participants.

The analysis of interview data

The manner in which interview data may be analysed is determined in part by how the data have been recorded and, in part, by the theoretical orientation of the researcher. In the previous discussion, we have seen that these formats include videotapes, audiotapes, completed response sheets and free-form summary interviewer notes.

The basis for many analyses of interview data is the interview transcript. The transcript of an interview is a verbatim written version of the conversation that took place between the participants. To provide an example, an excerpt from an interview transcript produced by Janet Doyle at La Trobe University follows (Doyle & Thomas 2000). The transcript is of an interview between a clinician and a client, concerning the client's hearing loss.

Clinician:	Okay. So what are you noticing with your hearing?
Client:	Well, in a crowded area I can't, you know, understand the other people.
Clinician:	Right, sound's a bit jumbled up.
Client:	And when I am in the next room I can't even hear the phone.
Clinician:	Right.
Client:	I am not bad, it is like I am not that bad but still at times.
Clinician:	Right.
Client:	There is a lot of times I can't hear it.
Clinician:	If people speak directly to you like this you are fairly good?
Client:	Yes I am alright.
Clinician:	But in a group have a bit of trouble?
Client:	Have trouble.
Clinician:	Right, does one ear seem better than the other ear?
Client:	Yes, this one seems better than this.
Clinician:	Right.
Clinician:	How long have you been noticing your difficulty?
Client:	Oh, about 12 to 18 months I suppose.
Clinician:	Just gradual was it?
Client:	Yes.
Clinician:	Okay. Do you get any ringing or buzzing in your ears?
Client:	Oh, now and again, very seldom though.
Clinician:	It doesn't bother you?
Client:	No.
Clinician:	Okay. Have you had medical trouble with your ears like infection or anything?
Client:	No, no.
Clinician:	Do you know of any family history of hearing loss?
Client:	No, only the older brother, he has got a hearing aid.
Clinician:	Right.
Client:	That's all.
Clinician:	Have you been exposed to excessive noise?
Client:	Yes.
Clinician:	… machinery or?
Client:	Yeah. I worked down the car plant, you know, with the heavy machinery.
Clinician:	The assembly line?
Client:	Right.
Clinician:	Were you doing that sort of work for a long time?
Client:	Oh yes, 30 years.
Clinician:	Yeah, that's a fair …
Client:	I wasn't on the line all the time but.
Clinician:	Right.

And so the interview continued.

Let us now consider some of the analysis options under the quantitative and qualitative headings.

Quantitative analysis of interview transcripts

A number of quantitative analyses possibilities are presented with interview transcripts. For example, the researcher might count the number of words spoken by each participant to obtain a quantitative measure of their relative contributions to the conversational process. Another possibility would be to count the number of questions asked by the clinician. These quantitative measures could then be used to test various hypotheses. Analyses of interview transcripts similar to the example shown above, in the study from which it was taken, have demonstrated substantial sex differences between the number of questions asked by male and female clients. It seems that the male clients asked many more questions than the females. Thus, the quantitative researcher might use interview transcripts to count and analyse certain features of the transcripts.

Qualitative analysis of interview transcripts

Under the qualitative heading there is a broad variety of approaches to the collection and analysis of interview data. Such approaches may, however, be broadly categorized as *descriptive* or *theoretical*.

A descriptive qualitative study is often termed an ethnography. They are often written from the perspective of the participant(s) in the first person. The purpose of the ethnography is to provide a detailed description of a particular set of circumstances and to encourage readers to make their own interpretations. A celebrated example of such an ethnography is found in Bogdan & Taylor's (1976) description of Ed Murphy's life. Ed Murphy was a former resident of a home for the intellectually disabled in the USA.

Many qualitative studies, however, are theoretical in nature. That is, they attempt to develop theories and concepts and, often, to verify these concepts and theories.

A key approach to theoretical qualitative research is provided by Glaser & Strauss' (1967) grounded theory (see also Strauss 1987, Strauss & Corbin 1998). Glaser & Strauss advocate two methods for the development of grounded theory: the constant comparative method in which the researcher codes and analyses data to develop concepts, and the theoretical sampling method in which cases are selected purposively to refine the 'theory' previously developed. Glaser & Strauss provide highly detailed examples of their analytic methods in the above references and the interested reader is referred to them for further detail. Glaser & Strauss' approach is not universally accepted in that some qualitative researchers argue for the necessity both to develop and verify their theories. Notwithstanding these theoretical differences, many qualitative researchers share common analysis tools such as coding and thematic analysis.

Coding and thematic analysis

Coding is used to organize data collected in an interview and, for that matter, in other types of documents such as field notes. Different qualitative researchers advocate different approaches to coding but it typically involves the following steps. The researchers closely study their materials, in this case the interview transcripts, and develop a close familiarity with the material. During this process, all the concepts, themes and ideas are noted to form major categories. For example, in interviews of nursing home residents, some themes that arise might include personal safety, autonomy and decision making, personal hygiene and so on. Often, the researcher will then attach a number or label to each category and record their positions in the transcript. Coding is an iterative process, with the researcher coding and recoding, as the scheme develops. Some computer programs are now available to assist with the coding analysis of machine-readable transcripts and these ease some of the clerical burden, although most qualitative researchers still employ manual coding methods. The researchers, having developed the codes and coded the transcripts, then attempt to interpret their meanings in the context in which they appeared. The reporting of this process typically involves 'thick' or detailed description of the categories and their context, with liberal use of examples from the original transcripts. The process of analysis of qualitative research materials is examined in more detail later in this book.

Summary

Interviews may be defined as a conversation between interviewers and interviewees with the purpose of eliciting certain information. Structured interviews generally involve a fixed set of questions or schedule, the use of preplanned response sheets, a greater proportion of closed-response questions and direction from the interviewer. Unstructured interviews tend not to have these attributes, with less structure and control. Interviews may be conducted face to face or by telephone and both these methods have certain advantages and disadvantages. The focus group is a valuable alternative to the individual interview. Interview data may be recorded in a number of different ways, but the transcript is often used. Transcripts may be analysed using quantitative or qualitative techniques.

Self-assessment

Explain the meaning of the following terms:

coding
ethnography
grounded theory
interview
response schedule
structured interview
transcript
unstructured interview

True or false

1. A structured interview always involves a written questionnaire.
2. In an unstructured interview, the questions are asked in a fixed order.
3. In an interview, it is important for interviewers to express their feelings.
4. In a response schedule, the interviewer records his/her interpretation of the interviewee's statements.
5. Coding is a method of qualitative analysis of interview transcripts.
6. An ethnography is generally written in the third person.
7. A transcript is a summary of the interviewer's interpretation of the questions.
8. Video recording of an interview may affect the honesty of the interviewee's answers.

Multiple choice

1. One of the problems with unstructured interviews is that:
   a the same questions may not be asked of all interviewees
   b the answers are recorded in the interviewee's own words
   c the questions are all asked in the same order
   d the interviews are too brief.
2. One of the problems with structured interviews is that:
   a the same questions may not be asked of all interviewees
   b the answers are not recorded in the interviewee's own words

   c the questions are all asked in the same order
   d the interviews are often too long.
3. One of the advantages of a face-to-face interview is that:
   a the interviewer can take an audio recording of the interview
   b non-verbal cues can be ignored
   c interviewers can minimize their influence on the answers
   d the interviewer has more credibility than a telephone interviewer.
4. A qualitative analysis of an interview transcript is likely to include:
   a counting the number of words spoken by each participant
   b the use of a checklist
   c coding of recurrent themes and ideas
   d checks on the quality of the interviewer's speech.
5. A quantitative analysis of an interview transcript is likely to include:
   a the use of unstructured field notes
   b coding of recurrent themes and ideas
   c counting the number of words spoken by each participant
   d checks on the quality of the interviewer's speech.
6. To record the age, sex, height and weight of a patient, it would be best to use:
   a a video recorder
   b an audiotape recorder
   c a transcript of the interview
   d a response checklist.
7. An ethnography is:
   a an interview with a non-English-speaking person
   b an interview with a foreign-born but English-speaking person
   c a type of descriptive qualitative study of someone's experiences
   d a type of quantitative study.
8. Coding is:
   a a qualitative method of analysing interview data
   b a method of keeping interview data confidential
   c a quantitative method of analysing interview data
   d usually performed without a written transcript.

Chapter **Eleven**

11

Observation

Introduction

Observation is a common method for data collection in both health research and clinical practice. Observation involves being close to things, such that the observer is in a position directly to perceive and record the phenomena under study. The advantage of observational data collection over questionnaires and interviews in research is that the researcher is in a position directly to see and hear what people actually do, rather than relying on the participants' interpretations and perceptions of their actions.

The aims of this chapter are to:

1. Outline different approaches to conducting observations and examine their relative advantages.
2. Discuss the different roles observers may adopt.
3. Examine observation in the context of qualitative and quantitative approaches.

Overview of different approaches to observation

Depending on the phenomenon being studied and the research questions being asked, one or more of a number of different observational approaches may be employed in the data collection. Each of these approaches has associated advantages and disadvantages. The basic issues are:

- who is to make the observations
- the settings in which the observations are made
- the use of instrumentation.

Who is to make the observations?

When research involves the observation of human subjects, self-observation becomes feasible and, at times, desirable. As an example, consider the study of pain. Here the patients themselves are uniquely positioned to provide subjective evidence concerning the intensity and location of pain over a period of time. Figure 11.1 shows a typical chart for guiding self-recorded pain observations in chronic pain patients, which is used in both research and clinical assessment.

The self-observations of the patients provide data for understanding how patients' pain experiences change over time, events correlating with the onset and offset of the pain and also evidence for evaluating the relative effectiveness of pain management strategies. Given that the experience of pain may be expressed in the sufferer's overt behaviour, we may observe such pain-related behaviours when assessing pain. For instance, in a study involving comparison of pain behaviours of surgical patients with different cultural backgrounds, independent observers recorded pain-related behaviours in patients at agreed time intervals during physiotherapy treatments. Figure 11.2 is based on whether the observers recorded a yes or no for each category for each time interval in which the behaviours were sampled.

There are probable relative advantages and disadvantages to using self-observation or outside observers, as shown in Table 11.1.

	On average, what was your level of pain during today
Monday	0 1 2 3 4 5 6 7 8 9 10 no pain very intense
Tuesday	0 1 2 3 4 5 6 7 8 9 10 no pain very intense
Wednesday	0 1 2 3 4 5 6 7 8 9 10 no pain very intense

Figure 11.1 • Typical chart for self-recorded pain observations.

| Behaviours | Time | | |
	t1	t2	t3
Verbal complaint			
Vocalization			
Protective response			

Figure 11.2 • Observation guide for recording pain behaviours.

Table 11.1 Advantages and disadvantages of using self-observation or outside observers

	Advantages	Disadvantages
Self-observation	Greater access to subjective experience (introspection) Less intrusive Less expensive	Greater bias Less likely to record accurately Less likely to carry out observation as agreed
Outside observer	Greater objectivity Less bias More likely to record accurately More likely to carry out observations as agreed	Cannot directly access subject's perceptions More intrusive More expensive and time-consuming

Settings in which observation is conducted

Some disciplines, such as astronomy or geography, focus on phenomena which are best studied as they occur, in their natural settings. Other disciplines, such as anatomy or chemistry, are more likely to be studied in a laboratory. In the broad range of health sciences research, phenomena are studied in either laboratory or natural settings, and observational data collection may be appropriate in both of these settings.

The general advantage of laboratory environments is that we can impose a considerable degree of control over extraneous variables which may systematically influence our observations. In addition, equipment for facilitating or recording observations is more readily available. For example, in the 1960s, Masters & Johnson began a series of studies to examine the physiology of the human sexual response. The controlled laboratory setting and the use of appropriate instrumentation enabled these researchers to observe and accurately record poorly understood aspects of human sexual functioning. This work was thought to be fundamental for developing clinically useful interventions aimed at helping people with sexual dysfunction, although it must be noted that this work has not been without controversy.

The disadvantage with laboratory settings is that the phenomenon being observed may change when it is being observed in an artificial setting. This is particularly true for human behaviour, where the social contexts are fundamental determinants of the behaviours and experiences. Indeed, the discipline of social psychology is devoted to the study of these effects. In other words, laboratory research sometimes has problematic ecological validity in that the findings discovered in this context may not generalize well to other contexts. Table 11.2 summarizes some of the relative advantages and disadvantages of laboratory and natural settings for making observations.

Unaided observation or the use of instrumentation

The accurate observation of a variety of phenomena is possible through the unaided senses; for example, observing aspects of human behaviour or clinical symptoms such as abnormal postures, discoloration of the skin, or abnormalities in patients' eye movements. Other phenomena may be inaccessible to unaided observation such as, for example, very small objects and events, where we might need to use a microscope for accurate observations. Some events are also extremely complex and occur relatively quickly in relation to the observer. An example of this is human locomotion where recording the event using a device such as a video camera greatly enhances the accuracy of the observation. A fundamental reason for the advancement of science and clinical practice has been the development of sophisticated instrumentation.

Table 11.2 Advantages and disadvantages of laboratory and natural settings for making observations

	Advantages	Disadvantages
Laboratory setting	Better control over extraneous variables Observation aids and recording equipment available	Distortion of phenomena in artificial environments Problematic ecological validity
Natural setting	Increased ecological validity Observation of phenomena as they occur naturally	Little control over extraneous variables Observation aids and recording equipment may be more difficult to use

There are, however, certain disadvantages associated with using instrumentation. These issues are discussed later in this book, when we review instrumentation and measurement. We can note here, however, that the use of instruments may distort the event being observed; for example, the preparation of tissue for electron microscopy changes to some extent the internal organelles of a cell being observed. It requires considerable expertise to use more complex instruments, and a strong theoretical background to separate the artefacts from useful data and interpret the observations. Human subjects also react to being observed. The more intrusive the observer is with equipment and instruments, the more likely that the subjects' behaviour will change.

The use and relative advantages and disadvantages of recording techniques were discussed in the context of interviewing techniques earlier in the book. Table 11.3 represents the relative advantages and disadvantages of using instruments for aiding observations.

Observer roles

Whether or not instrumentation is used as an adjunct, observation involves a person perceiving and recording an event. There are various positions observers may take in relation to observing human behaviour in health care settings. The fundamental issue is the extent to which the observer becomes involved or participates in the events being observed. There are generally considered to be four main roles that an observer may take. These are: complete participant, participant as observer, observer as participant and complete observer. These are discussed below.

The *complete participant* assumes the role of participant in the setting under investigation and does not normally disclose his or her intent to the other participants. Thus, the researcher actively participates in the setting without the knowledge or consent of the other participants. The purpose behind this approach is to minimize any changes in behaviour of the other participants as a result of their being observed. It can, however, border on the edge of unethical practice and must be used with caution. An example of the use of the complete participant method is provided by Rosenhan's (1975) classic study of 'pseudo-patients' in psychiatric hospitals. Here, the observers posed as (and were admitted as) psychiatric patients in order to study the experiences of psychiatric patients. The pseudo-patients were not recognized as impostors by the staff or the institutions. In this way, they could make and record observations about the interpersonal interactions between the staff and patients. However, in order to be admitted, the observers deliberately misled the staff, who were in fact under study.

The *participant as observer* participates fully in the situation under study, but discloses his or her identity and purpose to the other participants. Examples of this can be seen in anthropological

Table 11.3 The advantages and disadvantages of using instruments for aiding observations

	Advantages	Disadvantages
Unaided observations	Less disruptive Best suited for observing human behaviour Relatively simple and inexpensive	Insufficient for observing some phenomena Insufficient accuracy and detail
Instrumentation	Access to events outside unaided human senses Increased accuracy and detail	May distort phenomena May be complex and expensive to use

studies, where the observer attempts to participate as an active member of a cultural group.

The *observer as participant* makes no pretence of participation but interacts with the other participants. When using this method in a health setting, the observer obtains permission to record events and observe patients, while interacting with the staff and the patients. An example of this method is provided by a study performed by a PhD student with a nursing background, supervised by one of the authors. The student's objective was to investigate how psychiatric nurses working in the community make decisions to act in a crisis situation with a disturbed person. He accompanied the nurses on their crisis visits. While travelling to the crisis scene, he interviewed the nurses about their expectations. He observed the crisis scene and its participants and, immediately following its conclusion, interviewed the nurses about it.

The *complete observer* does not interact with the other participants at all and, as with complete participation, does not disclose his or her identity or purpose. As an example, one might investigate therapist–patient interactions by observing from behind a one-way mirror. Observers can, if they wish, use a structured schedule for making the observations.

The level of participation chosen involves a tension between the requirements of objective and independent analysis, and the proximity from which the social and clinical phenomena can be studied. Clearly, the participation of the observer introduces changes in the phenomenon under study. It is a question of whether these changes are so large as to negate the benefits obtained by closer observation afforded by actual participation. This question has generated much discussion in the social, behavioural and clinical sciences.

Observation in qualitative field research

Observation data collection in the context of qualitative field research requires providing authentic pictures and reports of individuals functioning in their natural environments. Lofland (1971) outlined the following four important principles for conducting field research:

1. The investigator should establish proximity with the subjects in both a physical and a social sense. It is desirable that this involvement should be long-term, both to enable understanding and to reduce the subjects' reactivity to the presence of the investigator.

2. The report should be truthful. The reporter should not allow ideological biases to distort or censor their observations or deliberately lie to place their subjects in a good or bad light.

3. The data should contain a large amount of 'pure description of action, people, activities and the like. The reality of the place should be conveyed through representation of its mundane aspects in a straightforward manner' (Lofland 1971, p. 4).

4. The data should contain direct quotations from the participants. Note-taking, audio and video recordings are appropriate for conveying the actual situation. The obtrusiveness of the data collection methods is a major factor. It would not do to assume the role of a complete participant and turn up with a movie camera, while denying any other motives.

Lofland (1971) suggested that, when observing subjects in the context of field research, the investigator might focus on the following categories:

1. *Acts and activities*. These are actions constituting brief or major involvements of an individual:

All pseudo patients took extensive notes publicly. Under ordinary circumstances, such behaviour would have raised questions in the minds of observers, as, in fact, it did among patients. Indeed, it seemed so certain that the notes would elicit suspicion that elaborate precautions were taken to remove them from the ward each day. But the precautions proved needless. The closest any staff member came to questioning these notes occurred when one pseudo-patient asked his physician what kind of medication he was receiving and began to write down the response. 'You needn't write it', he was told gently. 'If you have trouble remembering, just ask me again.'

Rosenhan (1975)

2. *Meanings*. These are verbal productions, defining or explaining the subject's activities: holding her breath, standing still, sniffing, and coughing were all means of countering what she felt as her mother's impingements.

Mary:	*I used to hold my breath because my mother used to go on so quick and (pause).*
Interviewer:	*Moving you mean?*
Mary	*Yes.*
Interviewer:	*You mean your mother was moving about the house quickly?*
Mary:	*Yes and everything.*
Interviewer:	*And what did you do?*
Mary:	*Sort of stand like that.*
Interviewer:	*Can you demonstrate to me – sitting in a chair?*
Mary:	*Yes. I just sort of (shows what she did).*
Interviewer:	*With your elbows?*

Laing & Esterson (1970)

3. *Participation*. This describes the subjects' involvement in a particular setting:

The pseudo-patient behaved afterward as he normally behaved. The pseudo-patient spoke to patients and staff as he might ordinarily. Because there is uncommonly little to do on a psychiatric ward, he attempted to engage others in conversation. When asked by staff how he was feeling, he indicated that he was fine, that he no longer experienced symptoms. He responded to instructions from attendants, to calls for medication (which was not swallowed), and to dining-hall instructions. Beyond such activities as were available to him on the admissions ward, he spent his time writing down his observations about the ward, its patients, and the staff. Initially these notes were written secretly, but as it soon became clear that no one much cared, they were subsequently written on standard tablets of paper in such public places as the day-room. No secret was made of these activities.

Rosenhan (1975)

4. *Relationships*. These are descriptions of the nature of the interrelationships among several people:

Her absence of social life, her withdrawal, appears to be an unwitting invention of her parents that never seems to have been called into question.

Ruth:	*Well the places I like to go to my parents don't like me to go to.*
Mother:	*Such as?*
Ruth:	*Eddie's club.*
Mother:	*Oh, goodness. You don't really –*
Father:	*?*
Ruth:	*I do.*
Interviewer:	*What is 'Eddie's'?*
Mother:	*It's a drinking club. She doesn't really drink. It's just that she likes to meet different types.*
Interviewer:	*She sounds as though the people that she does want to go out with are people she feels you disapprove of.*
Mother:	*Possibly.*
Father:	*Yes.*
Mother:	*Possibly.*

Her parents' attitude to the life Ruth actually leads involves both the negation of its existence and the perception of mad or bad behaviour on Ruth's part. Thus, she is said to drink excessively, while, simultaneously, she is said not to drink at all.

Laing & Esterson (1970)

5. *Settings*. These are descriptions of the entire setting for the investigation:

A stranger entering an ICU is at once bombarded with a massive array of sensory stimuli, some emotionally neutral but many highly charged. Initially, the greatest impact comes from the intricate machinery, with its flashing lights, buzzing and beeping monitors, gurgling suction pumps, and whooshing respirators. Simultaneously, one sees many people rushing around busily performing lifesaving tasks. The atmosphere is not unlike that of the tension-charged strategic bunker. With time, habituation occurs, but the ever-continuing stimuli decrease the overload threshold and contribute to stress at times of crisis.

As the newness and strangeness of the unit wears off, one increasingly becomes aware of a host of perceptions with specific stressful emotional significance. Desperately ill, sick, and injured human beings are hooked up to that machinery. And, in addition to mechanical stimuli, one can discern moaning, crying, screaming and the last gasps of life. Sights of blood, vomitus and excreta, exposed genitalia, mutilated wasting bodies, and unconscious and helpless people assault the sensibilities. Unceasingly, the ICU nurse must face these affect-laden stimuli with all the distress and conflict that they engender.

Hay & Oken (1977)

Observations of the above classes of behaviours and settings will provide a report representing individuals' experiences and their interactions in a natural setting.

Observation in quantitative research

Research involving human subjects may be conducted using either qualitative or quantitative approaches. With non-human phenomena, quantitative approaches are obviously more relevant. The following are common features of observations in the context of quantitative research.

1. *Observer roles*. In quantitative research, the observer attempts to be as objective and detached as possible. Therefore, the observer as participant or the complete observer roles are most suited for quantitative approaches.
2. *Definition of relevant variables*. Considerable effort is made in quantitative research to specify precisely what aspect of an object, event or human behaviour the investigator intends to study and observe. In studies where several observers are involved in data collection it is appropriate to

discuss and demonstrate that there is a substantial degree of agreement among the observers. The above issues will be discussed in more detail in the context of operational definitions, validity and reliability in the next chapter.

3. *Observation and structure*. For quantitative studies, we prefer the maximum level of control and structure. Bailey (1987, p. 243) suggested that there were two types of 'structures' relevant for observational data collection. The first is the degree of structure in the environment in which the observations are made. We have examined this point earlier, where we compared laboratory and natural settings with laboratory settings having a higher degree of structure or predictability. The degree of structure for observation may be further increased by using explicit, previously prepared observation guides or protocols. This is quite similar to how degrees of 'structure' or 'formality' are determined in the context of interview techniques, as outlined in the previous chapters.

We have examined two different types of observation guides (shown in Figs 11.1 and 11.2). If they are to be useful for conducting observational data collection, considerable effort must be made in the design of such guides and in establishing their reliability and validity, as we shall see in the next chapter.

The advantages of an observation guide are that the recording of the observations is made simple, and the data are easily summarized and evaluated using descriptive and inferential statistics, as discussed in later chapters of this book. The disadvantage of highly structured observations (as with interview and questionnaire techniques) is that the spontaneity and uniqueness of certain events may be lost, to the extent that only predetermined categories are recorded.

Summary

Data collection based on observation is appropriate for a wide range of research designs, ranging from laboratory-based experiments to qualitative field research. A basic issue is the extent to which a structure is imposed on the observer. Highly structured observational frameworks are most suited for quantitative research while more loosely structured participant observation is better suited for qualitative research. In general, when making observations involving human subjects, researchers attempt to minimize subject reactivity and enhance the accuracy of recording the evidence. When appropriate, instrumentation may be used to enhance or record observations. It is worth noting that data collection using questionnaires, interviews and observations may well be used in combination in both research and clinical case work.

Self-assessment

Explain the meaning of the following terms:

acts
complete observer
complete participant
meanings
natural setting
observer as participant
participation
relationships
settings

True or false

1. By 'meanings' Lofland was referring to verbal explanations of a person's behaviours.
2. Of the variety of observer roles, the 'complete participant' is the least likely to create ethical problems.
3. In a study involving changes in sleep patterns, self-observation would be an appropriate data collection strategy.
4. Detailed personal diaries of life events and their personal implications are suitable for qualitative research.
5. In the context of modern health sciences research, researchers must use instrumentation to facilitate and record their observations.
6. Anatomic research is well suited for the participant observer role.
7. 'Settings' refers to the physical and social environment in which field observations are conducted.
8. The 'observer as participant' attempts to create interesting, novel situations in the setting in which they carry out field research.
9. Laboratory settings require minimal structure for observational data collection.

10. Observational and interview data collection may be carried out simultaneously in clinical case work.

Multiple choice

1. The advantage of observation over interview as a data collection technique is that:
   a observations may be recorded and scrutinized later
   b observations enable the recording of actual behaviours, rather than subjects' interpretations
   c observation is scientific, unlike interviews which necessarily involve personal interactions
   d observations are unbiased and do not elicit reactions in human subjects.
2. You design an investigation to examine therapist–patient interaction in a hospital setting. Your suggested data collection involves a peep-hole and a hidden microphone for observing specific interactions unknown to the subjects. This study:
   a may well be rejected on ethical grounds
   b involves participant observation
   c would probably maximize subject reactivity
   d both a and c.
3. In order to reduce subjects' reactivity in the context of qualitative observational studies, the researcher should:
   a use subjects who do not react to being observed
   b inform the subjects of the detailed aims of the study, to reduce ambiguity
   c carry out the observations over a prolonged period of time
   d use video-recording equipment to minimize reactivity.
4. Participant observation may be defined as:
   a the observation of participants in the study
   b the observation of the researcher's input to a study
   c participation in a group while studying it
   d the study of observational and clinical techniques.
5. One of the major problems associated with the use of participant observation as a research strategy is that:
   a it is more expensive than experimental approaches to implement

b it does not allow 'in-depth' study of any phenomena

c the results cannot be replicated

d participation may alter the phenomena under study.

6. Observation in the context of qualitative field research:

a involves the use of well-designed and pre-defined observation guides

b depends on the precise definition of the variables being observed

c requires physical and social proximity with the subjects

d both a and b.

7. The advantage of observational data collection in laboratory settings is that:

a extraneous events disrupting observations are more easily controlled

b the ecological validity of the study as a whole is improved

c there is less distortion of the phenomena because of the improved structure

d there is no need to use expensive equipment for recording observations.

8. Which of the following would represent an 'observer as participant' role?

a A researcher pretends to be a non-English-speaking migrant to observe doctors' responses to reports of low back pain.

b A physiotherapist carries out observations of patients while carrying out normal clinical practice.

c A researcher is given permission to attend clinical sessions in order to observe doctor–patient interactions.

d A neurologist suffers a stroke and keeps detailed records of her observed cognitive and sensory changes.

Chapter Twelve

12

Measurement

Introduction

The term *measurement* refers to the procedure of attributing qualities or quantities to specific characteristics of objects, persons or events. Measurement is a key process in quantitative research, evaluation and in clinical practice. If the measurement procedures in a study are inadequate its usefulness will be limited. Similarly, in clinical practice, the validity of diagnoses and treatment decisions can be compromised by inadequate measurement processes and tools.

The aims of this chapter are to:

1. Discuss key issues in measurement procedures.
2. Describe good practice in measurement in both research and clinical settings.
3. Evaluate and discuss the different types of measurement scales.

Operational definitions and measurement

Sometimes researchers start off with rather vague views of how to measure the variables included in a study. For instance, if researchers are interested in measuring 'levels of pain' experienced by patients, then the researchers must convert their general ideas about measuring pain to a tightly defined statement of how this is to be measured.

Depending on their theoretical interpretation of the concept of 'pain', and the practical requirements of the investigation, one of the many possible approaches to measurement of pain will then be selected.

The process of converting theoretical ideas to a tightly defined statement of how variables are to be measured is called operationalization. It is important that researchers give exact details of how the measures were taken in order that others may judge their adequacy and appropriateness and be in a position to repeat the procedures in a new study. A study that is adequate in terms of design, sampling methods and sample size may nevertheless have poor validity due to the use of inadequate measurement techniques. Let us now discuss operationalization.

The *operational definition* of a variable is a statement of how the researcher in a particular study chooses to measure the variable in question. It should be unambiguous.

At the outset, let us note that in most circumstances there is no single best way of taking measurements. If a researcher claimed that her therapeutic techniques significantly increased 'motor control' in her sample of patients, the obvious question that arises is 'What was meant by 'motor control' and how was it measured?' If our researcher replied that she was interested in motor control as measured by the Plunkett Motor Dexterity Task scores, she has, in fact, supplied her operational definition. Another researcher may challenge the adequacy of this definition and substitute her own, stating that patients' self-ratings of control in various tracking tasks is a more appropriate definition.

A good operational definition will contain enough information to enable another researcher or clinician to replicate the measurement techniques used in the original study. Similarly, a good operational definition of a clinically relevant variable will enable a fellow professional to replicate the original diagnostic or assessment procedures. An operational definition can be an unambiguous description, a photograph or diagram, or the specification of a brand name of a standard tool. In describing a piece of research, one must include operational definitions of the measuring apparatus and all procedures, so that readers are quite clear as to what has been done and with whom and when.

Objective and subjective measures

A distinction is commonly drawn between objective and subjective measures, often with overtones of suspicion directed towards so-called 'subjective' measures. Let us make a much less value-laden distinction and define them as follows: objective measurements involve the measurement of physical quantities and qualities using measurement equipment; subjective measures involve ratings or judgments by humans of quantities and qualities.

One should not confuse the distinction between objective and subjective measures as corresponding to good or bad measurement techniques. Equipment might be improperly calibrated, complicated to use, or become damaged during an investigation. For instance, a researcher might have an absolutely terrible set of weight scales that give results far at variance with the correct measures. With the sophistication and complexity of much current measurement equipment, it is often difficult to calibrate equipment accurately without a complex calibration procedure. Just because a machine is involved in measurement does not mean that the results will be accurate. Furthermore, many quantities and qualities associated with persons and clinical phenomena are difficult to measure objectively, such as the personal attractiveness of individuals, or aspects of patient–therapist relationships, or the 'quality' of a patient's gait.

Desirable properties of measurement tools and procedures

Measurement tools and procedures ought to yield measurements that are reproducible, accurate, applicable to the measurement task in hand and practical or easy to use. These properties are often given the technical terms of reliability, validity, applicability and practicability. These properties will be reviewed in detail in the following sections. Measurement theory and method are concerned with the development of measurement tools that maximize these properties.

Before these specific test properties are reviewed, it is useful to review some basic concepts in test theory. In any measurement, we have three related concepts: the observed value or test score, the true value or test score and measurement error. Thus if I could be weighed on a completely accurate set of weighing scales, my true score might be 110 kg. However, the scales that I use in my bathroom might give me a reading of 100 kg. The difference between the observed score and my true score is the measurement error. This relationship can be expressed in the form of an equation such that:

Observed value = true value ± error

Thus, measurement tools are designed with a view to minimize measurement error so that the observed value we obtain from our assessment process is close to the true value.

Reliability

Reliability is the property of reproducibility of the results of a measurement procedure or tool. There are several different ways in which reliability can be assessed. These include test–retest reliability, inter-observer reliability and internal consistency. Let us examine each.

Test–retest reliability

A common way to assess test reliability is to administer the same test twice to the same participants. The results obtained from the first test are then correlated with the second test. Reliability is generally measured by a correlation coefficient that may vary from −1 to +1 in value. A test–retest reliability of +0.8 or above is considered to be sound. When the measurement process involves clinical ratings, e.g. a clinician's rating of the dependency level of a cerebrovascular accident (CVA) patient, test–retest reliability is sometimes

termed *intra-observer* reliability, i.e. the same observer rates the same patients twice and the results are correlated.

Inter-observer (inter-rater) reliability

A common issue in clinical assessment is the extent to which clinicians agree with each other in their assessments of patients. The extent of agreement is generally determined by having two or more clinicians independently assess the same patients and then comparing the results using correlations. If the agreement (correlation) is high then we have high inter-observer or inter-rater reliability.

Table 12.1 illustrates examples of both high and low inter-observer reliability on ratings of patients on a 5-point scale. Let's imagine that this scale measures the level of patient dependency and need for nursing support. As we mentioned earlier, the degree of reliability is quantitatively expressed by correlation coefficients. However, by inspection you can see that in Table 12.1 there is a high degree of disagreement in the two observers' ratings in the 'Low reliability' column. In this instance the clinical ratings would be unreliable, and inappropriate to use in the research project. However, the outcome shown in the 'High reliability' column in Table 12.1 shows a high level of agreement.

An example of a classic study of inter-rater and intra-rater reliability is provided by Coppleson et al (1970). Over an 11-month period, 29 biopsy

Table 12.1 Inter-observer reliability

| Subjects | Observers' ratings | | | |
| | Low reliability | | High reliability | |
	A	B	A	B
1	4	3	4	4
2	2	5	2	3
3	3	4	4	5
4	1	4	2	2
5	3	1	1	1
6	4	4	5	5

slides with suspected Hodgkin's disease were presented to three pathologists. The pathologists were asked to make a number of judgments about features of the specimens. The specimens were unlabelled and over the year of the study were presented on two occasions to each of the three observers. This permitted an assessment of the test–retest or intra-rater reliability of each observer. The three observers disagreed with themselves on 7, 8 and 9 occasions, respectively, out of the total number of specimens. Overall, inter-rater agreement was calculated at 76% or 54%, depending on the diagnostic classification system used by the observers. Studies of clinical judgment often find low levels of agreement between raters (see, for example, Doyle & Thomas 2000, Thomas et al 1991).

Internal consistency

Measurement tools will often consist of multiple items. For example, a test of your knowledge of research methods might include 50 items or questions. Similarly, a checklist designed to measure activities of daily living might have 20 items. The internal consistency of a test is the extent to which the results on the different items correlate with each other. If they tend to be highly correlated with each other, then the test is said to be internally consistent. Internal consistency is also measured by a form of correlation coefficient known as Cronbach alpha and an alpha of above 0.8 is considered to be a desirable property for a test.

Thus, the reliability or reproducibility of an assessment or test can be determined in several different ways including the test–retest, intra-rater, inter-rater and internal consistency methods.

Validity

Validity is concerned with accuracy of the test procedure. Just because one keeps getting the same result upon repeated administrations, or agreement among independent observers, doesn't mean that the results are accurate. If I jump on the bathroom scales and get a result of 40 kg and then jump off the scales and then get back on and it is still reading 40 kg, this reading is certainly reliable, but obviously it is an error (for readers who do not know us, 40 kg as an observed score for our weight entails major measurement error!). Thus the adequate reproducibility or reliability of a test or assessment process is essential, but we also need the results to be accurate or valid.

A case study in clinical test validity

The early detection of breast cancer in women has been recognized as an important public health initiative in many countries. Common ways of detecting suspicious lumps include breast self-examination and mammography, an X-ray of the breasts. Mammography is a common screening procedure and some countries such as Australia have funded large-scale programmes to promote it.

However, commendable as these initiatives may be, there are some doubts about the validity of mammography as a diagnostic tool. Walker & Langlands (1986), in their classic research project, studied the mammography results of 218 women, who, through the use of a diagnostic biopsy, were known to have breast cancer. Of the 218 women with cancer, 95 (43.6%) had recorded a (false) negative mammography test result. Of these patients, 47 had delayed further investigation and treatment for almost a year, no doubt relieved and reassured by their 'favourable' test results. The delays in treatment, given what we know about the relationship between early intervention and improved prognosis, in all likelihood seriously compromised the health and ultimate survival of these women. In this instance, the accuracy (or lack of it) of the test results has very important consequences for the people concerned. Test quality is of profound importance in research and clinical practice, as is demonstrated by this example.

Types of test validity

As with reliability, test validity may be assessed in a number of different ways. These include content validity, sensitivity and specificity, and predictive validity.

Content or face validity

In many contexts it is difficult to find external measures to correlate with the measure to be validated. For example, an examination in a particular academic subject may be the sole measure of the student's performance available to determine grades. How can it be determined whether the tests administered will be valid or not? One way is to write down all the material covered in the subject and then make sure that there is adequate sampling from the overall content of the material delivered in the subject. If this criterion is satisfied it can be said that the test has content or face validity. You may have had an experience where you felt that a subject assessment task had low content validity in that it did not reflect the material presented in the subject.

Sensitivity and specificity

The concepts of sensitivity and specificity are most commonly applied to diagnostic tests, where the purpose of the test is to determine whether the patient has a particular problem or illness. There are four possible outcomes for a test result, as shown in Table 12.2.

Table 12.2 Possible outcomes of test results

Test result	Real situation	
	Disease present	Disease not present
Disease present	True positive	False positive
Disease not present	False negative	True negative

Sensitivity refers to the proportion of people who test as positive who really have the disease (i.e. the proportion of true positives out of all positives). Specificity refers to the proportion of individuals who test as negative who really do not have the disease (i.e. the proportion of true negatives out of all negative test results). If a diagnostic test has a sensitivity of 1.0 and specificity of 1.0 it is a perfectly accurate or valid test. Most clinical tests are not perfect and some have unknown or quite low sensitivity and specificity.

Predictive validity

Predictive validity is concerned with the ability of a test to predict values of it or other tests in the future. Some tests are designed to assist with prognostic decisions, i.e. what is going to happen in the future; and for these tests high predictive validity is an important quality.

Let us examine an example of predictive validity. Say a researcher devised a screening rating scale, X, for selecting patients to participate in a rehabilitation programme. The effectiveness of the rehabilitation programme is assessed with rating scale Y. Say that each rating scale involves assigning scores of 1–10 to the patients' performance. Table 12.3 illustrates two outcomes: low predictive validity and high predictive validity.

Although the calculation of correlation coefficients is needed to examine quantitatively the predictive validity of test X, it can be seen in Table 12.3 that in the 'Low predictive validity' column, the scores on X are not clearly related

Table 12.3 Predictive validity

Subjects	Low predictive validity		High predictive validity	
	Score on X	Score on Y	Score on X	Score on Y
1	4	3	3	3
2	4	8	4	3
3	5	2	5	5
4	5	7	5	5
5	6	4	6	6
6	8	5	8	7

to the level of scores on Y. On the other hand, in the 'High predictive validity' column, scores on the two variables correspond quite closely. Within the limits of the fact that only six subjects were involved in this hypothetical study, it is clear that only the results in the 'High predictive validity' column are consistent with rating scale X being useful for predicting the outcome of the rehabilitation programme, as measured on scale Y.

At this point we should again refer to the concepts of internal and external validity. The concepts of predictive and content validity apply to the specific tests and measures a researcher or clinician uses. Internal and external validity refer to characteristics of the total research project or programme. Test validity should not be confused with other forms of research design validity such as external and internal validity.

External validity is concerned with the researcher's ability to generalize her or his findings to other samples and settings, i.e. the generalizability of the study findings. The external validity or generalizability of a study is affected by the sample size, the method of sampling, and the design characteristics and measures used in the study. If we say a study has high external validity, we mean that its findings generalize to other settings and samples outside the study. It does not make sense to talk about the external validity of a particular test.

Similarly, internal validity is concerned with the design characteristics of experimental studies. If a study is internally valid, any effects/changes or lack thereof in the dependent (outcome) variable can be directly attributed to the manipulation of the independent variable. It is important not to confuse the meanings of these terms.

Standardized measures and tests

Because reliability and validity of measures are so important, many researchers have devoted considerable time and energy to the development of measuring instruments and procedures that have known levels of reliability and validity.

The development of measurement standards for physical dimensions such as weight, length and time has been fundamental for the growth of science. That is, we have standards for comparing our measurements of a variable and we can meaningfully communicate our findings to colleagues living anywhere in the world. There are a variety of clinical measures, for instance the Apgar tests for evaluating the viability of neonates, that represent internationally recognized standards for communicating information about attributes of persons or disease entities.

Furthermore, there are standards relevant to populations, in terms of which assessments of individuals become meaningful. For instance, there are standards for the stages of development of infants: levels of physical, emotional, intellectual and social development occurring as a function of age.

Some tests have been trialled on large samples, and reliability and validity levels recorded. Tests that have been trialled in this way are known as standardized measures or tests. A large variety is available, particularly in the clinical and social areas. Bowling's *Measuring Health* (1997) is a very useful source of descriptions of such tests. Many US firms and cooperatives market standardized tests. However, many researchers use tests and measures that have not been standardized, and do not report levels of reliability in their literature. This is of particular concern in studies where subjective measures with incomplete operational definitions are employed.

Measurement scale types

Measurement can produce different types of numbers, in the sense that some numbers are assigned different meanings and implications from others. For instance, when we speak of Ward 1 and Ward 2, we are using numbers in a different sense from when we speak of infant A being 1 month old, and infant B being 2 months old. In the first instance, we used numbers for naming; in the second instance the numbers indicate quantities. There are four scale types, distinguished by the types of numbers produced by the measurement of a specific variable.

1. Nominal scales

The 'lowest' level of the measurement scale types is the nominal scale, where the measurement of a variable involves the naming or categorization of possible values of the variable. The measurements produced are 'qualitative' in the sense that the categories are merely different from each other. If numbers are assigned to the categories they are merely labels and do not represent real quantities; for example, Ward 1 and Ward 2 might be renamed St. Agatha's Ward and St. Martha's Ward without conveying any less information. Table 12.4 shows some other examples of nominal scaling.

The only mathematical relationship pertinent to nominal scales is equivalence or non-equivalence; that is, $A = B$ or $A \neq B$. A specific value of a variable either falls into a specific category, or it does not. Thus, there is no logical relationship between the numerical value assigned to its category and its size, quantity or frequency of occurrence. The arbitrary values of a nominal scale can be changed without any loss of information.

2. Ordinal scales

The next level of measurement involves rank ordering values of a variable. For example, 1st, 2nd or 3rd in a foot race are values on an ordinal scale. The numbers assigned on an ordinal scale signify order or rank.

With ordinal scales, statements about ranks can be made. Where A and B are values of the variable, we can say $A > B$ or $B > A$. For instance, we can say Mrs Smith is more cooperative than Mr Jones ($A > B$), or Mr Jones is more cooperative than Ms Krax ($B > C$). We cannot, however, make any statements about the relative sizes of these differences. Examples of ordinal scales are shown in Table 12.5.

3. Interval scales

Examples of interval scales are shown in Table 12.6. For these scales, there is no absolute zero point; rather, an arbitrary zero point is assigned. For instance, 0°C does not represent the point at which there is no heat, but the freezing point of water. An IQ of zero would not mean no intelligence at all, but a serious intellectual or perceptual problem in using the materials of the test.

Table 12.4 Some examples of nominal scaling

Variable	Possible values
Patients' admission numbers	3085001, 3085002
Sex	Male, female
Religion	Catholic, Protestant, Jewish, Muslim, Hindu
Psychiatric diagnosis	Manic-depressive, schizophrenic, neurotic
Blood type	A, B, AB, O
Cause of death	Cardiac failure, neoplasm, trauma

Table 12.5 Some examples of ordinal scales

Variable	Possible values
Severity of condition	Mild=1, moderate=2, severe=3, critical=4
Patients' satisfaction with treatment	Satisfied=1, undecided=2, dissatisfied=3
Age group	Baby, infant, child, adult, geriatric
Cooperativeness with nurse or patients in a ward	(In decreasing order) Mrs Smith, Mr Jones, Ms Krax

Table 12.6 Some examples of interval scales

Variable	Possible values
Heat (Celsius or Fahrenheit)	−10°C, +20°C, +5°C, +10°F
Intelligence (IQ)	45, 100, 185

The use of an interval scale enables identification of equal intervals between any two values of measurements: we can say A − B = B − C. For example, if A, B and C are taken as IQ scores, and A = 150, B = 100, and C = 50, then it is true that A − B = B − C. However, we cannot say that A = 3C (that A is three times as intelligent as C).

4. Ratio scales

Ratio scales have what is called a meaningful or non-arbitrary zero point. For example, in the Kelvin temperature scale, 0°K (or absolute zero) represents an absence of heat, in that the molecules have stopped vibrating completely; whereas 0°C is simply the freezing point of water. The Centigrade or Celsius zero is an arbitrary one tied to the freezing point of a particular compound. Thus °K is a ratio scale and °C is an interval scale. Examples of variables measured on ratio scales are shown in Table 12.7.

Table 12.8 compares the characteristics of different scales or levels of measurement.

Interval and ratio scales represent quantitative measurements. A ratio scale is the 'highest' scale of measurement, in the sense that it involves all the characteristics of the other scales, as well as having an absolute zero. A measurement on a higher level can be transformed into one on a lower level in this framework, but not vice versa, because the higher scale measurement contains more information and the values can be put to more use by permitting more mathematical operations than those on a lower level.

Also, a given variable might be measured on one of several types of scales, depending on the needs of the investigator. Consider, for instance, the variable 'height'. This variable could be measured on any of the four scales, as follows:

1. *Ratio scale*. The height of individuals above the ground, for example, 180 cm.
2. *Interval scale*. The height of individuals above an *arbitrary* surface; for example 100 cm above the surface of a bench.
3. *Ordinal scale*. The comparative heights of individuals, for example, rank-ordered from tallest to shortest.
4. *Nominal scale*. Categorizing individuals as, for example, 'normal' or 'abnormal'.

The different types of measurement scales are important when considering statistical analysis of data. Statistics are numbers with special properties from data. The type of measurement scale determines the type of statistic that is appropriate for its analysis. This issue is taken up later in this book.

Table 12.7 Variables measured on ratio scales

Variable	Possible values
Weight	10 kg, 20 kg, 100 kg
Height	50 cm, 150 cm, 200 cm
Blood pressure	110 mmHg, 120 mmHg, 160 mmHg
Heart beats	10 per minute, 30 per minute, 50 per minute
Rate of firing of a neurone	10 per millisec, 20 per millisec, 30 per millisec
Protein per blood volume	2 mg/cc, 5 mg/cc, 10 mg/cc
Vocabulary	100 words, 1000 words, 30 000 words

Table 12.8 Characteristics of levels of measurement

Characteristic	Level of measurement			
	Nominal	Ordinal	Interval	Ratio
Distinctiveness	•	•	•	•
Ordering in magnitude		•	•	•
Equal intervals			•	•
Absolute zero				•

Distinctiveness: different numbers assigned to different values of property.
Ordering in magnitude: larger values represent more of the property.
Equal intervals: same distance between points on a scale.
Absolute zero: zero value represents absence of property.

Summary

This section defines good measurement practice and its importance in research and clinical practice.

In good measurement practice we need to define concepts operationally, so that other investigators can also carry out or assess the measurement procedure. We also need to establish the reliability and validity of our measurements. A high degree of reliability and validity is necessary for minimizing measurement error. We have noted that measures involving the exercise of human judgment (i.e. 'subjective' measures) are not necessarily unreliable or invalid.

Four different scale types were discussed: nominal, ordinal, interval, and ratio. These scales have different characteristics, particularly in relation to the permissible mathematical operations. In subsequent sections, we shall see that the scale type involved in our measurements determines the descriptive and inferential statistics appropriate for describing and analysing the data.

Self-assessment

Explain the meaning of the following terms:

content validity
inter-observer reliability
interval scale
measurement
nominal scale
objective measures
operational definition
ordinal scale
predictive validity
ratio scale
standardized measures
standardized tests
subjective measures
test–retest reliability

True or false

1. The term 'measurement' refers to the assignment of qualities or quantities to specific aspects of objects or events.

2. An operational definition of a variable entails an explicit statement of how the variable is to be measured.

3. An objective measure is produced by the use of a measuring instrument.

4. A reliable test or measure will tend to produce accurate results.

5. A test–retest reliability as indicated by a correlation coefficient of 0.9 indicates a rather low reliability.

6. When an instrument is valid, we mean that it is measuring the characteristic which it is supposed to be measuring.

7. To establish the predictive validity of a test, we correlate the scores of individuals on the test with scores on other relevant measures.

8. A high correlation for scores between a college entrance examination and the subsequent examination results of students indicates that the entrance examination lacks predictive validity.

9. One of the advantages of using a standardized test is that its validity and reliability are already known.

10. Ordinal measures involve rank-ordering the values of a variable.

11. An interval scale has an absolute zero.

12. All arithmetical operations are permissible with measurements based on interval scales.

13. The levels of measurement which have the properties of distinctiveness, ordering of magnitude and equal intervals are the ordinal and nominal scales.

14. The statement 'Anxiety is a feeling of impending injury' is an example of an operational definition.

15. 'Operationalization' is defined as a statement specifying how a variable should be measured.

16. For a general concept like 'intelligence' only one operational definition is possible.

17. Subjective measures are necessarily unreliable.

18. Objective measures can be invalid and unreliable.

19. A correlation coefficient of 1.0 indicates an excellent test–retest reliability.

20. If a measurement is valid, then it is necessarily reliable.

21. A test may be highly reliable but invalid.

22. A low inter-observer reliability implies that the observed scores for a set of subjects on repeated tests tend to be unrelated to one another.

23. High predictive validity necessarily implies high content validity.

24. With a nominal scale, we can only make statements about the distinctiveness of scores.
25. The mathematical statement A – B=B – C is in correct form, given an ordinal scale.
26. Nominal scales do not have the characteristic of 'distinctiveness'.
27. The variable 'motor functioning' could be measured on either an ordinal or a nominal scale.
28. The variable 'blood sugar level' could be measured on either an ordinal or a ratio scale.
29. Ordinal scales are generally preferable to interval scales.
30. Statements such as $y=zx$ can be made validly with ratio measures.

Multiple choice

1. Which of the following does not include an operational definition?
   a Patients were encouraged to eat healthy food.
   b Males under 60 who were currently in full-time employment were the population for study.
   c Anxiety was measured by the Spielberger Anxiety Scale.
   d Patients who did not return for a scheduled follow-up appointment four weeks after initial treatment were classified as dropouts.
   e Students who get over half the test items correct will be classified as having passed.

2. Subjective measures:
   a are not operationally defined
   b are always less valid than objective measures
   c involve measuring physical attributes
   d are not reliable because everybody's subjective experience is different
   e none of the above.

3. Which of the following statements does not include an operational definition of the dependent variable?
   a In the present study, intelligence was measured on the Stanford Binet IQ test.
   b In the present study, intelligence was measured in terms of the level of subjects' knowledge of their cultures.
   c In the present study, intelligence was measured by the number of hairs on the subjects' heads.
   d b and c
   e a and c.

4. Objective measures:
   a are always more valid and reliable than subjective measures
   b involve extensive human intuition for interpretation
   c are always more reliable, but not necessarily more valid, than subjective measures
   d are used in experimental, but not in non-experimental, investigations
   e involve the measurement of physical qualities and quantities using measuring equipment.

5. A test is assessed for its reliability and its predictive validity. Both these measures are expressed as correlation coefficients, with the reliability coefficient being 0.9 and the predictive validity coefficient being 0.2. This indicates that:
   a the test is not reliable
   b the test has face validity
   c the test is reliable but does not appear to measure the variable of interest
   d the test is reliable, so it must measure the variable of interest
   e the test is a good one.

6. If the test–retest reliability of a measure is low, then it follows that:
   a the scores for different people tend to be different
   b the validity must be high
   c the scores for different people tend to be the same
   d the same person measured twice tends to produce different results.

7. If a test is valid then:
   a it might be reliable
   b it must be reliable
   c the reliability is unaffected
   d it must be unreliable.

8. The reading '64 kilograms' is a value on a(n):
   a ratio scale
   b interval scale
   c ordinal scale
   d nominal scale.

9. In a study of weight problems in a sample of pre-adolescent children, the relevant variable was expressed as 'percentage overweight' or 'underweight', given the child's height. This is an example of a(n):
   a ordinal scale
   b ratio scale
   c nominal scale
   d interval scale.

10. The gender of patients is an example of a(n):
a   ratio scale
b   nominal scale
c   ordinal scale
d   interval scale.

11. Which of the following variables has been labelled with an incorrect measuring scale?
a   The number of heart beats per minute: interval.
b   Platform numbers at a railway station: nominal.
c   Finishing order in a horse race: ordinal.
d   Self-rating of anxiety levels on a five-point scale: ordinal.

12. '10th' is a value on a(n):
a   ratio scale
b   interval scale
c   ordinal scale
d   nominal scale.

13. Response delay in milliseconds is an example of a(n):
a   ratio scale
b   ordinal scale
c   interval scale
d   nominal scale.

14. In a patient records system, patients are randomly assigned a unique identification number. These numbers represent a(n):
a   nominal scale
b   ratio scale
c   interval scale
d   ordinal scale.

Therapists assess levels of clients' 'independence' using the following scale:

0: Totally dependent on assistance from other/s for the activity.

1: Maximum assistance from other/s; can assist in a limited way.

2: Minimum assistance from one person; contributes significantly in carrying out the activity.

3: Supervised by another person due to mental/physical limitations and/or to ensure safety.

4: Independent with aids. Safe and consistent; would need assistance/supervision without aids.

5: Independent. Safe and consistent without aids, supervision or assistance.

Questions 15–17 refer to this scale.

15. The above scale is:
a   ratio
b   interval
c   nominal
d   ordinal.

16. If the subjects are assigned scores by the therapist's clinical judgment, then the measurement process is:
a   subjective
b   objective
c   unreliable
d   invalid
e   a and b.

17. Given the following three interval scale independence scores for three clients, A, B and C:
A: 4
B: 2
C: 0
which of the following statements is (are) true?
a   Client A is twice as independent as B.
b   The difference in independence between clients A and B is the same as that between clients B and C.
c   Client A is more independent than either B or C.
d   b and c.

18. Which of the following measures of the variable 'weight' is nominal?
a   Weight in kg.
b   Weight as percentage overweight in relation to 'healthy' weight.
c   Weight as obese/overweight/normal/underweight/grossly underweight.
d   Weight as 'normal against pathological' (obese or grossly underweight).

19. If a variable is not defined operationally, then:
a   the investigation of the variable might be difficult to replicate
b   it might be difficult to explain how the variable was measured
c   a and b
d   neither a nor b.

20. The terms 'external' and 'internal' validity refer to:
a   complete investigations
b   specific measurements
c   measurement scales, as a whole
d   characteristics of standardized, objective measures.

Section Four

Discussion, questions and answers

The same research questions may be answered by the use of a variety of different research methodologies. There is no single 'correct' research method to answer a research question. Indeed the 'triangulation' of methods is sometimes used to try and answer the same research question, so that the answer can be demonstrated not to be an artefact of the method used. Just as in land surveying, in which several reference points are used to fix better the position of the object being surveyed, researchers may study the same question or phenomenon using a variety of research techniques. The results may then be compared to get a better 'fix' on the question. The use of a single reference point or methodology gives one perspective of the object under study.

To illustrate this point it is proposed to consider a research issue of some importance and much contention in modern health care – the allocation of donated organs to transplant recipients. Despite the advances in transplantation techniques, there is a chronic worldwide under-supply of donor organs, to the extent that, in some countries, over one-third of patients accepted for transplantation die while on the waiting list due to the unavailability of suitable organs. A consequence of the chronic under-supply of donor organs is the necessity for transplantation teams to choose the most 'worthy' candidate to receive the donated organ from a panel of potential recipients. How these decisions are made and how they ought to be made have been the subjects of substantial research.

Many transplantation units around the world use a points system to assist with decisions concerning the priority of the people on their waiting lists. The points are typically based on tissue and blood type match (methods of measuring donor–recipient compatibility), time on the waiting list, 'urgency' (the extent to which the patient can wait) and prognosis (the quality of the expected outcome). This is in addition to certain technical requirements that vary with the organ system being replaced. For example, the size of the donor's and recipient's organ systems is a factor in heart–lung transplants. However, in recent years many commentators have presented data that indicate that 'social' criteria (such as the age, sex, education, race and wealth of the potential recipient) as well as 'medical' criteria are highly influential in the allocation of organs to recipients. These findings have generated considerable controversy.

How might one discover what criteria are used in the allocation of organs? One method might be to conduct a survey of those people involved in the decisions. The survey could take the form of an individual or group interview, or a written questionnaire. Alternatively, one could examine the written policies of various transplantation units or examine the medical records of the potential recipients for transplantation in the units and follow up the actual outcomes for each candidate.

Let us consider the questions we may wish to ask of people involved in the organ transplant decisions. They might include:

In your opinion, what criteria should be used in deciding who should receive an organ transplant?

In your opinion, what criteria are actually used in deciding who should receive an organ transplant?

These questions could be asked directly of the respondents in person and their comments recorded on tape and/or in the form of notes for subsequent analysis. In other words, the respondents could be interviewed. Excerpts of typical responses to these questions when the authors have asked them of members of transplant teams include:

We have an unwritten policy that we won't transplant into patients over 60. We think they have had their turn. Also their prognosis is often poorer than younger patients.

A consequence of the HLA emphasis is that people with unusual tissue types never get a transplant. I have a problem with this. In my area, there is only slim evidence that it makes much difference. Fifteen per cent max (sic) between best and worst case match. Most people fall in the middle so the actual difference would be even smaller. This means a lot of people miss out. I think it should be a strict queue.

Another method of collecting the data would involve getting people to use a structured response question in a questionnaire. The following might be an example:

In your opinion, what criteria should be used in deciding who should receive an organ transplant. Please circle as many as you like.

Age   Urgency of need
Sex   Prognosis

Education level   Whether recipient is
                       a parent
Race   Citizenship status
Occupation   Other, please specify
Wealth
Blood type match between donor and
recipient
HLA match between donor and recipient
tissues

A follow-up question might include something like:

When you have selected the criteria you consider should be used in allocating organs to recipients, please write a number alongside each one to indicate your opinion of its importance in the decision. For example, the one you consider the most important should have a '1' placed alongside it, the second a '2' and so on until you have exhausted all the ones you selected.

In this type of exploratory study, the use of fixed-response questions may send a clear signal to the respondent as to what the researcher considers to be acceptable criteria. Therefore, respondents may not be inclined to reveal their true answer if it is not included in the list of available answers, because of fear of disapproval or perhaps disinclination for the effort to do so. Thus, before a structured response question is used, the clinical researcher needs to ensure that all possible and likely answers are included. The current authors advocate the use of unstructured questions with a small sample prior to the use of structured questions in a large-scale survey.

It is interesting to note that, in a study of 310 Australian people from the community recently conducted by the authors, the respondents consistently nominated the age of recipients, their prognosis, the length of time they spent on the waiting list and whether they had children as the four factors they considered ought to be used to determine recipient priority in transplantation decisions.

Thus, clinical researchers could use interview or questionnaire approaches in the conduct of their survey. A further approach would involve the auditing of potential recipient medical files over a period in the various transplantation units in order to check whether those who actually received the transplants were representative of the potential recipient pool. For example, if it were found that women were less likely to receive transplants than men, taking into account their relative proportions in the recipient pool, then this would be of major concern. Unfortunately, as mentioned above, there is strong evidence in the US (where most such research has been performed) that social factors have an important impact upon the actual transplantation decisions. These findings reflect the situation in the delivery of health care in areas other than transplantation.

Questions

1. What are some of the possible disadvantages of using structured-response questions when the researcher is unsure as to what answers respondents may want to use?
2. When are structured-response questions best used?
3. If you wanted to study the outcomes of transplant patients at a hospital, how would you go about gaining access to the records?
4. In the case where a researcher uses a structured questionnaire, to what extent does the respondent have the opportunity to contribute to the research agenda?
5. How can a researcher avoid bias in designing a questionnaire?

Answers

1. If the researcher is unsure as to what answers the respondents wish to give, structured-response questions will probably not do the job required. In fact, even an open-ended response written question will not do the job, if the answer is complicated, because people are often a lot more fluent in their speech.

2. If the questions being asked are straightforward, e.g. 'what is your sex?' or 'what is your age?' or 'how often did you go to the doctor last month?' then structured-response questions will give structured data cheaply and quickly.
3. Access to confidential data requires a lot of work, although you may find that some of the data you require may be published in the annual report for the hospital or agency. Typically, one starts by contacting the head of the unit concerned and then progressing through the ethics committees and procedures laid down by the agency. If access is granted at all, it can be many months before permission is given, as the rights of patients to their data are now strictly enforced in most countries.
4. Most structured research questionnaires are designed wholly by the researcher, without input from the respondents to be studied. What questions are asked, how these are asked and what is not asked can send clear messages to the respondents about the researcher's agenda and assumptions. In this context, it is rare that respondents challenge the researcher, even if they believe that the researcher has missed the point. The typically low level of respondent input avoids anarchy (imagine every single respondent to a survey questionnaire designing his or her own questions!). However, if the researcher has a totally different understanding of the situation under study from the respondents, then he/she may ask the 'wrong' questions. The data may then be invalid because they do not reflect the true positions of the respondents.
5. It depends upon the type of bias. With adherence to principles of question design, problems such as the use of leading questions should be avoided. However, since the researchers select their questions, which may number 30 or so, from a range of several billion possible, selection bias is unavoidable. Every study is not a study of the universe. Focus and selectivity are unavoidable and are inherent to the reductionist scientific process. A problem of 'bias' may arise when the researcher does not ask the questions the respondents believe they should be answering.

Section **Five**

Descriptive statistics

Depending on the complexity of the research design and the number of measurements obtained during data collection, we will have generated a set of scores called 'raw data'. Section 5 is concerned with the principles of descriptive statistics, which include mathematical principles for organizing and summarizing the raw data.

In Chapter 13 we outline techniques used for tabulating and graphing data. These techniques enable us to visualize trends and identify differences across levels of the independent variables. When the data have been appropriately organized we may calculate statistics, such as the percentages and proportions of scores found in the groups being studied.

Another important use for descriptive statistics is to 'crunch' or condense data into typical values for representing scores. The statistics are discussed in Chapter 14 and include 'measures of central tendency' (mode, median and mean) and also measures of variability (range, semi-interquartile range and standard deviation). Using these statistics enables us to condense the raw data and to convey to the reader information about the research findings.

Statistics such as the mean and the standard deviation can also be applied to calculating standard scores. Standard scores are used to establish the position of a particular score relative to a population. In Chapter 15 we examine how the standardized normal distribution can be used to calculate the position of any specific score within a population and how to interpret the clinical implications of these scores.

In Chapter 16 we examine another important class of statistics called correlation coefficients. The correlation coefficient is used to express the degree and direction of association between two or more variables. For example, we could use correlation coefficients to demonstrate if there is an association between the variables 'level of exercise' and 'body weight'. The closer the calculated correlation coefficient is to 1.0 (the maximum value), the more precisely we may predict from one variable to the other. Although correlation coefficients are extremely important for showing how different variables are associated, they do not necessarily indicate causal relationships between the variables. Showing causal effects requires appropriate research designs, as we suggested in Section 3.

Chapter Thirteen

Organization and presentation of data

Introduction

The summary and interpretation of data from quantitative research entail the use of *statistics*. We use statistics to organize and interpret research observations and measurements. A statistic is also a number that is obtained by the mathematical manipulation of the research data. Descriptive statistics describe characteristics of the researcher's data.

In previous chapters we examined how interviews, observations and measurement are used to produce data in clinical investigations or research. It can be difficult to make sense of raw data when they consist of a large number of measurements. Before we can interpret or communicate the information provided by a research project, the raw data must be organized and presented in a clear and intelligible fashion. We do this using statistics. The aim of this chapter is to outline methods used in descriptive statistics for the organization, tabulation and graphic presentation of data. We will also examine the use of some simple statistics directly derived from the tabulation of the data.

The aims of this chapter are to:

1. Outline methods for organizing and representing data in the form of frequency distributions, tables or graphs.
2. Demonstrate how the measurement scale used for data collection influences the organization and presentation of the evidence.

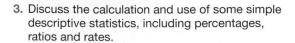

3. Discuss the calculation and use of some simple descriptive statistics, including percentages, ratios and rates.

The organization and presentation of nominal or ordinal data

A fundamental consideration in selecting appropriate statistics is the question of whether the data are discrete or continuous. Nominal and ordinal data are necessarily discrete, so that the organization of the data involves counting the number (frequency) of cases falling into each category of measurement. Let us examine two simple examples as an illustration.

Organization of discrete data

Example 1: nominal data

We are interested in the sex of patients (nominal data) undergoing gall bladder surgery (cholecystectomy) at a public hospital over a period of one year. The raw data indicating the sex (M or F) of the patients is simply read off the patients' records, as follows:

F, M, M, F, F, F, M, F, M, F, M, F, F, F, F, F, F, F, F, F, F, M, F, F, F, M, M, F, M, F, M

Grouping the above nominal data involves counting the number of cases (or measurements) falling into each category. The total is M = 10 and F = 20. The data can be presented in tabular form. Table 13.1 shows the following conventions in tabulating data:

Table 13.1 Frequency distribution of gender of patients undergoing cholecystectomy at a hospital over a period of 1 year

Gender	f
Males (M)	10
Females (F)	20
	n = 30

1. Tables must be clearly and fully labelled – both the table as a whole and the categories – so that readers can interpret unambiguously what they are observing.
2. *f* represents frequency of cases or measurements falling into a given category.
3. *n* represents the total number of cases or measurements in a sample.
4. *N* represents the number of cases in a population. (See Section 3 for the difference between samples and populations.)

Example 2: ordinal data

Ordinal data are presented by counting the number of cases (frequency) of each ordered rank making up the scale.

An investigator intends to evaluate the effectiveness of a new analgesic versus placebo treatment. A post-test only control group design is used: the experimental group receives the analgesic and the control group the placebo. Twenty patients are randomly assigned into each of the two groups. Pain intensity is assessed by the patients' pain reports five hours after minor surgery, on the following scale:

 5: Excruciating pain
 4: Severe pain
 3: Moderate pain
 2: Mild pain
 1: No pain

The raw data are:

Experimental group: 3,4,5,3,3,3,4,2,1,3,2,1,3,4,5, 2,3,3,3,3

Control group: 5,4,4,4,5,3,4,3,2,4,4,2,4,5,3,4,4,4, 5,5

After tallying the results, the above data can be presented as a frequency distribution, as shown in Table 13.2. This demonstrates that when the data have been tabulated, we can see the outcome of the investigation. Here, the pain reported by the experimental group is less than that of the control group.

Graphing discrete data

Once a frequency distribution of the raw data has been tabulated, a variety of techniques is available for the pictorial or graphical presentation of a given set of measurements. Frequency distributions of qualitative data are often plotted as bar graphs (also termed 'column' graphs), or shown pictorially as pie diagrams.

A bar graph involves plotting the frequency of each category and drawing a bar, the height of which represents the frequency of a given category. Figure 13.1 graphs the data given in Table 13.1.

Figure 13.1 demonstrates conventions in plotting bar graphs:

1. The y-axis, also called the ordinate, is used to plot frequencies.

2. The x-axis, also called the abscissa, is used to indicate the categories.

3. The bars do not touch each other, reflecting the discontinuity of the measurement categories.

It should be noted that care must be exercised in interpreting graphs, as the axes may be translated or compressed causing a false visual impression of the data. Make sure that you inspect the values along the axes, so that you are not misled. It is also acceptable to calculate the percentage of scores falling into each category and to display the percentages instead of frequencies.

It can be seen in Figure 13.2 that by presenting the data for the experimental and control groups on the same graph, the reader gains a visual impression of the possible effectiveness of the analgesic treatment in contrast to that of the control intervention or treatment. Nominal data can also be meaningfully presented as a pie chart, where the percentage of each category is converted into a proportional part of a circle or 'pie'. For example, in a given hospital we have the hypothetical spending patterns shown in Table 13.3.

Figure 13.3 represents a pie chart of the information. In constructing Figure 13.3, we converted the numbers into percentages and then into degrees (out of a total of 100% = 360°), that is, each 1% of the total is represented by 3.6° in the circle.

Table 13.2 Reported pain intensity of patients following placebo and analgesic treatments

Pain intensity	Experimental group (analgesic) f	Control group (placebo) f
1	2	0
2	3	2
3	10	3
4	3	10
5	2	5
	$n = 20$	$n = 20$

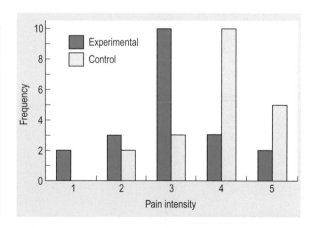

Figure 13.1 • Bar (column) graph of patients undergoing cholecystectomy.

Figure 13.2 • Bar (column) graph of patients' pain intensity.

Table 13.3 Hypothetical spending patterns

Item	Cost ($)	Percentage of total
Wages and salaries	1 500 000	50.00
Medical supplies	500 000	16.67
Food and provisions	500 000	16.67
Administrative costs	500 000	16.67
Total	$3 000 000	100.00

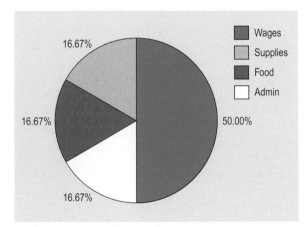

Figure 13.3 • Pie diagram of a hospital's spending pattern.

Organization and presentation of interval or ratio data

Previously we have noted that interval and ratio scales of measurement produce real numbers that can be processed according to the standard rules of arithmetic. Interval and ratio measurements typically produce continuous data (such as weight, length, time, IQ), implying that increasingly accurate values of the variable are possible to obtain, depending on the precision of the measurement process. For example, the weight of a neonate could be measured as 4, 4.2, 4.18 or 4.183 kg.

Grouped frequency distributions

When the continuous data are made up of a large number of varied measurements, it is useful to present the data as grouped frequency distributions. When drawing up a grouped frequency distribution, the following conventions should be taken into account:

1. The table of grouped frequency distributions should have no more than nine groups of values, otherwise it is too difficult to inspect. However, if too few groups are used, the meaning of the data is obscured, as varied measurements are combined into too few equivalent categories.
2. There should be equally sized class intervals, the *width* of which is represented by i.
3. Individual scores within a given class interval 'lose' their precise identity. The midpoint of each class interval is taken to represent the class interval.

Example

On admission to hospital, patients are routinely weighed. You are asked to summarize the weights of 50 male patients who were admitted in your ward over a period of time. The weights (raw data) are as follows (to nearest kg):

75, 67, 76, 71, 73, 86, 72, 77, 80, 75, 80, 96, 93, 75, 73, 83, 81, 82, 73, 92, 81, 87, 76, 84, 78, 79, 99, 100, 88, 77, 71, 76, 75, 83, 66, 79, 95, 85, 77, 87, 90, 73, 72, 68, 84, 69, 78, 77, 84, 94

The steps in constructing a grouped frequency distribution are:

1. Organize data into an ordered array, and find the frequency of each score (see Table 13.4).
2. Find the range of scores. The range is the difference between the highest and lowest score plus 1. We add 1 to include the real limits for continuous data. In this case the range is $100 - 66 + 1 = 35$.
3. Decide on the width (i) of the class intervals; i can be approximated by dividing the range by the number of groups or class intervals. In this instance, if we decide on seven classes, i will be $35 \div 7 = 5.0$. When i is a decimal, it should be rounded up to the nearest whole number: here, $i = 5$. As stated earlier, the number of class intervals is arbitrary and will be chosen by the researcher, depending on the properties of the

Table 13.4 Ordered array of data

Score	f	Score	f	Score	f	Score	f
100	1	91	0	82	1	73	4
99	1	90	1	81	2	72	2
98	0	89	0	80	2	71	2
97	0	88	1	79	2	70	0
96	1	87	2	78	2	69	1
95	1	86	1	77	4	68	1
94	1	85	1	76	3	67	1
93	1	84	3	75	4	66	1
92	1	83	2	74	0		

Figure 13.4 • Real limits of a class interval.

Table 13.5 Grouped frequency distribution of patients' weight in a given ward

Class interval	f
66–70	4
71–75	12
76–80	13
81–85	9
86–90	5
91–95	4
96–100	3
	$n = 50$

However, some precision in the data has been lost as somewhat different scores have been assigned into the same class intervals.

Graphing frequency distributions

The two common types of graphs used to graph frequency distribution of quantitative data are histograms and frequency polygons.

Histograms

A histogram resembles a bar graph but the bars are drawn to touch each other. The fact that the bars touch each other reflects the underlying continuity of the data. The height of the bars along the y-axis represents the frequency of each score or class interval plotted along the x-axis. With grouped data, the midpoint of each class interval becomes the midpoint of each bar, and the width of the bar corresponds to the real limits of each class interval.

For example, consider the lowest class interval 66–70 on Table 13.5. Because the data are continuous, the real upper and lower limits of the class interval are 65.5 and 70.4 (Fig. 13.4). Although all the weights are given as whole numbers of kilograms, these will in most cases be the result of rounding off by the nursing staff to the nearest whole number. Thus, someone who actually weighed 70.2 kg would have been recorded as weighing 70 kg and would fall into the 66–70 class. As Figure 13.4 shows, $i = 5$, and the midpoint of the class interval is 68.

Frequency polygons

Any data which can be represented by a histogram can also be graphed as a frequency polygon. For this type of graph, a point is plotted over the midpoint of each class interval, at a height

data. By convention, more than nine class intervals are rarely employed.

4. The next step is to determine the lowest class interval, and then list the limits of each class interval. Clearly, the lowest class interval must include the lowest score in the distribution.

5. Then, the frequency of scores is determined from each class interval and tabulated, as in Table 13.5.

It is easier to understand the data by inspecting Table 13.5 than by looking at the raw data.

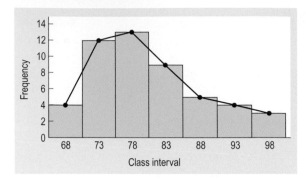

Figure 13.5 • Combined histogram and frequency polygon for the same data (see Table 13.5).

representing the frequency of the scores. Figure 13.5 represents a histogram and a frequency polygon for the data in Table 13.5.

Frequency polygons allow the reader to interpolate, that is, to estimate the frequency of values in between those actually measured or graphed. Of course, interpolation cannot be done for discrete data (for example, Fig. 13.1), as values between categories have no meaning. When a frequency polygon is plotted, it can take on a variety of shapes. The shapes which are of particular importance for frequency polygons are shown in Figure 13.6.

Figure 13.6A represents a bell-shaped, normal distribution. It is symmetrical, in the sense that one-half is the mirror image of the other. The curve indicates that most of the scores fell in the middle, with relatively few scores towards either 'tail'. Figure 13.6B represents a negatively skewed distribution, with most of the scores being high and spreading out toward the lower end of the distribution. Figure 13.6C represents a positively skewed distribution, with most of the scores being low, but with some scores spreading out towards the upper end of the distribution.

An easy way to remember the direction of the skew is to consider the region where the 'tail' or portion of the graph with lower frequencies falls. For example, if the tail is located at the low score end of the x-axis, the graph is negatively skewed. The significance of the skew or a symmetrical, normal distribution will be discussed in subsequent sections.

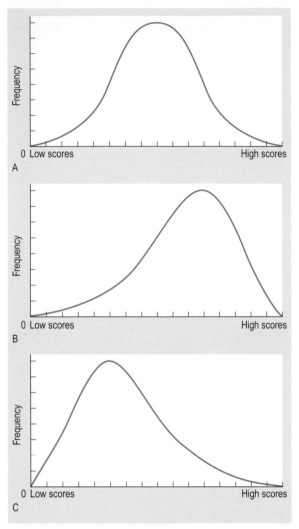

Figure 13.6 • Shapes of frequency polygons: (A) normal distribution; (B) negative skewing; (C) positive skewing.

Simple descriptive statistics

Once the data have been summarized in frequency distribution, it is often useful to make comparisons concerning the relative frequencies of scores falling into specific categories. The following statistics are useful for understanding comparative trends in the data, and can be used for measurements on any scale: nominal, ordinal, interval or ratio. A statistic is a number resulting from a computation based upon the raw data. The calculation of statistics is essential for 'crunching' the raw data into single numbers that represent the characteristics of the full data set.

Ratios

Ratios are statistics which express the relative frequency of one set of frequencies, A, in relation to another, B. The formula for ratios is:

$$\text{Ratio} = \frac{A}{B}$$

Therefore, the ratio of males to females for the data presented in Table 13.1 is:

$$\text{Ratio (males to females)} = \frac{10}{20} = 0.5$$

or

$$\text{Ratio (females to males)} = \frac{20}{10} = 2.0$$

Ratios are useful in the health sciences when we are interested in the distribution of illnesses or symptoms or the categories of subjects requiring or benefiting from treatment. The ratio calculated above tells us about the relative frequency of gall bladder surgery for males and females.

Proportions

Proportions are statistics which are calculated by putting the frequency of one category over that of the total numbers in the sample or the population:

$$\text{Proportion of } A = \frac{A}{A + B}$$

Therefore, the proportion of males in the sample represented in Table 13.1 is:

$$\text{Proportion of males} = \frac{f(\text{males})}{n} = \frac{10}{30} = 0.33$$

Percentages

Proportions can be transformed into percentages, by multiplying by 100. Of course, this is how we obtained the values of the y-axis for Figure 13.2. To illustrate, patients scoring 5 (excruciating pain) in the control group:

$$\% \text{ scoring } 5 = 5/20 \times 100 = 25\%$$

The values of the pie chart (Fig. 13.3) also involved such calculations.

Rates

When summarizing the results of epidemiological investigations it is often useful to use this statistic to represent the level at which a disorder is present in a given population. The two rates which are commonly used in the health sciences are:

- *Incidence rates*, which represent the number of new cases of a disorder reported within a time period.

$$\text{Incidence rate} = \frac{\begin{array}{c}\text{number of new}\\ \text{cases of a disorder}\end{array}}{\begin{array}{c}\text{total population at}\\ \text{risk of the disorder}\end{array}} \times \text{base}$$

- *Prevalence rates*, which represent the total number of cases suffering from a disorder.

$$\text{Prevalence rate} = \frac{\begin{array}{c}\text{number of existing}\\ \text{cases of a disorder}\end{array}}{\begin{array}{c}\text{total population at}\\ \text{risk of the disorder}\end{array}} \times \text{base}$$

Let us illustrate the above equation by applying it to hypothetical data. Let us consider the condition herpes, a nasty little condition associated with the virus herpes simplex that attacks various parts (lips, etc.) of the body. Assume that an epidemiologist is interested in the spread of the condition in a given community.

1. Assume that all the population above the age of 15 years ($N = 1\,000\,000$) is at risk of herpes.
2. In 2005, 5000 new cases were reported.
3. In 2005, there was a total (old and new active cases) of 15 000 known cases.

Table 13.6 Incidence of herpes

Year	Incidence of herpes (per 1000)
1982	8
1983	15
1984	17
1985	16
1986	10

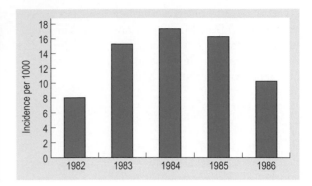

Figure 13.7 • Incidence rate of genital herpes 1982–1986.

Here, substituting into the equation:

Incidence rate for herpes $= 5000/1\,000\,000 \times$ base $= 0.005 \times$ base

The statistic 0.005 is not seen as the best way to represent a rate.

Often, epidemiologists select a base to make the statistic more understandable. The base represents a number for transforming the rate. The base selected depends on the magnitude of the rate; conventionally a multiple of 10, such as 1000, 10000 or 100000 is selected. In this instance we select 1000 as the base. Therefore, substituting into the equation, we obtain:

Incidence rate for herpes simplex
$$= \frac{0.005 \times 1000}{1} = 5 \text{ per } 1000$$
Prevalence rate for herpes simplex
$$= \frac{15\,000}{1\,000\,000} \times \frac{1000}{1} = 15 \text{ per } 1000$$

The above statistics can be graphed. For example, we may wish to represent pictorially the incidence of herpes simplex in the community over a period of 5 years. The (fictitious) evidence is shown in Table 13.6.

The graph of the time-series for the incidence over time (Fig. 13.7) gives us a visual impression of the changing incidence rate of the problem in question.

Summary

We outlined several techniques for organizing, tabulating and graphically presenting both discontinuous (nominal, ordinal) and continuous (interval, ratio) data. It was shown that raw data can be organized and tabulated as a frequency distribution, by counting the number of cases falling into specific categories or class intervals. Data composed of a large number of highly varied measurements were shown to be best presented by grouping the scores into class intervals.

Several techniques of graphing data were discussed: bar graphs and pie charts for discontinuous data, and histograms and frequency polygons for continuous data. The possible shapes of frequency polygons were also examined. It was shown that data grouped in frequency distributions could also be represented as ratios, proportions, percentages or rates. These statistics were obtained by computations based upon the raw data, and were shown to be useful for representing the characteristics of all the raw data. In the next chapter, we will examine further techniques of 'crunching' or condensing data by using appropriate descriptive statistics.

Self-assessment

Explain the meaning of the following terms:

bar graph
bell-shaped curve
continuous data
cumulative frequency
discontinuous data
frequency distribution

frequency polygon
histogram
incidence rate
negative skew
ordered array
pie diagram
positive skew
proportion
rate
ratio
real limit

True or false

1. The organization of nominal or ordinal data involves counting the number of scores falling into discrete categories.
2. Nominal and ordinal data are best graphed as histograms.
3. It is useful to organize interval or ratio data into ordered arrays before constructing frequency distributions.
4. Given a large number of varied scores, we can construct a grouped frequency distribution, usually with about seven class intervals.
5. The midpoint of a given class interval is i
6. Frequency distributions of continuous data can be presented graphically as histograms or frequency polygons.
7. In a negatively skewed distribution most of the scores are low, with a few high scores spread along the x-axis.
8. With a bell-shaped or normal distribution, most of the scores are located at the two extreme ends of the distribution.
9. 'Incidence rates' are statistics which represent the number of active cases of a disorder within a specific time period.
10. For a chronic condition like arthritis, we would expect the prevalence rates to be smaller than the incidence rates.
11. A 'base' represents a number for transforming a rate into a more easily understandable statistic.
12. The wider i is, the more specific information is lost about the actual data.
13. A frequency polygon is appropriate for graphing continuously distributed variables.
14. The percentile rank of a score is equal to the frequency of the scores falling up to and including the score.

15. If a curve is negatively skewed, the distribution of the scores has a 'tail' towards the lower values of the variable.
16. The height of a bar (column) represents the frequency, rather than the value, of a variable.
17. A pie diagram is inappropriate for representing nominally scaled data.
18. Incidence rates represent the number of new cases of a disorder reported within a time period.
19. The 'base' for calculating incidence rates is always 10 000.
20. We cannot construct frequency tables for nominally or ordinally scaled data.
21. Ratios are the same as proportions.
22. We can only calculate proportions for nominally scaled data.

Multiple choice

1. Patients indicate their satisfaction with treatment by responding to a question with four options:
   (1) very dissatisfied
   (2) dissatisfied
   (3) satisfied
   (4) very satisfied.
   This is an example of a(n) (I) scale, and the resulting frequency distribution should be plotted as a (ii):
   a (i) nominal (ii) bar graph
   b (i) ordinal (ii) bar graph
   c (i) interval (ii) histogram
   d (i) ordinal (ii) histogram
   e none of the above.
2. Interval or ratio data should be graphed as a:
   a histogram
   b bar graph
   c frequency polygon
   d a and b
   e a and c.
3. Your class is asked to do an exam in theoretical physics. Given that only a few students know anything about this subject, the distribution of scores would be:
   a symmetrical
   b negatively skewed
   c positively skewed
   d bell-shaped
   e both a and b.

4. If a curve is symmetrical:
   a most of the scores fall at the higher values of the x-axis
   b most of the scores fall at the lower end of the x-axis
   c most of the scores fall at the higher end of the y-axis
   d most of the scores fall at the lower end of the y-axis
   e if folded in half, the two sides of the curves will coincide.

5. The percentile rank of a person's score on a test is 35. This means that:
   a the person got 35% of the items correct
   b the person performed better than 65% of the sample doing the test
   c both a and b
   d the person's score was equal to or better than 35% of the sample doing the test.

6. You are interested in calculating the incidence rate for Huntington's disease, which is a very rare disorder. Which of the following numbers would be your best 'base'?
   a 10
   b 100
   c 1000
   d 10 000

7. A continuous scale of measurement is different from a discrete scale in that a continuous scale:
   a is an interval scale, not a ratio scale
   b never provides exact measurements
   c can take an infinite number of intermediate possible values
   d never uses decimal numbers
   e b and c.

A researcher wished to study the effectiveness of a new treatment, A, upon the severity of migraine. A random sample of 50 subjects ($n = 50$) was selected from a group of migraine sufferers attending a pain clinic. Patients were randomly allocated to be treated either with A, or with a currently available biofeedback treatment, B. A pre-test/post-test experimental design was used. Level of pain was assessed using a standardized pain questionnaire, measuring pain responses on a scale between 1–100.

Questions 8–14 refer to the above information.

8. The independent variable in this study was:
   a the new treatment A
   b the type of treatment used
   c the migraine
   d the patients' scores on the pain questionnaire.

9. The dependent variable in the above study was:
   a the new treatment A
   b the type of treatment used
   c the migraine
   d the patients' scores on the pain questionnaire.

10. The scale of measurement used to assess the pain responses was:
    a nominal
    b ordinal
    c interval
    d ratio.

The data for the post-test pain scores for the two groups are summarized in the table below.

Pain ratings	Treatment A	Treatment B
31–40	1	1
41–50	2	2
51–60	3	–
61–70	10	3
71–80	4	4
81–90	3	10
91–100	2	5

Questions 11–14 refer to this table.

11. What would be an appropriate way for this information to be graphed?
    a frequency polygon
    b histogram
    c bar graph
    d either a or b.

12. What are the real limits of the lowest category?
    a 31–40
    b 31.5–40.4
    c 30.5–40.4
    d 30.5–39.5.

13. Which of the following statements is (are) true?
    a The post-test scores for treatment B are skewed.
    b i is equal to 9.

c 6% of treatment A post-test scores are under 50.5.

d All of the above statements are true.

14. Which of the following statements is supported by the data, assuming that the pre-test scores were equivalent for the two groups?
   a Treatment A appears to be more effective than B.
   b Treatment B appears to be more effective than A.
   c The two treatments appear to be equivalent.
   d Treatment B appears to be harmful.
   e a and d.

The total number of deaths reported in a hypothetical country for a given year was 120 000. The following lists 'deaths by cause' as a percentage of all deaths:

Heart disease	35%
Cancer	25%
Cerebrovascular disease	15%
Trauma	10%
Respiratory illness	5%
Infections	5%
Other causes	5%

Questions 15–20 refer to these data.

15. Data such as the above are compiled by asking hospitals, physicians, etc. to report deaths to a central agency. This type of information collection is best described as:
   a a survey
   b an experiment
   c a mathematical model
   d field research.

16. The variable 'cause of death' is measured on a(n):
   a nominal scale
   b ordinal scale
   c interval scale
   d ratio scale.

17. The above table should be graphed as a:
   a frequency polygon
   b histogram
   c bar graph
   d a and b.

18. The number of people who died of either heart disease or cancer was:
   a 35 000
   b 60 000
   c 72 000
   d 90 000.

19. Which of the following statements is false?
   a The proportion of all deaths caused by cancer is 0.25.
   b 5000 persons died of respiratory illnesses.
   c Twice as many persons died of trauma than of infections.
   d 18 000 persons died of cerebrovascular disease.

20. Of the people who died of trauma, the male: female ratio was 2:1. How many females died of trauma?
   a 4000
   b 8000
   c 12 000
   d Insufficient information to calculate answer.

21. Which of the following statements is true?
   a A graph of continuous data enables the reader to interpolate.
   b When constructing a frequency distribution for grouped scores, i should be equal to the number of class intervals.
   c A histogram is like a bar graph, except that with a histogram the bars do not touch each other.
   d A bell-shaped curve is an example of a skewed distribution.

22. Descriptive statistics:
   a are used to make inferences about populations from small samples
   b are only appropriate in non-experimental designs
   c summarize data about samples or populations
   d are derived from probability theory.

A researcher has collected data concerning the amount of time in seconds that it took a group of normal and a group of brain-damaged subjects to complete a standard motor task. The data are shown in the table at the top of page 154, arranged in a grouped frequency distribution. Questions 23–29 refer to these data.

23. The total number of subjects used in this study was:
   a 7
   b 26
   c 46
   d 50.

24. The class interval width i is:
   a 2
   b 3
   c 4
   d 7.

Class interval	Time in seconds Normals	Brain-damaged
12–14	1	0
15–17	2	0
18–20	5	1
21–23	10	2
24–27	4	4
28–30	3	10
31–33	1	3

25. The real limits for the class interval 15–17 are:
 a 14.5–17.4
 b 15 + 0.5
 c 14–18
 d 2.
26. The scale of measurement used for the dependent variable was:
 a nominal
 b ordinal
 c interval
 d ratio.
27. Which of the following statements is (are) true?
 a The distribution of scores for the normals approximates a normal distribution.
 b The scores for the brain-damaged subjects was highly skewed.

c The above investigation should not be classified as an experiment.
d All the above are true.
28. On the basis of previous evidence, the score of 27.4 is taken as demonstrating adequate motor function, while longer times for completing the task demonstrate some motor impairment. The proportion of normals who scored under 27.4 is X while the proportion of brain-damaged who scored under this score was Y (insert values for X and Y).
 a 4, 13
 b 0.85, 0.35
 c 0.80, 0.17
 d 0.26, 0.20.
29. Assuming external validity, which of the following statements is supported by the evidence?
 a Brain-damaged subjects take longer to complete the standard task.
 b The greater the degree of brain damage, the slower the task completion.
 c The task is valid for discriminating subjects with brain damage.
 d a and c.
30. The selection of appropriate descriptive statistics for organizing quantitative data is most influenced by the:
 a design of the research project
 b scales of measurement used to collect data
 c number of research participants
 d expected magnitude of the differences among the groups.

Chapter Fourteen

14

Measures of central tendency and variability

Introduction

In the previous chapter we examined how raw data can be organized and represented by the use of statistics in order that they may be easily communicated and understood. The two statistics that are necessary for representing a frequency distribution are measures of central tendency and variability.

Measures of central tendency are statistics or numbers expressing the most typical or representative scores in a distribution. *Measures of variability* are statistics representing the extent to which scores are dispersed (or spread out) numerically. The overall aim of this chapter is to examine the use of several types of measures of central tendency and variability commonly used in the health sciences. As quantitative evidence arising from investigations is presented in terms of these statistics, it is essential to understand these concepts.

The aims of this chapter are to:

1. Discuss the selection and use of measures of central tendency.
2. Discuss the selection and use of measures of variability.
3. Outline the relationship between the skew of frequency distributions and the selection of appropriate descriptive statistics.

Measures of central tendency

The mode

When the data are nominal (i.e. categories), the appropriate measure of central tendency is the mode. The mode is the most frequently occurring score in a distribution. Therefore, for the data that was shown in Table 13.1 the mode is the 'females' category. The mode can be obtained by inspection of grouped data (with the largest group being the mode). As we shall see later, the mode can also be calculated for continuous data.

The median

With ordinal, interval or ratio scaled data, central tendency can also be represented by the median. The median is the score that divides the distribution into half: half of the scores fall under the median, and half above the median. That is, if scores are arranged in an ordered array, the median would be the middle score. With a large number of cases, it may not be feasible to locate the middle score simply by inspection. To calculate which is the middle score, we can use the formula $(n + 1)/2$, where n is the total number of cases in a sample. This formula gives us the number of the middle score. We can then count that number from either end of an ordered array.

In general, if n is odd, the median is the middle score; if n is even, then the median falls between the two centre scores. The formula $(n + 1)/2$ is again used to tell us which score in an ordered array will be the median. For example:

5, 8, 9, 10, 28. Median = 9 (n is odd)
6, 17, 19, 20, 21, 27. Median = 19.5 (n is even)

For a grouped frequency distribution, the calculation of the median is a little more complicated. If we assume that the variable is continuous (for example, time, height, weight or level of pain), we can use a formula for calculating the median. This formula (explained in detail below) can be applied to ordinal data, provided that the variable being measured has an underlying continuity. For example,

in a study of the measurement of pain reports we obtain the following data, where $n = 17$:

1, 1, 2, 2, 2, 2, 2, 3, 3, 3, 3, 4, 4, 4, 5, 5, 5

The above data can be represented by a bar graph (Fig. 14.1).

Here we can obtain the mode simply by inspection. The mode = 2 (the most frequent score). For the median, we need the ninth score, as this will divide the distribution into two equal halves (see Table 14.1). By inspection, we can see that the median will fall into category 3. Assuming underlying continuity of the variable and applying the previously discussed formula, we have:

$$Mdn \text{ (median)} = X_L + i\left[\frac{(n/2) - \text{cum } f_L}{fi}\right]$$

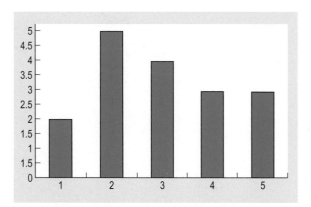

Figure 14.1 • Distribution of pain scores.

Table 14.1 Table of sample data

Score	Real class interval	f	cum f
1	0.5–1.4	2	2
2	1.5–2.4	5	7
3	2.5–3.4	4	11*
4	3.5–4.4	3	14
5	4.5–5.4	3	17
		$n = 17$	

*class interval containing median

where X_L = real lower limit of the class interval containing the median, i = width of the class interval, n = number of cases, cum f_L = cumulative frequency at the real lower limit of the interval and fi = frequency of cases in the interval containing the median.

Substituting into the above equation:

$$Mdn = 2.5 + 1 \left| \frac{(17/2) - 7}{4} \right|$$

$$= 2.5 + 1 \left[\frac{1.5}{4} \right]$$

$$= 2.875$$

The mean

The mean, $\bar{X}$ or μ, is defined as the sum of all the scores divided by the number of scores. The mean is, in fact, the arithmetic average for a distribution. The mean is calculated by the following equations:

$$\bar{X} = \frac{\Sigma x}{n} \text{ (for a sample)}$$

$$\mu = \frac{\Sigma x}{N} \text{ (for a population)}$$

where Σx = the sum of the scores, $\bar{X}$ = the mean of a sample, μ = the mean of a population, x = the values of the variable, that is the different elements in a sample or population, and n or N = the number of scores in a sample or population.

The formula simply summarizes the following 'advice':

To calculate the average or mean of a set of scores ($\bar{X}$), add together all the scores (Σx) and divide by the number of cases (n).

Therefore, given the following sample scores:

2, 3, 5, 6, 7

To calculate the mean:

$$\bar{X} = \frac{\Sigma x}{n} = \frac{23}{5} = 4.6$$

When n or N is very large, the average is calculated with the formula above but usually with the assistance of computers.

Comparison of the mode, median and mean

The mode can be used as a measure of central tendency for any level of scaling. However, since it only takes into account the most frequent scores, it is not generally a satisfactory way of presenting central tendency. For example, consider two sets of scores, A and B, shown in Table 14.2. It can be seen, either by inspection or by sketching a graph, that the two distributions A and B are quite different, yet the modes are the same, i.e. 1.

The median divides distributions into two equal halves, and is appropriate for ordinal, interval or ratio data. For interval or ratio data, however, the mean is the most appropriate measure of central tendency. The reason for this is that in calculating this statistic, we take into account all the values in the study sample. In this way, it gives the best representation of the average score. Clearly, it is inappropriate to use the mean with nominal data, as the concept of 'average' does not apply to discrete categories. For example, what would be the average of 10 males and 20 females?

There is some justification for using the median as a measure of central tendency when the variable being measured is continuous. However this is controversial, and the mean should be preferred. Alternatively, when a distribution is highly skewed, the median might be more appropriate than the mean for representing the 'typical' score. Consider the distribution:

2, 2, 2, 5, 7, 8, 9
mode = 2

Table 14.2 Example data sets

A		B	
x	f	x	f
1	16	1	8
2	1	2	7
3	1	3	6
4	7	4	4
	n = 25		n = 25

median = 5
$\bar{X}$ = 5

Let us change the 9 to 44:

2, 2, 2, 5, 7, 8, 44
mode = 2
median = 5
$\bar{X}$ = 10

Clearly, the median and the mode are less sensitive to extreme scores, while the mean is pulled towards extreme scores. This might be a disadvantage. For example, there are seven people working in a small factory, with the following incomes per week:

$100; $200; $200; $300; $400; $400; $1900

median = $300

$\bar{X}$ = $500

The distribution of wages is highly skewed by the high income of the owner of the factory ($1900). The mean, $500, is higher than six of the seven scores; it is in no way typical of the distribution. In cases like this the median is more representative of the distribution.

Figure 14.2 illustrates the relationships between the skew of frequency distributions and the three measures of central tendency discussed in this chapter. We should remember that the mode will always be at the highest point, the median will divide the area under the curve into halves, and the mean is the average of all the scores in the distribution. Also, the greater the skew in distribution, the more the measures of central tendency are likely to differ.

Measures of variability

We have seen that a single statistic can be used to describe the central tendency of a frequency distribution. This information is insufficient to characterize a distribution; we also need a measure of how much the scores are dispersed or spread out. The variability of discrete data is of little relevance, as the degree of variability will be limited by the number of categories defined by the investigator at the beginning of measurement.

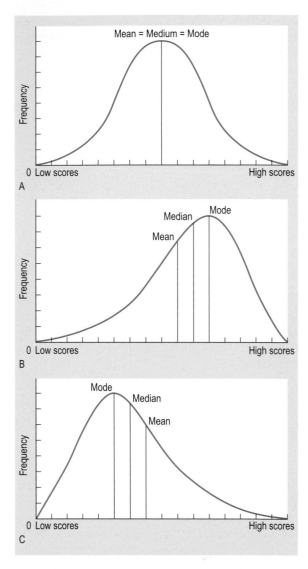

Figure 14.2 • Measures of central tendency in (A) normal distribution; (B) negative skewing; (C) positive skewing.

Consider the following two hypothetical distributions representing the IQs of two groups of intellectually disabled children:

Group A: 45, 50, 55, 60, 60, 70, 80
Group B: 57, 58, 59, 60, 61, 62, 63

It is evident that although $\bar{X}_A = \bar{X}_B = 60$, the variability of the scores of Group A is greater than that of Group B. Insofar as IQ is related to the activities appropriate for these children, Group A will provide a greater challenge to the therapist working with the children.

The three statistics commonly used to indicate the numerical value of variability are the *range*, the *variance* and the *standard deviation*.

The range

The range is the difference between the highest and lowest scores in a distribution. As we mentioned, given the IQ data above, the ranges are:

Group A: $80 - 45 + 1 = 36$
Group B: $63 - 57 + 1 = 7$

Although the range is easy to calculate, it is dependent only on the two extreme scores. In this way, we are not representing the typical variability of the scores. That is, the range might be distorted by a small number of atypical scores or 'outliers'. Consider, for instance, the differences in the range for the data given. The earlier example of the distribution of wages shows that just one outlying score in a distribution has an enormous impact on the range ($1900 - $100 = $1800). Obviously, some measure of average variability would be a preferable index of variability.

The average deviation

A convenient measure of variability might be average deviation about the mean. Consider Group B shown previously. Here $\bar{X} = 60$. To calculate the average variability about the mean, we subtract the mean from each score, sum the individual deviations, and divide by n, the number of measurements (see Table 14.3).

$$\text{Average deviation} = \frac{\Sigma(x - \bar{X})}{n}$$

Therefore: $\Sigma (x - \bar{X}) = (-3) + (-2) + (-1) + (0) + (1) + (2) + (3) = 0$

This is a general result; the sum of the average deviations about the mean is always zero. You can demonstrate this for the average deviation of Group A. The problem can be solved by squaring the deviations, as the square of negative numbers is always positive. This statistic is called the sums of squares (SS) and is always a positive number. This leads to a new statistic called the variance.

The variance

The variance (σ^2 or s^2) is defined as the sum of the squared deviations about the mean divided by the number of cases.

$$\sigma^2 = \frac{\Sigma(x - \mu)^2}{N}$$

(for a population)

$$s^2 = \frac{\Sigma(x - \bar{X})^2}{n - 1}$$

(for a sample)

Divide by $n - 1$ when calculating the variance for a sample, when we use s^2 as an estimate of population variance. Dividing by n results in an estimate which is too small, given that a degree of freedom has been lost calculating $\bar{X}$.

For the IQ example shown above, the variance is calculated as shown in Table 14.4.

Substituting into the formula:

$$\sigma^2 = \frac{\Sigma(x - \bar{X})^2}{n - 1} = \frac{28}{6} = 4.67$$

The problem with this measure of variability is that the deviations were squared. In this sense,

Table 14.3 Average variability about mean for Group B

x	x − $\bar{X}$
57	−3
58	−2
59	−1
60	0
61	+1
62	+2
63	+3

Table 14.4 Calculation of variance

x	$x - \bar{X}$	$(x - \bar{X})^2$
57	−3	9
58	−2	4
59	−1	1
60	0	0
61	+1	1
62	+2	4
63	+3	9
$\bar{X} = 60$		$\Sigma(x - \bar{X})^2 = 28$

we are overstating the spread of the scores. In taking the square root of the variance, we arrive at the most commonly used measure of variability for continuous data; the standard deviation.

The standard deviation

The standard deviation (σ or s) is defined as the square root of the variance:

$$\sigma = \sqrt{\sigma^2} = \frac{\sqrt{\Sigma(x - \mu)^2}}{N}$$

$$s = \sqrt{s^2} = \frac{\sqrt{\Sigma(x - \bar{X})^2}}{n - 1}$$

Therefore, the standard deviation for Group B is:

$$s = \sqrt{s^2} = \sqrt{4.67} = 2.16$$

The size of the standard deviation reflects the spread or dispersion of the frequency distribution representative of the data. Clearly, the larger σ or s, the relatively more spread out the scores are about the mean in a distribution. Calculation of the variance or the standard deviation is extremely tedious for large n using the method shown above. Statistics texts provide a variety of calculation formulae to derive these statistics. However, the common use of computers in research and administration makes it superfluous to discuss these calculation formulae in detail.

The semi-interquartile range

We have seen previously that if we are summarizing ordinal data, or interval or ratio data which is highly skewed, then the median is the appropriate measure of central tendency. The statistic called interquartile and semi-interquartile range is used as the measure of dispersion when the median is the appropriate measure of central tendency for a distribution. The interquartile range is the distance between the scores representing the 25th (Q1) and 75th (Q3) percentile ranks in a distribution.

It is appropriate to define what we mean by percentiles (sometimes called centiles). The percentile or centile rank of a given score specifies the percentage of scores in a distribution falling up to and including the score. As an illustration, consider Figure 14.3, in which:

- 25% of cases or scores fall up to and including Q1
- 50% of cases or scores fall up to and including the median
- 75% of cases or scores fall up to and including Q3
- 25% of cases or scores fall above Q3.

The distances A and B represent the distances between the median and Q1 and Q3. When a distribution is symmetrical or normal, the distances A and B will be equal. However, when a distribution is skewed, the two distances will be quite different. The semi-interquartile range (sometimes called the quartile deviation) is half of the distance between the scores representing the 25th (Q1) and 75th (Q3) percentile ranks in a distribution. Let us look at an example. If we have a sample where $n = 16$ and the values of the variable are:

1, 5, 7, 7, 8, 9, 9, 10, 11, 12, 13, 15, 19, 20, 20, 20.

clearly, a frequency distribution of these data is not even close to normal as the distribution is not symmetrical and the mode is at the maximum value. Therefore, the median is selected as the appropriate measure for central tendency, and we should use the interquartile range as the measure of dispersion.

Looking at the data, we find that:

1 5 7 7 * 8 9 9 10 † 11 12 13 15 ‡ 19 20 20 20

where * denotes the 25th centile (first quartile, Q1), † denotes the 50th centile: median (second

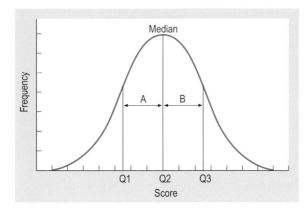

Figure 14.3 • Interquartile ranges.

quartile, Q2) and ‡ denotes the 75th centile (third quartile, Q3).

The score that cuts off the first 25% of scores (25th centile) is the first quartile (Q1). Since we have $n = 16$, Q1 will cut off the first four scores (25% of 16 is 4).

Thus: $Q1 = \dfrac{7 + 8}{2} = 7.5$

The third quartile (Q3) is the score which cuts off 75% of the scores. As $n = 16$, Q3 will cut off 12 scores (75% of 16 is 12).

$Q3 = \dfrac{15 + 19}{2} = 17$

Therefore, the semi-interquartile range is:

$\dfrac{Q3 - Q1}{2} = \dfrac{17.0 + 7.5}{2} = 4.75$

The larger the semi-interquartile range, the more the scores are spread out about the median.

Summary

In this section, we discussed two essential statistics for representing frequency distributions: measures of central tendency and variability. The measures of central tendency outlined were the mode and median for discrete data, and the mean for continuous data. Measures of variability were shown to be the range, average deviation, variance, and standard deviation. These statistics are appropriate for crunching the data together to the point that the distribution of raw data can be meaningfully represented by only two statistics. That is, the raw data representing the outcome of investigations or clinical measurements are expressed in this manner. We have seen that the mean and the standard deviation are most appropriate for interval or ratio data. The median and semi-interquartile range are used when the data were measured on an ordinal scale, or when interval or ratio data are found to have a highly skewed distribution. The mode represents the most frequent scores. The contents of the chapter focused on the use and meaning of these concepts, rather than stressing calculations involved. These calculations are now made by computers. In Chapter 15, we discuss the application of the mean and standard deviation for relating specific scores to an overall distribution.

Self-assessment

Explain the meaning of the following terms:

central tendency
descriptive statistics
dispersion
mean
median
mode
range
semi-interquartile range
standard deviation
statistic
variability
variance

True or false

1. Inferential statistics are used to describe specific characteristics of the data.
2. With nominal data, the mean should be used as a measure of central tendency.
3. The mode represents the most frequently occurring score in a distribution.
4. With ordinal data, we can use both the mode and the mean as a measure of central tendency.
5. When the data are interval or ratio, we can use the mean as a measure of central tendency.

6. With continuous data, the median is the most appropriate measure of central tendency.

7. If a continuous distribution is highly skewed, the median might be the appropriate measure of central tendency.

8. When a frequency distribution is positively skewed, the mean is greater than the median or the mode.

9. Given a normal distribution, the three measures of central tendency are equivalent.

10. The range is the simplest indicator of variability.

11. The range is calculated by adding the lowest score to the highest score in a distribution.

12. Given nominal or ordinal data, we should use the standard deviation as a measure of dispersion.

13. The square root of the variance is called the standard deviation.

14. s and σ indicate the extent to which scores are distributed about the mean.

15. When a distribution consists of very different scores, s or σ will be relatively large.

16. It is possible to have data with three different values for measures of central tendency.

17. The 50th percentile score and the median will always be the same value.

18. The median is less affected than the mean by extreme scores at one end of a distribution.

19. Central tendency describes the 'typical' value of a set of scores.

20. We use $n - 1$ in the denominator of the equation for calculating the sample standard deviation, because it provides us with an accurate estimate of the population standard deviation.

21. If the number of raw scores is odd, the median is the score in the middle position.

22. The mean must have a value equal to one of the scores in the distribution.

23. 25% of the scores fall between Q1 and the median.

24. The distance between Q1 and the median is always different to the distance between Q3 and the median.

25. The semi-interquartile range is inappropriate to use with skewed distributions.

Multiple choice

1. Given a set of nominally scaled scores, the most appropriate measure of central tendency is the:
   a mean
   b mode

   c standard deviation
   d range.

2. Which of the following statements is true?
   a The mode is the most useful measure of central tendency.
   b The variance is the square root of the standard deviation.
   c The median and the 50th percentile rank have different values.
   d The mean is more affected by extreme scores than the median.

Questions 3–6 refer to the following data:

2, 2, 3, 4, 6, 6, 7.

3. Σx is equal to:
   a 30
   b 40
   c 50
   d none of the above.

4. $(\Sigma x)^2$ is equal to:
   a 124
   b 128
   c 130
   d 900.

5. The median is equal to:
   a 6
   b 5
   c 4
   d 3.

6. The range for the above set of scores is:
   a 7
   b 5
   c 2
   d 1.

A clinic had 50 patients attending in a month. The number of times each patient visited the clinic is given in the table below in the form of frequency distribution.

Questions 7–9 refer to this information.

7. The total number of visits by the patients was:
   a 194
   b 28
   c 50
   d none of the above.

8. The mean number of visits by patients was:
   a 3.89
   b 3.50
   c 1.00
   d 3.88.

No. of visits (x)	No. of patients (f)
7	3
6	6
5	6
4	10
3	21
2	0
1	4

9. The median number of visits per patient was:
   a 3.88
   b 3.50
   c 3.00
   d 4.00.

10. The more dispersed, or spread out, a set of scores is:
    a the greater the difference between the mean and the median
    b the greater the value of the mode
    c the greater the standard deviation
    d the smaller the interquartile range.

11. The measure of central tendency which is most strongly influenced by extreme values in the 'tail' of the distribution is:
    a the mean
    b the median
    c the mode
    d the standard deviation
    e none of the above.

12. The mean height of a student group is 167 cm. Assuming height is normally distributed, this enables us to deduce that:
    a approximately half of all students are taller than 167 cm
    b being a student stunts your growth
    c approximately half of all students are shorter than 167 cm
    d a and c
    e none of the above.

13. If we subtract the value of the mean from every score in a set of scores the sum of the remaining values will be:
    a impossible to determine
    b equal to the mean

c a measure of the dispersion around the mean
d zero
e none of the above.

14. Given a normally distributed continuous variable, the best measure of central tendency is the:
    a mode
    b median
    c mean
    d standard deviation
    e none of the above.

15. If a distribution is negatively skewed, then:
    a the median is greater than the mean
    b the mode is greater than the median
    c the mean is greater than the median
    d both a and b are true
    e none of the above are true.

16. In a normal distribution, with regard to the mean, the median and the mode:
    a they always have the same value
    b the mean has the higher value
    c the mean has the lower value
    d they have no particular relationship
    e they cannot take the same value.

17. The measure of central tendency which is the most frequently occurring score is:
    a the mean
    b the median
    c the mode
    d the standard deviation
    e none of the above.

18. Given the group of scores 1, 4, 4, 4 and 7, it can be said of the mean, the median and the mode that:
    a the mean is larger than either the median or the mode
    b all are the same
    c the median is larger than either the mean or the mode
    d all are different
    e the mode is larger than either the median or the mean.

A nurse recorded the number of analgesic preparations taken by patients in a surgical ward. The resulting data were:

5, 2, 8, 2, 3, 2, 4, 12

Questions 19–23 refer to these data.

19. The mode for this distribution is:
    a 2
    b 3

c 8

d there is no mode.

20. The median is:

   a 2.00

   b 3.50

   c 3.00

   d 3.25.

21. The mean is:

   a 3.52

   b 5.43

   c 4.75

   d 4.15.

22. The range is:

   a 9

   b 10

   c 12

   d 2.

23. The standard deviation is:

   a 3.04

   b 5.81

   c 2.28

   d 3.58

Questions 24–28 refer to these data:

3, 3, 4, 5, 6, 7, 8, 9, 9, 10, 38, 60

24. The median is:

   a 7.0

   b 7.5

c 8.0

d 3 or 9.

25. Q1 is:

   a 4.5

   b 5.5

   c 8.0

   d 9.5.

26. Q3 is:

   a 4.5

   b 6.0

   c 7.5

   d 9.5.

27. The semi-interquartile range is:

   a 2.5

   b 4.5

   c 6.0

   d 9.0

28. The semi-interquartile range is preferred to the standard deviation as a measure of variability when:

   a the sample size is small

   b the distribution is standardized

   c the distribution is highly skewed

   d the range is small.

Chapter Fifteen

Standard scores and the normal curve

CHAPTER CONTENTS

Introduction

In this chapter we will discuss standard distributions. Standard scores represent the position of a score or measurement in relation to an overall set of scores. Standard distributions are also useful for comparing scores from different sets of measurements. Standard scores are used in both clinical practice and research in the health sciences. In clinical practice the score of a patient is often compared with a known distribution to interpret the score. Measures such as blood pressure or cholesterol measurements are compared with a distribution to interpret the patient's result.

The aims of this chapter are to:

1. Define 'standard' scores.
2. Describe the characteristics of normal and standard normal curves.
3. Show how standard normal curves can be used for calculating percentile ranks.
4. Show how standard normal curves can be used to compare scores from different distributions.

Standard scores (z scores)

Consider this example: infant A walked unaided at the age of 40 weeks, while infant B is 65 weeks old but still cannot walk. What sense can we make of these measurements? Could infant B need further clinical investigation in case he has some

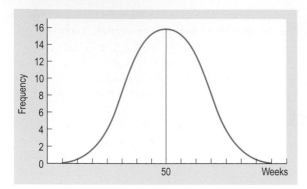

Figure 15.1 • Age at which children walk unaided.

neurological abnormality? The fact that infant B is unable to walk at the age of 65 weeks is not very informative in the absence of additional information about how this compares with norms for other children. However, say that it is known that the distribution of walking ages is such that $\mu = 50$ weeks and $\sigma = 5$. Assuming that the frequency distribution is normal, the frequency polygon representing the population would look something like that shown in Figure 15.1.

In this instance, infant B's score is clearly above the mean. In fact, by inspection, we can see the infant's score at this point of time was three standard deviations above ($+3$) the mean ($65 = 50 + (3 \times 5)$). In contrast, infant A began walking earlier than the mean, his score of 40 being two standard deviations below (-2) the mean. In general, any 'raw' score in a frequency distribution can be described in terms of its distance from the mean. The process of transforming a score into a measurement based on its distance from the mean in standard deviations is called *standardizing* the score. Such 'transformed' scores are called *z* scores or standard scores.

A *z* score represents how many standard deviations a given raw score is above or below the mean. The equation for transforming specific raw scores into *z* scores is given as:

$$z = \frac{x - \mu}{\sigma} \text{ (for a population)}$$

$$z = \frac{x - \bar{X}}{s} \text{ (for a sample)}$$

For the above equation, x is the raw score, $\bar{X}$ or μ is the mean of the distribution from which the score was drawn and s or σ is the standard deviation of the distribution. That is, when we know the mean and standard deviation of a distribution, we can transform any raw score into a *z* score. Conversely, when the *z* score is known, we can use the above equations to calculate the corresponding raw scores.

In the above example, the *z* scores corresponding to the infants' raw scores are:

$$\text{Infant A: } z = \frac{x - \mu}{\sigma}$$
$$= \frac{40 - 50}{5}$$
$$= -2$$

$$\text{Infant B: } z = \frac{x - \mu}{\sigma}$$
$$= \frac{65 - 50}{5}$$
$$= +3$$

These calculations support our previous observations that A's score was two standard deviations below the mean and B's score was three standard deviations above the mean. In other words, A walked very early and B was a very late starter. The particular value of standardizing scores for understanding clinical or research evidence will be discussed in the context of the concepts of normal and standard normal distributions.

Normal distributions

Many variables measured in the biological, behavioural and clinical sciences are approximately 'normally' distributed. What is meant by a normal distribution is illustrated by the normal curve (see Fig. 15.2), which is a frequency polygon representing the theoretical distribution of population scores. We assume here that the variable x has been measured on an interval or ratio scale and that it is a continuous variable such as weight, height or blood pressure.

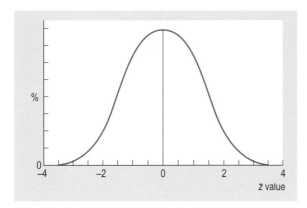

Figure 15.2 • Standard normal distribution.

The normal curve has the following characteristics:

1. It is symmetrical about the mean, so that equal numbers of cases fall above and below the mean (mean = median = mode).
2. Relatively few cases fall into the high or low values of x. Most of the cases fall close to the mean. (For the theoretical normal distribution, the arms of the curve do not intersect with the x-axis, allowing for a few extreme scores.)
3. The precise equation for the normal curve was discovered by the mathematician Gauss, so that it is sometimes referred to as a Gaussian curve.

We need not worry about the actual formula. Rather, the point is that, given that the functional relationship between f and x is known, integral calculus can be used to calculate areas under the curve for any value of x. All normal curves have the same general mathematical form; whether we are graphing IQ or weight, the same bell-shape will appear. The only differences between the curves are the mean value and the amount of variation. This is why the mean and the standard deviation provide us with important information about any particular normal distribution. Note that it is unlikely that any real data are exactly normally distributed. Rather, the normal distribution is a mathematical model that is useful for representing real distributions.

The standard normal curve

If we transform the raw scores of a variable into z scores and then plot the frequency polygon for the distribution, we will have a standard curve. If the original distribution was normal, then the frequency polygon will be a standard normal curve. Standard normal curves are identical regardless of the nature of the original variables.

By transforming raw scores into z scores we are adjusting for differences in means and standard deviations, which are the only things which distinguish between non-standardized normal curves.

The standard normal curve has the following additional properties:

1. The mean is always 0 (zero). For the previous example, the z score corresponding to $\mu = 50$ (as in the 'infants' walking age' example) is:

$$z = \frac{50 - 50}{5} = 0$$

2. The mean = median = mode, as the curve is symmetrical.
3. The standard deviation of z scores is always 1 (one). For instance, the z score for 55 (which is one standard deviation above the mean) is:

$$z = \frac{55 - 50}{5} = 1$$

4. It is assumed that the *total area under the curve adds up to 1.00*. Since the normal curve is symmetrical, 0.5 of the area falls above $z = 0$ and 0.5 falls below $z = 0$. This is another way of saying that 50% of the total cases fall below the mean, and 50% of the cases fall above the mean (which is equal to the median).
5. More generally, we can use appropriate *statistical tables* to estimate the area under the standard normal curve for any given z scores. These areas are available in table form (see Appendix A) so that for any value of z we can read off the corresponding area.
6. The area under the curve between any two points is directly proportional to the percentage of cases falling above, below or between those two points. We can use the standard normal curve to calculate the percentage of scores falling between any specified two scores.

In the next subsection, we will examine the use of the table of areas under the standard normal curve to understand the meaning of measurements in relation to distributions.

Calculations of areas under the normal curve

We have already examined the concept of percentile or centile ranks. The normal curve is useful for evaluating the percentile rank of scores in normal distributions. Appendix A gives the proportion of areas under the standard normal curve which lies:

- between the mean and a given z score
- beyond the z score.

Since normal distributions are symmetrical, the same proportions are also true for the area between the mean and any negative z score. Only the positive values are given in Appendix A.

Let us see how we can use this information to estimate the percentile ranks of the two infants' walking ages. We have shown previously in our hypothetical example that for infant A, $z = -2$. Let us now turn to Appendix A. In going down the column of z scores, we find that the area corresponding to $z = 2.00$ is 0.4772 (between) and 0.0228 (beyond).

We know that the area A1 under the curve in Figure 15.3 must be:

Shaded portion = 0.5000 – 0.4772
  = 0.0228 (as half the scores fall under the mean)

This proportion can be expressed as a percentage, so that 2.28% of the cases in the distribution fall below $z = -2$. We have defined percentile rank for a score as the percentage of cases in a distribution falling up to and including a specific score. Therefore, the percentile rank for infant A's walking is 2.28%. Of all children, only 2.28% learn to walk as early as or earlier than infant A. Clearly, he is doing well.

What then is the percentile rank for infant B's performance? As you remember, $z = +3$. Looking up the area corresponding to $z = 3.00$ in Appendix A we find the area (A1 in Fig. 15.4) is equal to 0.4987. Therefore, the proportion of scores falling up to and including $z = +3$ is 0.5 + 0.4987 = 0.9987.

Expressing this finding as a percentage, we find that 99.87% of children learn to walk by the age

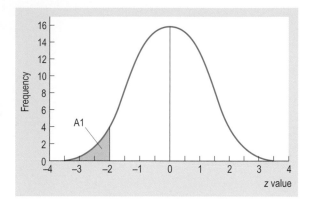

Figure 15.3 • Area (A1) corresponding to $z = -2$.

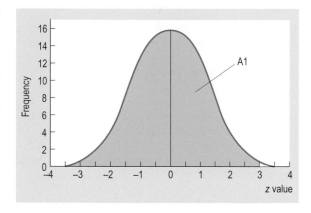

Figure 15.4 • Area (A1) corresponding to $z = +3$.

of 65 weeks. As we said earlier, infant B is still not walking. Perhaps further clinical tests are indicated, although we should keep in mind that an unusual or extreme score is not necessarily indicative of pathological states.

Critical values

We can work the other way by determining the raw scores corresponding to areas under the normal curve in Appendix A. For example, say that the slowest 5% of infants are offered some special exercises in learning to walk. What would be the age at which the exercises should be offered, should the child not be walking? The key here is

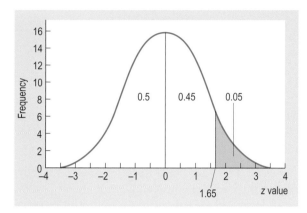

Figure 15.5 • Determining z score of 95th percentile.

Table 15.1 Scores for example in text

Raw scores	z scores	Percentile ranks
$x = 63$	-0.25	40.1
$x = 52$	$+1.50$	93.3

Table 15.2 Blood cholesterol

	Mean blood cholesterol (mg/cc)	Standard deviation
Meat eaters	0.6	0.15
Vegetarians	0.4	0.1

to determine the score that corresponds to the 95th percentile of the distribution. This can be represented as shown in Figure 15.5.

From Figure 15.5 we can see that we need to discover the z score that corresponds to an area of 0.45 above the mean. By consulting the normal distribution table (see Appendix A), it can be seen that the corresponding z score is $z = 1.65$. This is a critical value for the statistic in defining an area.

Given the z score, we can calculate the corresponding raw score from the formula:

$$z = \frac{x - \mu}{\sigma}$$

Therefore $1.65 = \dfrac{x - 50}{5}$

$$x = (5 \times 1.65) + 50$$
$$= 58.25$$

That is, if the slowest 5% are thought to be in need of help, then children somewhat over 58 weeks old and still not walking would be recommended for the remedial exercises. Of course, we can use the tables for reading off the z scores corresponding to any specified area or percentage.

Standard normal curves for the comparison of distributions

One of the uses of standard distributions is that we can compare scores from entirely different distributions. For example, if a student scored 63 on test A, and 52 on test B, on which test did the student do better? If we define 'better' as solely in terms of raw scores, then clearly the student did better on test A. However, test A might have been easier than test B, so that if the overall performances of all students on the tests are taken into account, the student's relative performance might be better on test B.

Say test A, $\bar{X} = 65$ and $s = 8$
    test B, $\bar{X} = 40$ and $s = 8$

Therefore, using the formula for calculating z scores, and looking up the corresponding areas in Appendix A (do this yourself) we obtain the results shown in Table 15.1. Thus, the student performed better on test B, by scoring higher than 93% of other students sitting for the test.

This example illustrates that in some circumstances the meaning of specific scores has to be interpreted against 'standards'.

Another use of standard distributions is in interpreting the meaning of the results of investigations in the health sciences. Let us examine the following hypothetical example. An investigator measured levels of blood cholesterol in a sample of 300 adults who are meat eaters, and 100 adults who are vegetarians. The results of the investigation are summarized in Table 15.2.

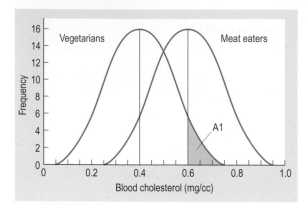

Figure 15.6 • Area A1 corresponds to the percentage of vegetarians with blood cholesterol higher than 0.6 mg/cc.

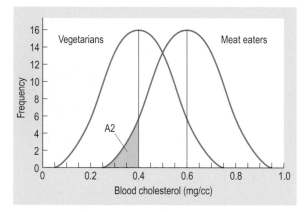

Figure 15.7 • Area A2 corresponds to the percentage of meat eaters with lower blood cholesterol than the mean for vegetarians.

Now, imagine that you are a clinician working with patients with cardiac disorders and you are interested in the following questions:

1. Approximately what per cent of vegetarians had blood cholesterol levels greater than the average meat eater?
2. Approximately what per cent of meat eaters had blood cholesterol levels lower than that of the average vegetarian?

The percentage of cases of vegetarians with blood cholesterol greater than 0.6 (the mean for the meat eaters) is represented by area A1 in Figure 15.6.

$$z = \frac{0.6 - 0.4}{0.1} = 2$$

Area A1 = 0.0228

Therefore, approximately 2.3% of vegetarians had blood cholesterol levels higher than the average for meat eaters.

Figure 15.7 demonstrates the area (A2) corresponding to the percentage of meat eaters with lower blood cholesterol than the average vegetarian.

$$z = \frac{0.4 - 0.6}{0.15} = -1.33$$

Area A2 = 0.0918

Therefore, approximately 9.2% of meat eaters had lower blood cholesterol levels than the average vegetarian.

Summary

We found that if the mean and standard deviation for a given distribution have been calculated, then we can transform any raw score into a standard (or z) score. The z score represents how many standard deviations a specific score is above or below the mean. We described how to calculate this transformed score for a population or a sample. Also, we outlined the essential characteristics of the normal and the standard normal curves.

It was pointed out that if the original frequency distribution was approximately normal, then the table of normal curves (Appendix A) could be used to calculate percentile ranks of raw scores, or the percentage of scores falling between specified scores. Also, z scores were shown to be useful in comparing scores arising from two or more different normal distributions. The above information is applicable to clinical practice, for example in interpreting the significance of an individual's assessment in relation to known population norms.

Self-assessment

Explain the meaning of the following terms:

normal curve

probability

standard normal curve

standard score

transformed score

z score

True or false

1. z scores express how many standard deviations a particular score is from the mean.
2. Negative z scores are further from the mean than positive z scores.
3. Even when the distribution of raw scores is skewed, the standardized distribution will be normal.
4. The mean of a standard normal distribution is always 1.0.
5. The total area under the standard normal curve is 1.0.
6. The area of a normal curve between any two designated z scores expresses the proportion or percentage of cases falling between the two points.
7. The greater the value of $\bar{X}$ and s, the greater the value of the z scores in corresponding standard distributions.
8. About 10% of scores fall 3 standard deviations above the mean.
9. A standardized distribution has the same shape as the distribution from which it was derived.
10. Notwithstanding the level of skewness in a distribution, the standard normal curve is useful for determining the percentile rank of a score.
11. In a normal distribution, the higher the z score, the higher will be the frequency of the corresponding raw score.
12. 50% of scores fall between $z = 0.5$ and $z = -0.5$.
13. In a normal curve, approximately 34% of the scores fall between $z = 0$ and $z = -1$.
14. A percentile rank represents the number of cases falling above a particular score.
15. Given a bimodal distribution of raw scores, the standard normal curve is inappropriate for calculating percentile ranks.
16. $z = -2.58$ has a percentile rank of 98 in a normal distribution.
17. $z = 1.28$ cuts off the highest 10% of scores in a normal distribution.
18. Numerous human characteristics are distributed approximately as a normal curve.
19. If 20% of scores fall into a given class interval, then the percentile rank of the upper real limit of the class interval is 20.
20. The percentile rank of $z = 0$ is always 50.

Multiple choice

1. Which of the following statements is true?
   a A z score indicates how many standard units or deviations a raw score is above or below the mean.
   b The mean of a standard normal distribution is always 0 (zero).
   c The distribution of z scores takes the same shape as that of the raw scores from which they have been derived.
   d All the above statements are true.

2. In an anatomy test, your result is equivalent to a standard or z score of 0.2. What does this z score imply?
   a You performed poorly when compared to others.
   b You performed very well when compared to others.
   c Your result was slightly above average.
   d Your result was slightly below average.

3. The z scores of three persons X, Y and Z in a statistical methods test were +2.0, +1.0 and 0.0, respectively. In terms of the original raw scores, which of the following statements is true?
   a The raw score difference between X and Y is greater than the raw score difference between Y and Z.
   b The raw score difference between X and Y is less than the raw score difference between Y and Z.
   c The raw score difference between X and Y is equal to the raw score difference between Y and Z.
   d No precise statement can be made about the relationships between the differences of the raw scores of X and Y and of Y and Z.

A group of patients has a mean weight of 80 kg, with a standard deviation of 10 kg. Questions 4 and 5 refer to these data.

4. What is the standard score (z) for a patient whose weight is 50 kg?
   - a +3
   - b +2
   - c −2
   - d −3

5. You are told that a patient's weight is two standard deviations below the mean. What is this patient's weight?
   - a 60 kg
   - b 55 kg
   - c 50 kg
   - d 45 kg

6. We develop a new method of treating spastic hemiplegia by giving weekly ultrasound massages to the affected muscles. In a consecutive study of 200 children treated by this method we find that the average number of weeks to full recovery is 8, with a standard deviation of 2 weeks. Therefore we conclude that (given a normal distribution):
   - a treatment may be stopped after 8 weeks
   - b half of all children will need treatment for longer than 8 weeks
   - c 90% of children will be fully recovered after 12 weeks of treatment.
   - d a and c.

7. A percentile rank:
   - a represents the frequency of occurrence of a particular category
   - b tells you whether or not a distribution is skewed
   - c can be used to estimate the range of distribution
   - d tells you what percentage of scores fall at or below a particular score.

Use this information in answering questions 8–12: a normally distributed set of scores has a mean of 40 and a standard deviation of 8.

8. A raw score of 24 corresponds to a z score of:
   - a 3.0
   - b −3.0
   - c 1.5
   - d −1.5
   - e −2.0

9. A z score of 1.25 corresponds to a raw score of:
   - a 50
   - b 10
   - c 30

   - d 56.4
   - e 40

10. The percentile rank of a raw score of 48 is:
    - a 34.13
    - b 15.87
    - c 84.13
    - d 65.87
    - e incalculable from information given.

11. The percentage of scores between 32–44 is:
    - a 68.26
    - b 53.28
    - c 46.82
    - d 32.74
    - e 43.32

12. The raw score which cuts off the lowest 5% of the population (rounded to the nearest whole number) is:
    - a 38
    - b 13
    - c 27
    - d 53
    - e 42

Questions 13–16 refer to a standard normal distribution.

13. The percentage of cases falling above $z = 0.35$ is:
    - a 16.8%
    - b 34.1%
    - c 84.1%
    - d 36.3%

14. The percentage of cases falling between $z = -1$ and $z = +1$ is:
    - a 16.8%
    - b 33.6%
    - c 34.1%
    - d 68.3%

15. The percentage of cases falling between $z = -0.5$ and $z = +2$ is:
    - a 85.0%
    - b 66.9%
    - c 28.6%
    - d 68.2%

16. The percentage of cases falling either below $z = -2$ or above $z = +2$ is:
    - a 95.5%
    - b 68.2%
    - c 47.7%
    - d 4.6%

The following information should be used in answering questions 17–20: a test of reaction times has a mean of 10 and a standard deviation of 4 in the normal adult population.

17. A person scores 8. That person's z score is:
   a 2
   b −2
   c −0.5
   d −1

18. What percentage of the population would have scores up to and including 14 on this test?
   a 84.13
   b 15.87
   c 65.87
   d 34.13

19. What is the percentile rank of a score of 8 on this test?
   a 19.15
   b 30.85
   c 80.85
   d 53.28

20. What score (to the nearest whole number) would cut off the highest 10% of scores?
   a 1
   b 14
   c 15
   d 18

Questions 21–25 refer to the following data: the mean for a population is 500, with a standard deviation of 90; the scores are normally distributed.

21. The percentile rank of a score of 667 is:
   a 4.14
   b 92.7
   c 3.22
   d 96.86

22. The proportion of scores which lie above 650 is:
   a 0.4535
   b 0.9535
   c 0.0475
   d 0.885

23. The proportion of scores which lie between 460 and 600 is:
   a 0.4394
   b 0.5365
   c 0.4406
   d 0.4635

24. The raw score which lies at the 90th percentile is:
   a 615.20
   b 384.80
   c 616.10
   d 383.90

25. The proportion of scores between 300–400 is:
   a 0.3665
   b 0.4868
   c 0.8533
   d 0.1203

Chapter Sixteen

Correlation

CHAPTER CONTENTS

Introduction

A fundamental aim of scientific and clinical research is to establish relationships between two or more sets of observations or variables. Finding such relationships or co variations is often an initial step for identifying causal relationships.

The topic of correlation is concerned with expressing quantitatively the degree and direction of the relationship between variables. Correlations are useful in the health sciences in areas such as determining the validity and reliability of clinical measures (Ch. 12) or in expressing how health problems are related to crucial biological, behavioural or environmental factors (Ch. 5).

The specific aims of this chapter are to:

1. Define the terms correlation and correlation coefficient.
2. Explain the selection and calculation of correlation coefficients.
3. Outline some of the uses of correlation coefficients.
4. Define and calculate the coefficient of determination.
5. Discuss the relationship between correlation and causality.

Correlation

Consider the following two statements:

1. There is a positive relationship between cigarette smoking and lung damage.
2. There is a negative relationship between being overweight and life expectancy.

You probably have a fair idea what the above two statements mean. The first statement implies that there is evidence that if you score high on one variable (cigarette smoking) you are likely to score high on the other variable (lung damage). The second statement describes the finding that scoring high on the variable 'overweight' tends to be associated with low measures on the variable 'life expectancy'. The information missing from each of the statements is the numerical value for degree or magnitude of the association between the variables.

A *correlation coefficient* is a statistic which expresses numerically the magnitude and direction of the association between two variables.

In order to demonstrate that two variables are correlated, we must obtain measures of both variables for the same set of subjects or events. Let us look at an example to illustrate this point.

Assume that we are interested to see whether scores for anatomy examinations are correlated with scores for physiology. To keep the example simple, assume that there were only five ($n = 5$) students who sat for both examinations (see Table 16.1).

To provide a visual representation of the relationship between the two variables, we can plot the above data on a *scattergram*. A scattergram is a graph of the paired scores for each subject on the two variables. By convention, we call one of the variables x and the other one y. It is evident from Figure 16.1 that there is a positive relationship between the two variables. That is, students who have high scores for anatomy (variable X) tend to have high scores for physiology (variable Y). Also, for this set of data we can fit a straight line in close approximation of the points on the scattergram. This line is referred to as a line of 'best fit'. This topic is discussed in statistics under 'linear regression'. In general, a variety of relationships is possible between two variables; the scattergrams in Figure 16.2 illustrate some of these.

Table 16.1 Examination scores

Student	Score (out of 10) Anatomy (X)	Physiology (Y)
1	3	2.5
2	4	3.5
3	1	0
4	8	6
5	2	1

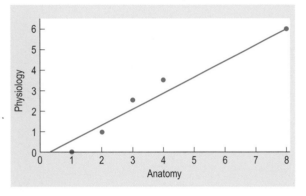

Figure 16.1 • Scattergram of students' scores in two examinations.

Figure 16.2A and B represent a linear correlation between the variables x and y. That is, a straight line is the most appropriate representation of the relationship between x and y. Figure 16.2C represents a non-linear correlation, where a curve best represents the relationship between x and y.

Figure 16.2A represents a *positive* correlation, indicating that high scores on x are related to high scores on y. For example, the relationship between cigarette smoking and lung damage is a positive correlation. Figure 16.2B represents a *negative* correlation, where high scores on x are associated with low scores on y. For example, the correlation between the variables 'being overweight' and 'life expectancy' is negative, meaning that the more you are overweight, the lower your life expectancy.

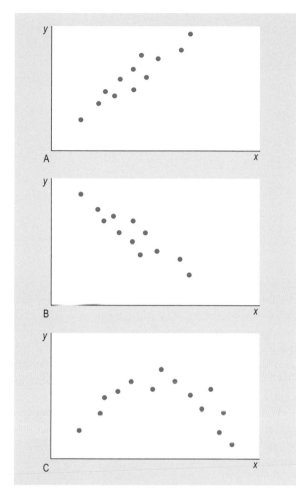

Figure 16.2 • Scattergrams showing relationships between two variables: (A) positive linear correlation; (B) negative linear correlation; (C) non-linear correlation.

Table 16.2 Correlation coefficient

Coefficient	Conditions where appropriate
ϕ (phi)	Both x and y measures on a nominal scale
ρ (rho)	Both x and y measures on, or transformed to, ordinal scales
r	Both x and y measures on an interval or ratio scale

correlation coefficients, and the conditions under which they are used. As the table indicates, the scale of measurements used determines the selection of the appropriate correlation coefficient.

All of the correlation coefficients shown in Table 16.2 are appropriate for quantifying linear relationships between variables. There are other correlation coefficients, such as η (eta) which are used for quantifying non-linear relationships. However, the discussion of the use and calculation of all the correlation coefficients is beyond the scope of this text. Rather, we will examine only the commonly used Pearson's r, and Spearman's ρ (rho).

Regardless of which correlation coefficient we employ, these statistics share the following characteristics:

1. Correlation coefficients are calculated from pairs of measurements on variables x and y for the same group of individuals.
2. A positive correlation is denoted by $+$ and a negative correlation by $-$.
3. The values of the correlation coefficient range from $+1$ to -1, where $+1$ means a perfect positive correlation, 0 means no correlation, and -1 a perfect negative correlation.
4. The square of the correlation coefficient represents the coefficient of determination.

Calculation of correlation coefficients

Pearson's r

We have already stated that Pearson's r is the appropriate correlation coefficient when both

Correlation coefficients

When we need to know or express the numerical value of the correlation between x and y, we calculate a statistic called the correlation coefficient. The correlation coefficient expresses quantitatively the magnitude and direction of the correlation.

Selection of correlation coefficients

There are several types of correlation coefficients used in statistics. Table 16.2 shows some of these

Table 16.3 Example calculations for correlation coefficient

Student	Raw scores		z scores		
	x	y	z_x	z_y	$z_x z_y$
1	3	2.5	−0.22	−0.04	+0.01
2	4	3.5	+0.15	+0.39	+0.06
3	1	0	−0.96	−1.12	+1.08
4	8	6	+1.63	+1.46	+2.38
5	2	1	−0.59	−0.69	+0.41
	$\bar{X} = 3.6$	$\bar{X} = 2.6$			$\Sigma z_x z_y = 3.94$
	$s_x = 2.7$	$s_y = 2.33$			

variables x and y are measured on an interval or a ratio scale. Further assumptions in using r are that both variables x and y are normally distributed, and that we are describing a linear (rather than curvilinear) relationship.

Pearson's r is a measure of the extent to which paired scores are correlated. To calculate r we need to represent the position of each paired score within its own distribution, so we convert each raw score to a z score. This transformation corrects for the two distributions x and y having different means and standard deviations. The formula for calculating Pearson's r is:

$$r = \frac{\Sigma z_x z_y}{n}$$

where z_x = standard score corresponding to any raw x score, z_y = standard score corresponding to any raw y score, Σ = sum of standard score products and n = numbers of paired measurements.

Table 16.3 gives the calculations for the correlation coefficient for the data given in the earlier examination scores example.

Therefore: $r = \dfrac{\Sigma z_x z_y}{n} = \dfrac{3.94}{5} = 0.79$

(The z scores are calculated as discussed in Ch. 15.)

This is quite a high correlation, indicating that the paired z scores fall roughly on a straight line.

In general, the closer the relationship between the two variables approximates a straight line, the more r approaches +1. Note that in social and biological sciences correlations this high do not usually occur. In general, we consider anything over 0.7 to be quite high, 0.3–0.7 to be moderate and less than 0.3 to be weak. The scattergrams in Figure 16.3 illustrate this point.

When n is large, the above equation is inconvenient to use to calculate r. Here we are not concerned with calculating r with a large n, although appropriate formulae or computer programs are available. For example, Coates & Steed (2003, Chapter 5) described how to use the program 'SPSS' for calculating correlation coefficients. The printouts provide not only the value of the correlation coefficients but also the statistical significance of the associations.

Assumptions for using r

It was pointed out earlier that r is used when two variables are scaled on interval or ratio scales and when it is shown that they are linearly associated. In addition, the sets of scores on each variable should be approximately normally distributed.

If any of the above assumptions are violated, then the correlation coefficient might be spuriously low. Therefore, other correlation coefficients should be used to represent association between two variables. A further problem may arise from the truncation of the range of values in

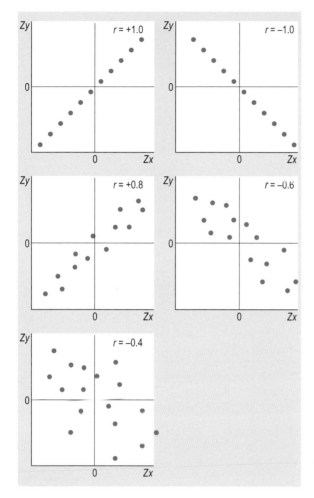

Figure 16.3 • Scattergrams and corresponding approximate *r* values.

Spearman's ρ

When the obtained data are such that at least one of the variables x or y was measured on an ordinal scale and the other on an ordinal scale or higher, we use ρ to calculate the correlation between the two variables. The higher scale can be readily reduced to an ordinal scale.

If one or both variables were measured on a nominal scale, ρ is no longer appropriate as a statistic.

$$\rho = 1 - \frac{6\Sigma d^2}{n^3 - n}$$

where d = difference in a pair of ranks and n = number of pairs.

The derivation of this formula will not be discussed here. The 6 is placed in the formula as a scaling device; it ensures that the possible range of ρ is from -1 to $+1$ and thus enables ρ and r to be compared. Let us consider an example to illustrate the use of ρ.

If an investigator is interested in the correlation between socioeconomic status and severity of respiratory illness, and assuming that both variables were measured on, or transformed to, an ordinal scale, the investigator rank-orders the scores from highest to lowest on each variable (Table 16.4).

Therefore:
$$\rho = 1 - \frac{6\Sigma d^2}{n^3 - n}$$
$$= 1 - \frac{6 \times 24}{8^3 - 8} = 0.71$$

Clearly, the association among the ranks for the paired scores on the two variables becomes closer the more ρ approaches $+1$. If the ranks tend to be inverse, then ρ approaches -1.

Uses of correlation in the health sciences

Prediction

When the correlation coefficient has been calculated it may be used to predict the value of one variable (y) given the value of the other variable (x).

one or both of the variables. This occurs when the distributions greatly deviate from normal shapes. The higher scale can be readily reduced to an ordinal scale.

If we measure the correlation between examination scores and IQs of a group of health science students, we might find a low correlation because, by the time students present themselves to tertiary courses, most students with low IQs are eliminated. In this way, the distribution of IQs would not be normal but rather negatively skewed. In effect, the question of appropriate sampling is also relevant to correlations, as was outlined in Chapter 3.

Table 16.4 Rank-ordering of scores				
Patient	Socioeconomic status (rank)	Severity of illness (rank)	d (difference between ranks)	d²
1	6	5	1	1
2	7	8	−1	1
3	2	4	−2	4
4	3	3	0	0
5	5	7	−2	4
6	4	1	3	9
7	1	2	−1	1
8	8	6	2	4
				$\Sigma d^2 = 24$

For instance, take a hypothetical example that the correlation between cigarette smoking and lung damage is $r = +1$. We can see from Figure 16.4 that, given any score on x, we can transform this into a z score (z_x) and then using the graph we can read off the corresponding z score on y (z_y). Of course, it is extremely rare that there should be a perfect ($r = +1$) correlation between two variables. In this case, the smaller the correlation coefficient, the greater the probability of making an error in prediction. For example, consider Figure 16.5, where the scattergram shown represents a hypothetical correlation of approximately $r = 0.7$. Here, for any transformed value on variable x (say Zx_1) there is a range of values of z_y that correspond. Our best guess here is Zy_1, the average value, but clearly a range of scores is possible, as shown on the figure.

That is, as the correlation coefficient approaches 0, the range of error in prediction increases. A more appropriate and precise way of making predictions is in terms of regression analysis, but this topic is not covered in this introductory book.

Reliability and predictive validity of assessment

As you will recall, reliability refers to measurements using instruments or to subjective

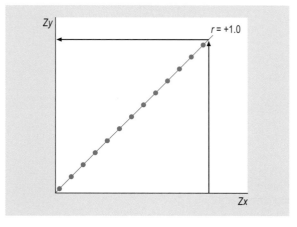

Figure 16.4 • Hypothetical relationship between cigarette smoking and lung damage. $r = +1.0$.

judgments remaining relatively the same on repeated administration (Ch. 12). This is called test–retest reliability and its degree is measured by a correlation coefficient. The correlation coefficient can also be used to determine the degree of inter-observer reliability.

As an example, assume that we are interested in the inter-observer reliability for two neurologists who are assessing patients for degrees of functional disability following spinal cord damage.

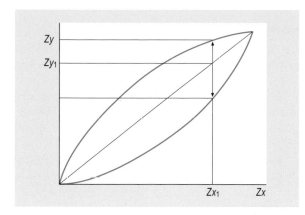

Figure 16.5 • Hypothetical relationship between cigarette smoking and lung damage. $r = +0.7$. With a correlation of <1.0 the data points will cluster around rather than exactly on the line and may vary between the range of values shown for any given values of x or y and their corresponding z scores.

Patient	Observer X	Observer Y	Rank X	Rank Y
1	85%	98%	1	1
2	75%	86%	2	2
3	74%	80%	3	3
4	72%	79%	4	4
5	69%	70%	5	5

Table 16.5 Assessment of disability (%) by observers X and Y

Table 16.5 represents a set of hypothetical results of their independent assessment of the same set of five patients.

Observer Y clearly attributes greater degrees of disability to the patients than observer X. However, as stated earlier, this need not affect the correlation coefficient. If we treat the measurement as an ordinal scale, we can see from Table 16.5 that the ranks given to the patients by the two observers correspond, so that it can be shown that $\rho = +1$.

Clearly, the higher the correlation, the greater the reliability. If we had treated the measurements as representing interval or ratio data, we would have calculated Pearson's r to represent quantitatively the reliability of the measurement.

Predictive validity is also expressed as a correlation coefficient. For example, say that you devise an assessment procedure to predict how much people will benefit from a rehabilitation programme. If the correlation between the assessment and a measure of the success of the rehabilitation programme is high (say 0.7 or 0.8), the assessment procedure has high predictive validity. If, however, the correlation is low (say 0.3 or 0.4), the predictive validity of the assessment is low, and it would be unwise to use the assessment as a screening procedure for the entry of patients into the rehabilitation programme.

Estimating shared variance

A useful statistic is the square of the correlation coefficient (r^2) which represents the proportion of variance in one variable accounted for by the other. This is called the *coefficient of determination*.

If, for example, the correlation between variable x (height) and variable y (weight) is $r = 0.7$, then the coefficient of determination is $r^2 = 0.49$ or 49%. This means that 49% of the variability of weight can be accounted for in terms of height. You might ask, what about the other 51% of the variability? This would be accounted for by other factors, say for instance, a tendency to eat fatty foods. The point here is that even a relatively high correlation coefficient ($r = 0.7$) accounts for less than 50% of the variability.

This is a difficult concept, so it might be worth remembering that 'variability' (see Ch. 14) refers to how scores are spread out about the mean. That is, as in the above example, some people will be heavy, some average, some light. So we can account for 49% of the total variability of weight (x) in terms of height (y) if $r = 0.7$. The other 51% can be explained in terms of other factors, such as somatotype. The greater the correlation coefficient, the greater the coefficient of determination, and the more the variability in y can be accounted for in terms of x.

Correlation and causation

In Chapter 4, we pointed out that there were at least three criteria for establishing a causal relationship. Correlation or co-variation is only one of these criteria. We have already discussed in Chapter 6 that even a high correlation between two variables does not necessarily imply a causal relationship. That is, there are a variety of plausible explanations for finding a correlation. As an example, let us take cigarette smoking (x) and lung damage (y). A high positive correlation could result from any of the following circumstances:

1. x causes y.
2. y causes x.
3. There is a third variable, which causes changes in both x and y.
4. The correlation represents a spurious or chance association.

For the example above, (1) would imply that cigarette smoking causes lung damage, (2) that lung damage causes cigarette smoking, and (3) that there was a variable (e.g. stress) which caused both increased smoking and lung damage. We need further information to identify which of the competing hypotheses is most plausible.

Some associations between variables are completely spurious (4). For example, there might be a correlation between the amount of margarine consumed and the number of cases of influenza over a period of time in a community, but each of the two events might have entirely different, unrelated causes. Also, some correlation coefficients do not reach statistical significance, that is, they may be due to chance (see Chs 18 and 19).

Also, if we are using a sample to estimate the correlation in a population, we must be certain that the outcome is not due to biased sampling or sampling error. That is, the investigator needs to show that a correlation coefficient is statistically significant and not just due to random sampling error. We will look at the concept of statistical significance in the next chapter.

While demonstrating correlation does not establish causality, we can use correlations as a source for subsequent hypotheses. For instance, in this example, work on carcinogens in cigarette tars and the causes of emphysema has confirmed that it is probably true that smoking does, in fact, cause lung damage (x causes y). However, given that there is often multiple causation of health problems, option (3) cannot be ruled out.

Techniques are available which can, under favourable conditions, enable investigators to use correlations as a basis for distinguishing between competing plausible hypotheses. One such technique, called path analysis, involves postulating a probable temporal sequence of events and then establishing a correlation between them. This technique was borrowed from systems theory and has been applied in areas of clinical research, such as epidemiology.

Summary

In this chapter we outlined how the degree and direction between two variables can be quantified using statistics called correlation coefficients. Of the correlation coefficients, the use of two were outlined: Pearson's r and Spearman's ρ. Definitional formulae and simple calculations were presented, with the understanding that more complex calculations of correlation coefficients are done with computers.

Several uses for r and ρ were discussed: for prediction, for quantifying the reliability and validity of measurements, and by using r^2 in estimating amount of shared variability. Finally, we discussed the caution necessary in causal interpretation of correlation coefficients. Showing a strong association between variables is an important step towards establishing causal links but further evidence is required to decide the direction of causality.

As with other descriptive statistics, caution is necessary when correlation coefficients are calculated for a sample and then generalized to a population. The question of generalization from a sample statistic to a population parameter will be discussed in the following chapters.

Self-assessment

Explain the meaning of the following terms:

coefficient of determination
correlation
correlation coefficient
curvilinear correlation
linear correlation
negative correlation
positive correlation
shared variance
zero correlation

True or false

1. Correlation is defined as the relative difference between two variables.
2. The association between two variables can be plotted on a scattergram.
3. If the distribution of paired scores is best represented by a curve, the relationship is non-linear.
4. When we speak of a positive (+) relationship, we mean that high scores on one variable are associated with high scores on the other variable.
5. In a negative (−) relationship, low scores on one variable are associated with low scores on the other.
6. There are several types of correlation coefficients, the selection of which is determined by the level of scaling of the two variables.
7. When both variables are measured on an interval or ratio scale, Pearson's r is the most appropriate correlation coefficient.
8. When both variables are measured on, or converted to, ordinal scales, we must use ϕ (phi) to express correlation.
9. For two variables measured on nominal scales, we use ρ (rho) to express correlation.
10. Pearson's r is calculated by a formula where $\Sigma z_x z_y$ stands for the sum of the z score pairs multiplied together.
11. When calculating Spearman's ρ, Σd_2 is the sum of the square of the differences between the means.
12. When we use Pearson's r, we assume that both variables are continuous and normally distributed.
13. The calculated values of correlation coefficients range between 0 and -1.

14. When there is no linear association between two variables, r or ρ will be close to zero.
15. A correlation coefficient of $+1$ represents a very low linear correlation.
16. Where there is a correlation of $r = +1$ between two variables, then the z scores of variable x will be equal to the z scores of variable y.
17. The coefficient of determination is the square of the correlation coefficient.
18. If $r = 0.3$, then the coefficient of determination will be 9.0.
19. If $r^2 = 0.36$ for a set of data, this implies that 36% of the variability of y is explained in terms of x.
20. As the correlation coefficient approaches zero, the possible error in linear prediction increases.
21. The closer the correlation coefficient is to zero, the greater the predictive validity of a test.
22. If a correlation coefficient for the test–retest reliability of a test is close to 1, then the test is unreliable.
23. Given a -1.00 correlation coefficient for two variables, a raw score of 50 on the first variable must be accompanied by a score of -50 on the second variable, for a given case.
24. Even a high correlation is not necessarily indicative of a causal relationship between two variables.
25. As the value of r increases, the proportion of variability of y that can be accounted for by x decreases.
26. Eta (η) is the appropriate correlation coefficient to use when two variables are nominally scaled.
27. If the relationship between two variables is non-linear, the value of the correlation coefficient must be negative.
28. Spearman's ρ is used where one or both variables are at least of interval scaling.
29. A scattergram is used to help to decide if the relationship between two variables is linear or curvilinear.
30. If the correlation between variables A and B is high, then there must be a direct causal relationship between A and B.

Multiple choice

1. Which of the following statements about correlations is false?

   a Spearman's ρ (rho) is appropriate to use when the relationship between two variables is non-linear.

   b A correlation coefficient of -0.8 represents a higher degree of association between two variables than a correlation coefficient of +0.6.

c The construction of a scattergram is useful for evaluating whether a relationship between two variables is linear or curvilinear.

d In a perfect positive correlation between two quantitatively measured variables, each individual obtains the same z scores on each variable.

e Negative correlation implies that high scores on one variable are related to low scores on another variable.

2. A scattergram:

a is a statistical test

b must be linear

c must be curvilinear

d is a graph of x and y scores

e is none of the above.

3. If the relationship between variables x and y is linear, then the points on the scattergram:

a will fall exactly on a straight line

b will fall on a curve

c must represent population parameters

d are independent of the variance

e are best represented by a straight line.

4. If the relationship between x and y is positive, as variable y decreases, variable x:

a increases

b decreases

c remains the same

d changes linearly

e varies.

5. In a 'negative' relationship:

a as x increases, y increases

b as x decreases, y decreases

c as x increases, y decreases

d both a and b

e none of the above.

6. The lowest strength of association is reflected by which of the following correlation coefficients?

a 0.95

b −0.60

c −0.33

d 0.29

e none of the above, as it cannot be determined.

7. The highest strength of association is reflected by which of the following correlation coefficients:

a −1.0

b −0.95

c 0.1

d 0.85

e none of the above, as it cannot be determined.

8. Which of the following statements is false?

a In a perfect positive correlation, each individual obtains the same z score on each variable.

b Spearman's ρ is used when one or both variables are at least of interval scaling.

c The range of the correlation coefficient is from −1 to +1.

d A correlation of $r = 0.85$ implies a stronger association than $r = -0.70$.

9. We can calculate the correlation coefficient if given:

a the top scores from one test and lowest scores from another test

b at least two scores from the same tests

c two sets of measurements for the same subjects

d either a or b.

10. The correlation between two variables x and y is −1.00. A given individual has a z score of $z_x = 1.4$ on variable x. We predict the z score on y is:

a 1.4 above the mean

b −1.4

c between 1.4 and −1.4

d −1.00.

11. Professor Shnook demonstrated a correlation of −0.85 between body weight and IQ. This means that:

a obesity decreases intelligence

b heavy people have higher IQs than light people

c people with high IQs are likely to be light

d malnutrition damages the brain

e none of the above.

12. A correlation coefficient of +0.5 was found between exposure to stressful life events and incidence of stress-induced disorders. A correlation of this direction and magnitude indicates that:

a a high level of exposure to stressful life events causes a high level of stress-induced disorders b a high level of stress-induced disorders causes a high likelihood of exposure to stressful life events

c either or both of *a* and *b* may be correct – we cannot be sure

d the levels of stress-induced disorders and of exposure to stressful life events are not causally related in any way.

13. You are told that there is a high inverse association between the variables 'amount of exercise' and 'incidence of heart disease'. A correlation coefficient consistent with the above statement is:

a $r = 0.8$

b $r = 0.2$

c $r = -0.2$

d $r = -0.8$.

14. Of the following measurement levels, which is at a minimum required for the valid calculation of a Pearson correlation coefficient?

a nominal

b ordinal

c interval

d ratio.

15. Of the following measurement levels, which is required for the valid calculation of the Spearman correlation coefficient?

a nominal

b ordinal

c interval

d ratio.

16. You are told that there is a high, positive correlation between measures of 'fitness' and 'hours of exercise'. The correlation coefficient consistent with the above statement is:

a 0.3

b 0.2

c −0.8

d −0.3

e none of these.

You are interested in selecting a test suitable for client assessment in a clinical situation. You find 4 tests in the literature, tests P, Q, R and S. Each of these tests has been validated against a clinically relevant variable. The test–retest and predictive validity of the four hypothetical tests are given in the table below.

Questions 17 and 18 refer to the above information.

Test	Test–retest reliability (r)	Predictive validity (r)
P	0.8	0.50
Q	0.9	0.18
R	0.5	0.40
S	0.2	0.03

17. Which test would you choose for clinical assessment?

a P

b Q

c R

d S

18. Which test has the best test–retest reliability?

a P

b Q

c R

d S

An investigation aims to establish for a sample of subjects the relationship between blood cholesterol levels (in mg/cc) and blood pressure (in mmHg).

Questions 19 and 20 refer to this investigation.

19. The correlation coefficient appropriate for establishing the degree of correlation between the two variables (assuming a linear relationship):

a is determined by the sample size

b depends on the direction of the causality

c is Spearman's ρ

d is Pearson's r

e both *b* and *c*.

20. Say that the correlation coefficient is calculated to be +0.7. A correlation of this direction and magnitude indicates that:

a high blood pressure causes high blood cholesterol

b high blood cholesterol causes high blood pressure

c there might be a third variable which causes both high blood pressure and high blood cholesterol

d none of the statements *a*, *b* or *c* is consistent with the evidence e any of the statements *a*, *b* or *c* might be correct; we cannot be sure from the available evidence.

21. When deciding which measure of correlation to employ with a specific set of data, you should consider:

   a whether the relationship is linear or non-linear

   b the type of scale of measurement for each variable

   c *a* and *b*

   d neither *a* nor *b*.

22. The proportion of variance accounted for by the level of correlation between two variables is calculated by:

   a $\bar{X}$

   b r^2

   c Σx

   d you cannot calculate this proportion under any circumstances.

23. If the correlation between two variables A and B is 0.36, then the proportion of variance accounted for is:

   a 0.13

   b 0.06

   c 0.60

   d 0.64.

24. We find that the correlation coefficient representing the outcome for the predictive validity of a test is $r = 0.2$. Such a finding would indicate that the test had:

   a low predictive validity

   b acceptable predictive validity

   c high predictive validity

   d 20% predictive validity.

Section Five

Discussion, questions and answers

Descriptive statistics are an integral part of everyday life and an important aspect of clinical practice. They are used to describe the essential characteristics of measurements for a sample of cases. Some descriptive statistics are quite familiar to the lay person. The mean or average is frequently used in discussions of public policy. For example, the question 'What has happened to the average household income in the UK over the last year?' uses this concept, as does a question such as 'What is the average length of stay in hospital for an orthopaedic patient with a fractured neck of femur in this ward?' Descriptive statistics are shorthand ways of conveying information about a sample of cases.

In recent years in the UK, Australia, Canada and the US, there has been a growing preoccupation with the effectiveness and efficiency of health services in particular, and government services in general. Economic conditions have resulted in the reduced availability of tax revenues and this has led to increased scrutiny of spending. Hospital services are an expensive component of health services in these countries. Much statistical information is collected concerning stays in hospital. The use of statistical information concerning case costs is heavily used to determine funding of hospitals by agencies such as government and insurers.

A key component of hospital costs is the length of time spent by the patient in the hospital. Each 'bed day' is very costly and most hospital services are under pressure to reduce the length of stay for their patients. However, one cannot reduce the length of stay for each patient too far, as this might be dangerous. Patients can come back unexpectedly because they require further hospitalization following discharge. This is termed an 'unplanned' readmission. Thus, the goal is to reduce lengths of stay but not increase unplanned readmissions.

Obviously, the expected length of stay for a woman giving birth ought to be much shorter than a man recovering from serious internal injuries and multiple compound fractures following a motor vehicle accident. How can these cases be compared without some adjustment for their differences? There is a large literature concerning how different types of patients might be compared. Comparability of types of patients is often achieved by the use of diagnosis-related groups (DRG) where patients of the same type are categorized together. This grouping enables hospitals and their funding agencies to compare how efficient and effective different hospitals are in treating the same types of patient.

Table D16.1 shows some data for patients admitted to an orthopaedics ward in a hospital.

Table D16.1 Details of patients admitted to an orthopaedics ward

Patient name	Diagnostic group	Length of stay in hospital (days)	Unplanned readmission within 14 days?
Jones	Fractured neck of femur	15	No
Ng	Fractured neck of femur	10	Yes
Thomas	Fractured neck of femur	19	No
Evans	Fractured neck of femur	12	No
Valperri	Fractured neck of femur	14	No
Hart	Fractured neck of femur	14	No
Elmahdy	Fractured neck of femur	13	No
Smith	Fractured neck of femur	11	Yes
Cairns	Fractured neck of femur	12	No
Eisenberg	Fractured neck of femur	12	No

Table D16.2 Lengths of stay and readmission rates for 30 consecutive patients with a fractured neck of femur at five hospitals

Hospital	Length of stay in hospital		Standard deviation (s)	Rate of unplanned readmissions per 100
	Number of cases (n)	Average ($\bar{X}$)		
A	30	13.0	2.6	6.7
B	30	12.3	2.4	10.0
C	30	13.4	2.8	6.7
D	30	14.4	3.3	3.3
E	30	14.8	3.0	3.3

All the cases with the same diagnostic category have been included.

For this sample of cases, the average length of stay was 13.2 days (standard deviation 2.5). The minimum stay was 10 days and the maximum stay was 19 days. The rate of unplanned readmissions within 14 days was 2 in 10 or 20%.

If one was to take larger samples of cases from a variety of hospitals (say a consecutive series of 30 cases for each), then it would be possible to compare their lengths of stay and the rates of readmissions. This has been done in Table D16.2, with hypothetical data from five hospitals.

Although the differences in average numbers of days spent in hospital between the five hospitals may not appear to be great, a difference of 2.5 days, for example between hospitals B and E, may represent over £500 for each case. In a busy hospital department, this would soon run into large sums of money. However, it is worrying that the hospital with the shortest period of stay also seems to be the one with the highest rate of readmissions within 14 days. Perhaps they are discharging some of their patients too soon. With such a small sample of hospitals (i.e. only five) and such a small number of readmissions (only three out of the 30 in the worst case), it would be difficult to conclude whether there is such a relationship. However, if these data were collected from a large number of hospitals with a larger number of cases, it would be possible to correlate these two variables to study the size of the relationship between them.

Correlation coefficients measure the size and direction of the statistical relationship between two variables. Following on from the above discussion, we might hypothesize that there is a negative correlation between the average length of stay and rate of readmission to hospital. In other words, we might expect that a shorter average stay in a hospital could result in a greater rate of readmission. Figure D16.1 shows the association between length of stay and rate of readmission for 30 hospitals, based on their 1993–1994 discharges for all their patients with a fractured neck of femur.

Each of the dots in the graph represents a different hospital. The graph shows that there is a tendency towards those hospitals with longer average lengths of stays having lower readmission rates for their patients.

The Pearson correlation between these variables is −0.52, which indicates a moderately sized negative correlation between average length of stay and readmission rate for the 30 hospitals.

Evidence such as discussed above is being continually collected by health administrators and the results of these analyses impact on the funding of your workplace and your opportunities for looking after your patients.

Questions

1. In Table D16.1, how many patients had a length of stay in hospital that was above the average of 13.2 days?
2. If a patient had a length of stay of 14 days, given that the sample mean was 13.2 days and the standard deviation 2.5, what would be that patient's standard or z score?
3. Is it appropriate to compare hospital lengths of stay for patients with different diagnoses?
4. From Figure D16.1, what is the longest average length of stay for this sample of hospitals? What is the shortest?
5. Why is the correlation between average length of stay and readmission rate negative in sign?

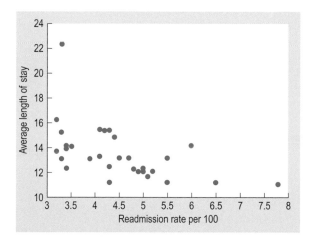

Figure D16.1 • Relationship between average lengths of stay and readmission rates for patients with fractured neck of femur at 30 hospitals.

Answers

1. Four: Jones, Thomas, Valperri and Hart.
2. The standard score is calculated using the following formula:

$$z = \frac{x - \bar{X}}{s}$$

Substituting into the equation, we find that:

$$z = \frac{14 - 13.2}{2.5} = 0.32$$

3. It is like comparing apples with oranges. It is quite reasonable to expect that an uncomplicated birth may involve a hospital stay of 3–4 days,

whereas this would be quite unreasonable for a heart transplant. Thus it does not make sense to compare the lengths of stay of different types of patients, because the averages or means are quite different. However, it would make sense to compare standard scores for different types of patients.

4. About 22.5 days; about 11 days.

5. Because an increase in average length of stay is associated with a decrease in readmission rate.

Section **Six**

Inferential statistics

The statistical analysis of the data is an essential stage in the process of quantitative research. The principles of inferential statistics, as introduced in this section, are applied for deciding if the obtained sample data show the differences and patterns we set out to demonstrate in the population. This is the case for all types of research where we are using sample data to make inferences concerning populations.

Quantitative research in the health sciences mostly involves working with samples drawn from populations. In order to generalize our findings, we must draw generalizations and inferences from sample statistics (e.g. $\bar{X}$, s) to the population parameters (e.g. μ, σ). Inferences are always probabilistic, because even with random samples there is always the chance of sampling error. The finite probability of sampling error implies that the differences or patterns identified in our sample data could represent random variations or chance patterns rather than 'real' ones which are true for the population as a whole.

As an illustration, imagine that we have collected data in a study aimed at identifying age-related differences in the use of sedatives and tranquillizers in a given population. Our participants ($n = 200$) kept diaries over a period of 1 year, recording each time they had taken a sedative or tranquillizer. The research question is: is there a difference between sedative or tranquillizer use in older and younger people? Assume that the following hypothetical data were obtained:

Sedative and tranquillizer consumption			
Age group	n	$\bar{X}$	s
20–39	100	20	5
40–59	100	30	5

Three important and interrelated questions are examined in Section 6 concerning the evidence provided by sample data such as those shown in the above table.

1. Even if we used an adequate sampling procedure (see Ch. 3), how confident are we to infer that the true population parameters (μ) are the same as, or are at least close to, $\bar{X}$? For example, is it true that the mean tranquillizer intake for the 20–39 age group is $\mu = 20$?

2. It appears that there is a large difference between the two sample means; but is this difference also true for the populations? In other words is this difference 'real' or significant, or is it simply due to sampling error?

3. What we are inferring is μ older $> \mu$ younger. In other words, are we justified in concluding that the mean sedative/tranquillizer intake for the older age group is greater than for the younger group in the population?

The key issue here is that we are using sample data for decision making. Sampling error refers to the difference between sample statistics and the actual state of the population.

We cannot eliminate sampling error even with large and well-chosen samples. Rather, as outlined in Section 6, we can apply the principles of inferential statistics to calculate the probability of error. We then use this information to minimize the probability of making errors when we generalize from sample statistics to population parameters.

In Chapter 17 we examine how sampling distributions are derived and used for calculating the probability of obtaining a given sample statistic. This information can be applied to the calculation of confidence intervals, which represent a range of scores which contain the true population parameter at a given level or probability.

In Chapter 18 we outline the logic of hypothesis testing, using single sample z and t tests as exemplars. Hypothesis testing is a procedure used to decide if a difference or pattern identified in our sample data is statistically significant. If the outcome of our analysis is significant, then we are in a position to decide that the patterns or differences found in our data may be generalized to the populations from which the samples were drawn.

There are numerous statistical tests available for analysing the significance of our data. In Chapter 19 we discuss basic criteria for selecting an appropriate statistical test, including (i) scale of measurement used to collect the data, (ii) the number of groups being compared and (iii) the dependence or independence of measurements. We will use the χ^2 (chi-squared) test to demonstrate how statistical tests are selected and used to analyse the data.

Ultimately, statistical decision making is probabilistic, implying that the possibility of making decision errors cannot be eliminated. Decisions may be correct, or involve what are called Type I and Type II errors. In Chapter 20, we examine how these errors may influence our interpretation of the obtained data in relation to the aims or hypotheses guiding our research, and we will examine strategies which can be employed to reduce the probability of making such errors. In this chapter we outline the relationship between effect size and the clinical or practical significance of research findings.

Chapter Seventeen

Probability and sampling distributions

Introduction

Sample statistics (such as $\bar{X}$, s) are estimates of the actual population parameters μ, σ. Even where adequate sampling procedures are adopted, there is no guarantee that the sample statistics are the exact representations of the true parameters of the population from which the samples were drawn. Therefore, inferences from sample statistics to population parameters necessarily involve the possibility of sampling error. As stated in Chapter 3, sampling errors represent the discrepancy between sample statistics and true population parameters. Given that investigators usually have no knowledge of the true population parameters, inferential statistics are employed to estimate the probable sampling errors. While sampling error cannot be completely eliminated, its probable magnitude can be calculated using *inferential statistics*. In this way investigators are in a position to calculate the probability of being accurate in their estimations of the actual population parameters.

The aims of this chapter are to examine how probability theory is applied to generating sampling distributions and how sampling distributions are used for estimating population parameters. Sampling distributions can be used for specifying confidence intervals, as discussed in this chapter, as well as for testing hypotheses, as further discussed in Chapter 18.

The specific aims of this chapter are to:

1. Define probability.
2. Demonstrate how sampling distributions are generated.
3. Show how sampling distributions of the mean are used to calculate the probability of a sample mean.
4. Explain how confidence intervals are calculated for continuous data.
5. Distinguish between z and t distributions.

Probability

The concept of probability is central to the understanding of inferential statistics. Probability is expressed as a proportion between 0 and 1, where 0 means an event is certain not to occur, and 1 means an event is certain to occur. Therefore if the probability (p) is 0.01 for an event then it is unlikely to occur (chance is 1 in a hundred). If $p = 0.99$ then the event is highly likely to occur (chance is 99 in a hundred). The probability of any event (say event A) occurring is given by the formula:

$$p(A) = \frac{\text{number of occurrences of A}}{\text{total number of possible occurrences}}$$

Sometimes the probability of an event can be calculated a priori (before the event) by reasoning alone. For example, we can predict that the probability of throwing a head (H) with a fair coin is:

$$p(H) = \frac{\text{number of occurrences of H}}{\text{total number of possible occurrences}}$$
$$= \frac{H}{H + T(\text{tails})} = \frac{1}{2} = 0.5$$

Or, if we buy a lottery ticket in a draw where there are 100 000 tickets, the probability of winning first prize is:

$$p(1\text{st prize}) = \frac{1}{100\,000} = 0.00001$$

This is true only if the lottery is fair, if all tickets have an equal chance of being drawn by random selection.

In some situations, there is no model which we can apply to calculate the occurrence of an event a priori. For instance, how can we calculate the probability of an individual dying of a specific condition? In such instances, we use previously obtained empirical evidence to calculate probabilities a posteriori (after the event).

For example, if it is known that the percentages (or proportions) for causes of death are distributed in a particular way, then the probability of a particular cause of death for a given individual can be predicted. Table 17.1 represents a set of hypothetical statistics for a community.

Given the data in Table 17.1, we are in a position to calculate the probability of a selected individual over 65 dying of any of the specified causes. For example, the probability of a given individual dying of coronary heart disease is:

$$p(\text{dying of heart disease})$$
$$= \frac{\% \text{ of cases dying of heart disease}}{100\%}$$
$$= \frac{50\%}{100\%} = 0.5$$

This approach ignores individual risk factors and assumes that the environmental conditions under which the data were obtained are still pertinent. However, the example illustrates the principle that once we have organized the data into a frequency distribution we can calculate the probability of selecting any of the tabulated values. This is true whether the variable was measured on a nominal, ordinal, interval or ratio scale. Here, we will

Table 17.1 Causes of death for persons over 65

Cause of death	Percentage of deaths
Coronary heart disease	50
Cancer	25
Stroke	10
Accidents	5
Infections	5
Other causes	5

examine how to calculate the probability of values for normally distributed, continuous variables.

We can use the normal curve model, as outlined in Chapter 15, to determine the proportion or percentage of cases up to, or between, any specified scores. In this instance, probability is defined as the proportion of the total area cut off by the specified scores under the normal curve. The greater the proportion, the higher the probability of selecting the specified values.

For example, say that on the basis of previous evidence we can specify the frequency distribution of neonates' weight. Let us assume that the distribution is approximately normal, with the mean ($\bar{X}$) of 5.0 kg and a standard deviation (s) of 1.5. Now, say that we are interested in the probability of a randomly selected neonate having a birth weight of 2.0 kg or under. Figure 17.1 illustrates the above situation.

The area A1 under the curve in Figure 17.1 corresponds to the probability of obtaining a score of 2 or under. Using the principles outlined in Chapter 15 to calculate proportions or areas under the normal curve, we first translate the raw score of 2 into a z score:

$$z = \frac{x - \bar{X}}{s} = \frac{2 - 5}{1.5} = -2$$

Now we look up the area under the normal curve corresponding to $z = -2$ (Appendix A). Here we find that A1 is 0.0228. This area corresponds

to a probability, and we can say that 'The probability of a neonate having a birth weight of 2 kg or less is 0.0228'. Another way of stating this outcome is that the chances are approximately 2 in 100, or 2%, for a child having such a birth weight.

We can also use the normal curve model to calculate the probability of selecting scores between any given values of a normally distributed continuous variable. For example, if we are interested in the probability of birth weights being between 6 and 8 kg, then this can be represented on the normal curve (area A2 on Fig. 17.2). To determine this area, we proceed as outlined in Chapter 15. Let $s = 1.5$.

$$z_1 = \frac{6 - 5}{1.5} = 0.67$$

$$z_2 = \frac{8 - 5}{1.5} = 2.0$$

Therefore: the area between z_1 and $\bar{X}$ is 0.2486 (from Appendix A) and the area between z_2 and $\bar{X} = 0.4772$ (from Appendix A). Therefore, the required area A2 is:

A2 − 0.4772 − 0.2486 = 0.2286

It can be concluded that the probability of a randomly selected child having a birth weight between 6 and 8 kg is $p = 0.2286$. Another way of saying this is that there is a chance of 23 in 100 or a 23% chance that the birth weight will be between 6 and 8 kg.

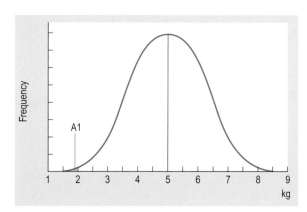

Figure 17.1 • Frequency distribution of neonate birth weights. Area A1 corresponds to $z \leqslant -2$.

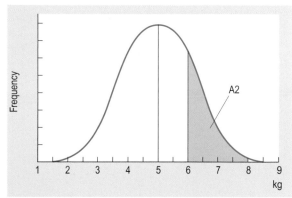

Figure 17.2 • Frequency distribution of neonate birth weights. Area A2 corresponds to probability of weight being 6–8 kg.

The above examples demonstrate that when the mean and standard deviation are known for a normally distributed continuous variable, this information can be applied to calculating the probability of events related to this distribution. Of course, probabilities can be calculated for other than normal data but this requires integral calculus which is beyond the scope of this text. In general, regardless of the shape or scaling of a distribution, scores which are common or 'average' are more likely to be selected than those which are atypical, being unusually high or low.

Sampling distributions

Probability theory can also be applied to calculate the probability of obtaining specific samples from populations.

Consider a container with a very large number of identically sized marbles. Imagine that there are two kinds of marbles present, black (B) and white (W), and that these colours are present in equal proportions, so that $p(B) = p(W) = 0.5$.

Given the above population, say that samples of marbles are drawn randomly and with replacement. (By 'replacement' we mean the samples are put back into the population, in order to maintain as a constant the proportion of B = W = 0.5.) If we draw samples of four (that is, $n = 4$) then the possible proportions of black and white marbles in the samples can be deduced a priori as shown in Figure 17.3.

Possible outcomes	Number black	Number white	Proportions black
● ● ● ●	4	0	1.00
● ● ● ○	3	1	0.75
● ● ○ ○	2	2	0.50
● ○ ○ ○	1	3	0.25
○ ○ ○ ○	0	4	0.00

Figure 17.3 • Characteristics of possible samples of $n = 4$, drawn from a population of black and white marbles.

Ignoring the order in which marbles are chosen, Figure 17.3 demonstrates all the possible outcomes for the composition of samples of $n = 4$. It is logically possible to draw any of the samples shown. However, only one of the samples (2B, 2W), is representative of the true population parameter. The other samples would generate incorrect inferences concerning the state of the population. In general, if we know or assume (hypothesize) the true population parameters, we can generate distributions of the probability of obtaining samples of a given characteristic.

In this instance, when attempting to predict the probability of specific samples drawn from a population with two discrete elements, the binomial theorem can be applied. The expansion of the binomial expression, $(P + Q)^n$, generates the probability of all the possible samples which can be drawn from a given population. The general equation for expanding the binomial expression is:

$$(P + Q)^n = P^n + \frac{n}{1} P^{n-1}Q + $$
$$\frac{n(n - 1)}{2} P^{n-2}Q^2 + \dots Q^n$$

P is the probability of the first outcome, Q is the probability of the second outcome and n is the number of trials (or the sample size).

In this instance, P = proportion black (B) = 0.5; Q = proportion white (W) = 0.5; $n = 4$ (sample size). Therefore, substituting into the binomial expression:

$$(B+W)^4 = B^4 + 4B^3W + 6B^2W^2 + 4BW^3 + W^4$$

Note that each part of the expansion stands for a probability of obtaining a specific sample. For the present case:

Sample 1 $p(4B0W)$	= B^4	= $(0.5)^4$	= 0.0625
Sample 2 $p(3B1W)$	= $4B^3W$	= $4 \times (0.5)^3(0.5)$	= 0.2500
Sample 3 $p(2B2W)$	= $6B^2W^2$	= $6 \times (0.5)^2(0.5)^2$	= 0.3750
Sample 4 $p(1B3W)$	= $4BW^3$	= $4 \times (0.5)^3(0.5)$	= 0.2500
Sample 5 $p(0B4W)$	= W^4	= $(0.5)^4$	= 0.0625

The calculated probabilities add up to 1, indicating that all the possible sample outcomes have been accounted for. However, the important issue here is not so much the mathematical details but the general principle being illustrated by the example. For a given sample size (n) we can employ a mathematical formula to calculate the probability of obtaining all the possible samples from a population with known parameters. The relationship between the possible samples and their probabilities can be graphed, as shown in Figure 17.4.

Taking the statistic 'number of black marbles in the sample', the graph in Figure 17.4 shows the probability of obtaining any of the outcomes. The distribution shown is called a 'sampling distribution'. In general, a sampling distribution for a statistic indicates the probability of obtaining any of the possible values of a statistic.

Therefore, having obtained our sampling distribution we can see that some sample outcomes have low probability while others are more likely. Although there is a finite chance of obtaining a sample such as 'all blacks', the probability of this happening is rather small ($p = 0.0625$). Conversely, a sample of 2B2W, which is equal to the true population proportions, is far more probable ($p = 0.375$). Generating sampling distributions for calculating the probability of given sample statistics is a basic practice in inferential statistics. The sampling distributions enable researchers to infer (with a determined level of confidence) the true population parameters from the sample statistics.

Sampling distribution of the mean

The binomial theorem is appropriate for generating sampling distributions for discontinuous nominal scale data. However, when measurements are continuous, the mean and standard deviations are appropriate as sample statistics and are measured on interval or ratio scales. The sampling distribution of the mean represents the frequency distribution of sample means obtained from random samples drawn from the population. The sampling distribution of the mean enables the calculation of the probability of obtaining any given sample mean ($\bar{X}$). This is essential for testing hypotheses about sample means (Ch. 18).

In order to generate the sampling distribution of the mean, we use a mathematical theorem called the central limit theorem. This theorem provides a set of rules which relate the parameters (μ, σ) of the population from which samples are drawn to the distribution of sample means ($\bar{X}$).

The central limit theorem states that if random samples of a fixed n are drawn from any population, as n becomes large the distribution of sample means approaches a normal distribution, with the mean of the sample means ($\bar{X}_{\bar{x}}$ or $\mu_{\bar{x}}$) being equal to the population mean (μ) and the standard error of estimate ($s_{\bar{x}}$ or $\sigma_{\bar{x}}$) being equal to $\sigma/\sqrt{n}$. The standard error of the estimate is the standard deviation of the distribution of sample means.

Let us follow the above step by step.

1. Imagine we have a population of continuous scores or measurements with a mean of μ and a standard deviation of σ.
2. We select a very large number of random samples, each sample being of a size n.
3. Having obtained our samples, for each sample we calculate the sample mean ($\bar{X}_1$, $\bar{X}_2$, ... and so on).
4. Each sample mean, $\bar{X}$, is a number. The sampling distribution of the mean is a frequency distribution representing the large number of sample means.
5. The central limit theorem predicts theoretically the shape (normal for large n), mean ($\bar{X}_{\bar{x}}$ or $\mu_{\bar{x}}$) and standard deviation ($s_{\bar{x}}$ or $\sigma_{\bar{x}}$) of a large number of sample means.

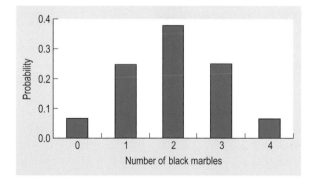

Figure 17.4 • Sampling distribution of black marbles; $n = 4$.

It should be noted that:

1. The sampling distribution of the mean is a frequency distribution of a large number of sample means of size n drawn from a given population. When n increases, the sampling distributions approach normal.
2. The mean of the sample means ($\mu_{\bar{x}}$ or $\bar{X}_{\bar{x}}$) is the mean of the distribution of sample means. $\bar{X}_{\bar{x}}$ and $\mu_{\bar{x}}$ are equal to μ, the population mean.
3. The standard error of the mean ($s_{\bar{x}}$ or $\sigma_{\bar{x}}$) is the standard deviation of the frequency distribution of sample means drawn from a population. The magnitude of $s_{\bar{x}}$ or $\sigma_{\bar{x}}$ is equal to $\sigma/\sqrt{n}$, the population standard deviation divided by the square root of the sample size.
4. $\mu_{\bar{x}}$ and $\sigma_{\bar{x}}$ are used in reference to a sampling distribution based on all the possible samples drawn from a population (a population of samples, would you believe?), while $\bar{X}$ and $s_{\bar{x}}$ are used when the sampling distribution is based on a 'sample' of samples.

Let us have a look at an example. Assume for a hypothetical test of motor function that $\mu = 50$ and $\sigma = 10$. What is the probability of drawing a random sample from this population with $\bar{X} = 52$ or greater (i.e. $\bar{X} \geqslant 52$) given that $n = 100$? The central limit theorem predicts that when we draw samples of $n = 100$ from the above population, the sampling distribution of the means will be as follows:

- The shape of the sampling distribution will be approximately normal.
- The mean of the sampling distribution will be equal to μ:

$$\mu_{\bar{x}} = \mu = 50$$

- The standard error of estimate ($\sigma_{\bar{x}}$) will be:

$$\sigma_{\bar{x}} = \frac{\sigma}{\sqrt{n}} = \frac{10}{\sqrt{100}} = 1$$

(We can show this as in Fig. 17.5.)

Previously, we saw how we can use normal frequency distributions for estimating probabilities. Using the same principles as in Chapter 15, we can calculate the z score corresponding to $\bar{X} = 52$, and look up Appendix A to find out the area representing the probability in question:

$$z = \frac{\bar{X} - \mu_{\bar{x}}}{\sigma_{\bar{x}}} = \frac{52 - 50}{1} = 2$$

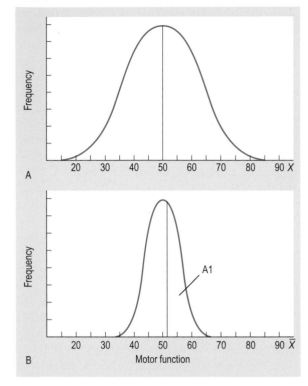

Figure 17.5 • Relationship between original population and sampling distribution of the mean, where $\mu = 50$ and $\sigma = 10$; (A) original population, (B) sampling distribution of the mean.

That is, $\bar{X} = 52$ is two standard error units above $\mu_{\bar{x}}$, the population mean for the sample means.

You may have noticed that the distribution of $\bar{X}$ is far less dispersed than X (i.e. the raw scores), as $\sigma_{\bar{x}} = 1$ and $\sigma = 10$.

Using Appendix A for establishing the probability, we find that the area representing $p(\bar{X} \geqslant 52)$, that is, area A1 in Figure 17.5B, is:

$$p(\bar{X} \geqslant 52) = 0.5000 - 0.4772 = 0.0228$$

Therefore the probability of drawing a sample of $\bar{X} \geqslant 52$ is 0.0228. We will apply this notion to hypothesis testing in Chapter 18, but you might have noticed that it is a rather low probability. That is, it is unlikely ($p = 0.0228$) randomly to draw a sample with $\bar{X} \geqslant 52$ where $n = 100$ and $\mu = 50$.

Application of the central limit theorem to calculating confidence intervals

Let us assume that you are asked to estimate the weight of a newborn baby. If you are experienced in working with neonates, you should be able to make a reasonable guess. You might say 'The baby is 6 kg'. Someone might ask 'How certain are you that the baby is exactly 6 kg?' You might then say 'Well, the baby might not be exactly 6 kg, but I'm very confident that it weighs somewhere between 5.5 and 6.5 kg'. This statement expresses a confidence interval – a range of values which probably include the true value. Of course, the more certain or confident you want to be of including the true value, the bigger the range of values you might give: you are unlikely to be wrong if you guess that the baby weighs between 4 and 8 kg.

Confidence intervals can be calculated for a large range of statistics such as proportions, ratios or correlation coefficients. In this chapter we will look at confidence intervals for single samples as an illustration for using confidence intervals.

We have seen previously that if we know the population parameters we can estimate the probability of selecting from that population a sample mean of a given magnitude. Conversely, if we know the sample mean we can estimate the population parameters from which the sample might have come, at a given level of probability. Let us take an example to illustrate this point.

A researcher is interested in the systolic blood pressure (BP) levels of smokers of more than 10 cigarettes per day. She takes a random sample of 100 10+ smokers in her district and finds that the mean BP = 148 mmHg for the sample, with a standard deviation of $s = 10$.

She wants to generalize to the population of smokers of more than 10 cigarettes per day in their district. The best estimate of μ (the population parameter) is 148, but it is possible that, because of sampling error, 148 is not the exact population parameter. However she can calculate a confidence interval (a range of blood pressures that will include the true population mean at a given level of probability). A confidence interval is a range of scores which includes the true population parameter at a specified level of probability. The precise probability is decided by the researcher and indicates how certain she can be that the population mean is actually within the calculated range. Common confidence intervals used in statistics are 95% confidence intervals, which offer a probability of $p = 0.95$ for including the true population mean, and 99% confidence intervals, which include the true population mean at a probability of $p = 0.99$.

Calculating the confidence interval requires the use of the following formula:

$$\bar{X} - zs_{\bar{x}} \leq \mu \leq \bar{X} + zs_{\bar{x}}$$

where $\bar{X}$ is the sample mean; z is the z score obtained from the normal curve table such that it cuts off the area of the normal curve corresponding to the required probability; $s_{\bar{x}}$ is the sample standard error, which is equal to the sample standard deviation divided by $\sqrt{n}$, that is, $s_{\bar{x}} = s/\sqrt{n}$.

Let us turn to the previous example to illustrate the use of the above equation. Here $\bar{X} = 148$, and $s_{\bar{x}} = 10/\sqrt{100}$. Assume that we want to calculate a 95% confidence interval. We are looking for a pair of z scores which have 95% of the standard normal curve between them. In this case, 1.96 is the value for z which cuts off 95% of a normal distribution. That is, we looked up the value of z corresponding to an area (probability) of 0.4750, since the 0.05 has to be divided among the two tails of the distribution, giving 0.025 at either end. Substituting into the equation above we have:

$$148 - (1.96)(10/\sqrt{100}) \leq \mu \leq 148 + (1.96)$$
$$\times (10/\sqrt{100}) = 146.04 \leq \mu \leq 149.96$$

That is, the investigator is 95% confident that the true population mean, the true mean BP of smokers, lies between 146.04 (lower limit) and 149.96 (upper limit). There is only a 5% or 0.05 probability that it lies outside this range. If we chose a 99% confidence interval, then using the formula as above, we have:

$$148 - (2.58)(10/\sqrt{100}) \leq \mu \leq 148 + (2.58)$$
$$\times (10/\sqrt{100}) = 145.42 \leq \mu \leq 150.58$$

Here, 2.58 is the value of z which cuts off 99% of a normal distribution (Fig. 17.6). That is, the investigator is 99% confident that the true population mean lies somewhere between 145.42 and 150.58. Clearly, the 99% interval is wider than the 95% interval; after all, here the probability of including the true mean is greater than for the 95% interval. Conventionally, health sciences publications report 95% confidence intervals.

Confidence intervals where *n* is small: the *t* distribution

It was previously stated that: 'as *n* becomes large, the distribution of sample means approaches a

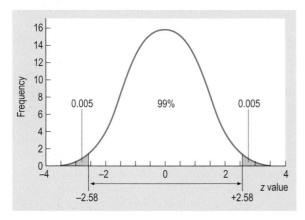

Figure 17.6 • z scores for 99% confidence interval.

normal distribution' (central limit theorem). The questions left to explain are:

- How large must the sample size, *n*, be before the sampling distribution of the mean can be considered a normal curve?
- What are the implications for the sampling distribution if *n* is small?

It has been shown by mathematicians that the sample size, *n*, for which the sampling distribution of the mean can be considered an approximation of a normal distribution is $n \geq 30$. That is, if *n* is 30 or more, we can use the standard normal curve to describe the sampling distribution of the mean. However, when $n < 30$, the sampling distribution of the mean is a rather rough approximation to the normal distribution. Instead of using the normal distribution, we use the *t distribution*, which takes into account the variability of the shape of the sampling distribution due to low *n*.

The *t* distributions (Fig. 17.7) are a family of curves representing the sampling distributions of means drawn from a population when sample size, *n*, is small ($n < 30$). A 'family of curves' means that the shape of the *t* distribution varies with sample size. It has been found that the distribution is determined by the *degrees of freedom* of the statistic.

The degrees of freedom (df) for a statistic represents the number of scores which are free to vary when calculating the statistic. Since the statistic we are calculating in this case is the mean,

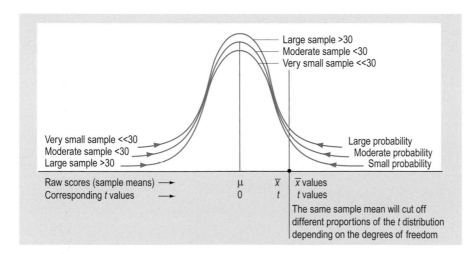

Figure 17.7 •
t distributions.

all but one of the scores could vary. That is, if you were inventing scores in a sample with a known mean, you would have a free hand until the very last score. There df is equal to $n - 1$ (the sample size minus one). Each row of figures shown in Appendix B represents the critical values of *t* for a given distribution.

1. The *t* distribution is symmetrical about the mean.
2. The values of *t* along the x-axis cut off specific areas under the curve, just as for *z*. These areas are given at the top of the page in Appendix B, under 'Directional' and 'Non-directional' probabilities.
3. The *t* distribution approaches a normal distribution as *n* becomes larger. As stated earlier, when $n \geq 30$, for all practical purposes the *t* and *z* distributions coincide.

The *t* distribution, just as the *z* distribution, can be used to approximate the probability of drawing sample means of a given magnitude from a population; *t* can also be used for calculating confidence intervals. Let us re-examine the example relating to the blood pressure of smokers presented earlier. Let us assume that $n = 25$, with the other statistics remaining the same: $\overline{X} = 148$, $s = 10$. The general formula for calculating the confidence intervals for small samples is:

$$\overline{X} - ts_{\overline{x}} \leq \mu \leq \overline{X} + ts_{\overline{x}}$$

You will note the similarity to the equation on page 199; here *t* replaces *z*. If we want to show the 95% confidence interval, then we use the same logic as for *z* distributions (Fig. 17.8).

To look up the *t* values from the tables (Appendix B) consider (i) direction, (ii) probabilities and (iii) degrees of freedom.

We are looking at a 'non-directional' or 'two-tail' probability in the sense that the *t* values cut off 95% of the area of the *t* curve between them, leaving 5% distributed at the two tails of the *t* distribution: $p = 0.05$; df $= 25 - 1 = 24$. Therefore $t = 2.064$ (from Appendix B). Substituting into the equation for calculating confidence intervals:

$$148 - (2.1)(10/\sqrt{25}) \leq \mu \leq 148 + (2.1)(10/\sqrt{25})$$
$$148 - 4.2 \leq \mu \leq 148 + 4.2$$
$$143.8 \leq \mu \leq 152.2$$

Consider the width of the confidence interval defined as the distance between the upper and lower limits. Note that this is a wider interval than that which was obtained when *n* was 100. As sample size, *n*, becomes smaller, our confidence interval becomes wider, reflecting a greater probability of sampling error.

To calculate the 99% confidence interval (Fig. 17.9) we need to look up $p = 0.01$, non-directional, df $= 24$ in Appendix B to obtain the critical value of *t*, which is 2.797.

$$148 - (2.8)(10/\sqrt{25}) \leq \mu \leq 148 + (2.8)(10/\sqrt{25})$$
$$142.4 \leq \mu \leq 153.6$$

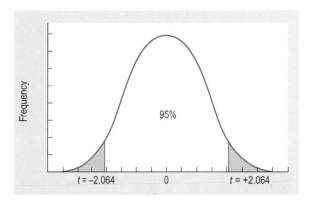

Figure 17.8 • The 95% confidence interval for sample size of 25.

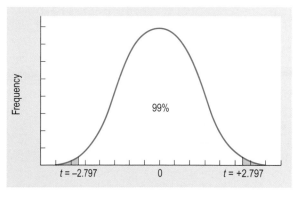

Figure 17.9 • The 99% confidence interval for sample size of 25.

We can see that, when $n = 25$, the 99% confidence interval is wider than for $n = 100$. That is, the bigger our sample size, the narrower (more precise) our estimate of the range of values (which includes the true population parameter) becomes when our sample size is large.

Summary

It was argued in this chapter that, even with randomly selected samples, the possibility of sampling error must be taken into account when making inferences from sample statistics to population parameters. It was shown that probability theory can be applied to generating sampling distributions, which express the probability of obtaining a given sample from a population. With discontinuous, nominal data the binomial theorem provides an adequate mathematical distribution for estimating the probability of obtaining possible samples. However, with continuous data, the central limit theorem is applied to generate the sampling distributions of the mean. The standard distribution of the mean enables the calculation of the probability-specified sample mean(s) by random selection. The sampling error of the mean ($s_{\bar{x}}$ or $\sigma_{\bar{x}}$), which expresses statistically the range of the sampling error, depends inversely on the sample size, such that the larger the n, the smaller the $s_{\bar{x}}$ or $\sigma_{\bar{x}}$.

One of the applications of sampling distributions is for calculating confidence intervals for continuous data. Confidence intervals represent a range of scores which specify, from sample data, the probability of capturing the true population parameters.

Health researchers usually report 95% confidence intervals. When sample sizes are small ($n < 30$), the t distribution is appropriate for representing the sampling distribution of the mean. With large sample sizes, the two distributions merge together. As the next chapter will demonstrate, sampling distributions are essential for testing hypotheses, a procedure which uses inferential statistics to calculate the level of probability at which sample statistics support the predictions of hypotheses.

Self-assessment

Explain the meaning of the following terms:

central limit theorem
confidence interval
degrees of freedom
population parameter
probability
sampling distribution
sampling distribution of the mean
sampling error
standard error of the mean
t distribution

True or false

1. If death and taxes are an absolute certainty, then the probability of their occurrence is infinite.
2. Probability values fall between 0 and 1.
3. When a score occurs at a relatively high level of frequency the probability of randomly selecting it from a distribution is $p = 1$.
4. The higher the corresponding z score, the lower the probability of randomly selecting the score from a distribution.
5. For a normal distribution, σ is the score which has the highest probability of random selection.
6. It is possible to have a negative z score but not a negative probability.
7. For a continuous normal distribution, the probability of selecting a score up to and including the mode is $p = 0.5$.
8. The probability of randomly selecting a score 2 standard deviations above the mean is $p = 0.2$.
9. We can generate appropriate sampling distributions for statistics derived from nominal or ordinal data.
10. Statistical inference involves the estimation of population parameters from sample statistics.
11. Statistical inference depends on knowing the true population parameters before beginning research.
12. The sampling distribution of the mean is a frequency polygon of mean scores.
13. Using the sample mean as an estimate for the population mean is an example of statistical inference.

14. The sampling distribution of the mean is always normally distributed.
15. As n increases, the variability of the sampling distribution of the mean increases.
16. $\mu_{\bar{x}} = \mu$ regardless of the shape of the sampling distribution of the mean.
17. The characteristics of the sampling distribution of the mean vary with the size of the sample.
18. If a random selection method is used, sampling error will be zero.
19. The bigger the sampling error, the smaller the confidence interval.
20. Generally speaking, the higher the level of confidence we have that an interval contains the population mean, the larger is that interval.

Multiple choice

1. The mean age of the Canadian population is known to be 31 years. A small randomly selected sample of Canadians is found to have a mean age of 32. This discrepancy is an example of:
   a a sampling error
   b a measurement error
   c a problem in ecological validity
   d failure to control for the effects of maturation.

At a large maternity hospital the following hypothetical data are compiled concerning the birth weights and survival of neonates.

Weight of neonates (g)	Numbers (n)	Percentage of neonates surviving
0–499	25	40
500–999	50	60
1000–1499	75	80
1500–1999	150	90
2000–2499	250	95
2500+	450	98

Questions 2–5 refer to this table.

2. What is the probability that a randomly selected neonate will weigh under 500 g?
   a 0.4000
   b 0.1700
   c 0.0250
   d 0.0025
3. What is the probability that a randomly selected neonate will have a birth weight of 2000 g or over?
   a 0.7000
   b 0.9638
   c 0.3000
   d 0.9500
4. What is the probability that a neonate weighing 499 g or under will survive?
   a 0.4000
   b 0.1700
   c 0.040
   d 0.025
5. What is the probability that a neonate weighing 2500 g or over will not survive?
   a 0.400
   b 0.300
   c 0.006
   d 0.020

A test of reaction times has a mean of 10 and a standard deviation of 4 in the normal adult population with a normal distribution. Questions 6–12 refer to this information.

6. A person scores 8. That person's z score is:
   a 2
   b 2
   c −0.5
   d −1
7. What percentage of the population would have scores up to and including 14 on this test?
   a 84.13
   b 15.87
   c 65.87
   d 34.13
8. What is the percentile rank of a score of 8 on this test?
   a 19.15
   b 30.85
   c 80.85
   d 53.28
9. What score (to the nearest whole number) would cut off the highest 10% of scores?
   a 1
   b 14

c 15

d 18

10. What is the probability that a randomly selected individual will score greater than 6 on this test?

a 0.4987

b 0.3413

c 0.8413

d 0.6587

11. What is the probability that a randomly selected individual will score between 8 and 14 on this test?

a 0.1498

b 0.5328

c 0.6816

d 0.4671

12. What is the probability that a randomly selected individual will score either more than 14 or less than 10 on this test?

a 0.6587

b 0.6816

c 0.3184

d 0.8184

13. Sampling error of the mean:

a occurs because of poor sampling techniques

b decreases as sample size increases

c is independent of the standard deviation

d is always equal to 1.

14. Samples of 100 are drawn from a normally distributed population with a mean of 50 and a standard deviation of 10. The distribution of sample means will:

a have a mean of 50

b have a standard deviation of 1

c be normally distributed

d all of the above.

15. Increasing the sample size, *n*:

a decreases sampling error

b increases sampling error

c has no effect on standard error of the mean

d requires increasing correction of sample estimates of population parameters

e none of these.

16. If the dispersion of the raw score population increases while *n* is held constant, $\sigma_{\bar{x}}$:

a decreases

b increases

c remains the same

d cannot be ascertained without more information.

17. The sampling distribution of the mean:

a is always positively skewed for continuous data

b is normally distributed if the population raw scores are not normally distributed

c is approximately normally distributed if sample size is large

d all of the above.

18. As the degrees of freedom decrease, the similarity between the *t* and *z* distributions:

a increases

b decreases

c remains the same

d approaches infinity.

19. The theoretical sampling distributions of the *t* statistics depend on:

a *p*

b *r*

c $s_{\bar{x}}$

d df.

A normally distributed population has a mean of 80 and a standard deviation of 12. Questions 20–24 refer to this information.

20. For samples of $n = 36$, what is the standard error of the mean?

a 12

b 0.33

c 2

d 3

21. A sample of 64 cases is found to have a mean of 83. What is the *z* score of this mean?

a 2

b 0.25

c 4

d 1.5

22. A sample of $n = 144$ has a mean of 77. What is the probability that a mean this low would occur by chance?

a 0.0300

b 0.0013

c 0.4989

d 0.9987

23. A sample of 36 cases is selected. What is the probability that its mean falls outside the range of 79–81?

a 0.6813

b 0.8085

c 0.3085

d 0.6170

24. Which is more likely: that a randomly selected sample of $n = 36$ will have a mean greater than 82 or that it will have a mean less than 77?
    a Greater than 82.
    b Less than 77.
    c Both are equally probable.
    d Impossible to tell.

25. The t distribution differs from the z distribution in which of these ways?
    a Its mean is not exactly equal to 0.
    b It is not quite symmetrical.
    c It is somewhat wider and flatter.
    d All of the above.

26. The 95% confidence interval arrived at from a particular experiment is 72–79. Therefore:
    a the probability is 0.05 that μ falls between 72–79
    b the probability is 0.95 that the interval 72–79 contains $\bar{X}$
    c the probability is 0.95 that the interval 72–79 contains μ
    d a and c.

27. Compared with a 99% confidence interval, a 95% confidence interval is:
    a larger
    b smaller
    c more likely to contain the population mean
    d less likely to contain the sample mean.

The following information should be used in answering questions 28–31: a random sample of 25 clients is selected, and their systolic blood pressures measured; the mean BP is 115 mmHg, with a standard deviation of 10.

28. This is an example of:
    a an experiment
    b a natural comparison study
    c a survey
    d field research.

29. What is the standard error of the mean for a sample of this size?
    a 10
    b 20
    c 2
    d 2.5

30. In order to calculate the 99% confidence interval of the mean, what t score will be used?
    a 2.492
    b 2.787
    c 2.797
    d 1.711

31. What is the 99% confidence interval of the mean in this example?
    a $110.0 \leqslant \mu \leqslant 120.0$
    b $109.4 \leqslant \mu \leqslant 120.6$
    c $111.6 \leqslant \mu \leqslant 118.4$
    d $113.0 \leqslant \mu \leqslant 117.0$

32. A random sample of 25 university students is found to have a mean IQ of 110, with a standard deviation of 10. Between what two possible scores can we be 99% confident that the true mean IQ for the students at the university lies?
    a 95.5–112.5
    b 85–135
    c 102.4–117.6
    d 104.1–115.9

In order to establish the mean weight of newborn babies at a large maternity hospital, a random sample of 64 babies is weighed. Their mean weight is 2500 g, with a standard deviation of 80 g.
    Questions 33–35 refer to this information.

33. What is the standard error of the mean?
    a 80
    b 10
    c 1.25
    d 0.1

34. In calculating the 95% confidence interval of the mean, what z value is used?
    a 1.96
    b 2.33
    c 2.58
    d 1.64

35. What is the 95% confidence interval of the mean in this example (to the nearest whole number)?
    a $2480 \leqslant \mu \leqslant 2520$
    b $2477 \leqslant \mu \leqslant 2523$
    c $2474 \leqslant \mu \leqslant 2526$
    d $2484 \leqslant \mu \leqslant 2516$

Chapter Eighteen

Hypothesis testing

Introduction

In the previous chapter we introduced the use of inferential statistics for estimating population parameters from sample statistics. In the case of some non-experimental research projects, such as surveys and descriptive statistics, parameter estimation is adequate for analysing the data. After all, these investigations aim at describing the characteristics of specific populations. However, other research strategies involve data collection for the purpose of testing hypotheses. Here the investigator has to establish if the data support or refute the hypotheses being investigated. The key issue is that hypotheses are generalizations addressing differences in patterns and associations in populations. Inferential statistics enables us to calculate the probability (level of significance) for asserting that what we are seeing in our sample data is generalizable to the population. This probability is related to the statistical significance of the sample data.

The aim of this chapter is to introduce the logical steps involved in hypothesis testing in quantitative research. Given that hypothesis testing is probabilistic, special attention must be paid to the possibility of making erroneous decisions, and to the implications of making such errors.

The specific aims of the chapter are to:

1. Examine the logic of hypothesis testing for retaining or rejecting null hypotheses.

2. Outline how decisions are made with directional and non-directional alternative hypotheses.
3. Define the concept of statistical significance.
4. Introduce the use of the single sample z and t test for analysing the statistical significance of the data.
5. Outline the probability and implications of making Type I and Type II decision errors.

A simple illustration of hypothesis testing

One of the simplest forms of gambling is betting on the fall of a coin. Let us play a little game. We, the authors, will toss a coin. If it comes out heads (H) you will give us £1; if tails (T) we will give you £1. To make things interesting, let us have 10 tosses. The results are:

Toss	1	2	3	4	5	6	7	8	9	10
Outcome	H	H	H	H	H	H	H	H	H	H

Oh dear, you seem to have lost. Never mind, we were just lucky, so send along your cheque for £10. What is that, you are a little hesitant? Are you saying that we 'fixed' the game? There is a systematic procedure for demonstrating the probable truth of your allegations:

1. We can state two competing hypotheses concerning the outcome of the game:
   (a) The authors fixed the game; that is, the outcome does not reflect the fair throwing of a coin. Let us call this statement the 'alternative hypothesis', H_A. In effect, the H_A claims that the sample of 10 heads came from a population other than P (probability of heads) $= Q$ (probability of tails) $= 0.5$.
   (b) The authors did not fix the game; that is, the outcome is due to the tossing of a fair coin. Let us call this statement the 'null hypothesis', or H_0. H_0 suggests that the sample of 10 heads was a random sample from a population where $P = Q = 0.5$.
2. It can be shown that the probability of tossing 10 consecutive heads with a fair coin is $p = 0.001$, as discussed previously (see Ch. 17). That is, the probability of obtaining such a sample from a population where $P = Q = 0.5$ is extremely low.
3. Now we can decide between H_0 and H_A. It was shown that the probability of H_0 being true was $p = 0.001$ (1 in a 1000). Therefore, in the balance

Table 18.1 Probability of obtaining all heads in coin tosses

n (number of tosses)	p (all heads)
1	0.5000
2	0.2500
3	0.1250
4	0.0625
5	0.0313

of probabilities, we can reject it as being true and accept H_A, which is the logical alternative. In other words, it is likely that the game was fixed and no £10 cheque needs to be posted.

The probability of calculating the truth of H_0 depended on the number of tosses (n = the sample size). For instance, the probabilities of obtaining all heads with up to five tosses, according to the binomial theorem (Ch. 17), are shown in Table 18.1. The table shows that, as the sample size (n) becomes larger, the probability at which it is possible to reject H_0 becomes smaller. With only a few tosses we really cannot be sure if the game is fixed or not: without sufficient information it becomes hard to reject H_0 at a reasonable level of probability.

A question emerges: 'What is a reasonable level of probability for rejecting H_0?' As we shall see, there are conventions for specifying these probabilities. One way to proceed, however, is to set the appropriate probability for rejecting H_0 on the basis of the implications of erroneous decisions.

Obviously, any decision made on a probabilistic basis might be erroneous. Two types of elementary decision errors are identified in statistics as *Type I* and *Type II errors*. A Type I error involves mistakenly rejecting H_0, while a Type II error involves mistakenly retaining H_0.

In the above example, a Type I error would involve deciding that the outcome was not due to chance when in fact it was. The practical outcome of this would be to accuse the authors falsely of fixing the game. A Type II error would represent the decision that the outcome was due to chance, when in fact it was due to a 'fix'. The practical outcome of this would be to send your hard-earned £10 to a couple of crooks. Clearly, in a situation like this, a Type II error would be more odious than a Type I error, and you would set a fairly high probability for rejecting H_0. However, if you were gambling with a villain, who had a loaded revolver handy, you would tend to set a very low probability for rejecting H_0. We will examine these ideas more formally in subsequent parts of this chapter.

The logic of hypothesis testing

Hypothesis testing is the process of deciding statistically whether the findings of an investigation reflect chance or real effects at a given level of probability. If the results do not represent chance effects then we say that the results are statistically significant. That is, when we say that our results are statistically significant we mean that the patterns or differences seen in the sample data are generalizable to the population.

The mathematical procedures for hypothesis testing are based on the application of probability theory and sampling, as discussed previously. Because of the probabilistic nature of the process, decision errors in hypothesis testing cannot be entirely eliminated. However, the procedures outlined in this section enable us to specify the probability level at which we can claim that the data obtained in an investigation support experimental hypotheses. This procedure is fundamental for determining the statistical significance of the data as well as being relevant to the logic of clinical decision making.

Steps in hypothesis testing

The following steps are conventionally followed in hypothesis testing:

1. State the alternative hypothesis (H_A), which is the prediction intended for evaluation. The H_A claims that the results are 'real' or 'significant', i.e. that the independent variable influenced the dependent variable, or that there is a real difference among groups. The important point here is that H_A is a statement concerning the population. A real

or significant effect means that the results in the sample data can be generalized to the population.

2. State the null hypothesis (H_0), which is the logical opposite of the H_A. The H_0 claims that any differences in the data were just due to chance: that the independent variable had no effect on the dependent variable, or that any difference among groups is due to random effects. In other words, if the H_0 is retained, differences or patterns seen in the sample data should not be generalized to the population.

3. Set the decision level, α (alpha). There are two mutually exclusive hypotheses (H_A and H_0) competing to explain the results of an investigation. Hypothesis testing, or statistical decision making, involves establishing the probability of H_0 being true. If this probability is very small, we are in a position to reject the H_0. You might ask 'how small should be the probability (α) for rejecting H_0?' By convention, we use the probability of $\alpha = 0.05$. If the H_0 being true is less than 0.05 we can reject H_0. We can choose an α of < 0.05, but not more, That is, by convention among researchers, results are not characterized as significant if $p > 0.05$.

4. Calculate the probability of H_0 being true. That is, we assume that H_0 is true and calculate the probability of the outcome of the investigation being due to chance alone, i.e. due to random effects. We must use an appropriate sampling distribution for this calculation.

5. Make a decision concerning H_0. The following decision rule is used. If the probability of H_0 being true is less than α, then we reject H_0 at the level of significance set by α. However, if the probability of H_0 is greater than α, then we must retain H_0. In other words, if:

p (H_0 is true) $\leq \alpha$; reject H_0

p (H_0 is true) $> \alpha$; retain H_0

It follows that if we reject H_0 we are in a position to accept H_A, its logical alternative. If we reject H_0, we decide that H_A is probably true.

Let us look at an example. A rehabilitation therapist devises an exercise programme which is expected to reduce the time taken for people to leave hospital following orthopaedic surgery. Previous records show that the recovery time for patients has been $\mu = 30$ days, with $\sigma = 8$ days. A sample of 64 patients are treated with the exercise programme, and their mean recovery time is found to be $\bar{X} = 24$ days. Do these results show that patients who had the treatment recovered significantly faster than previous patients? We can apply the steps for hypothesis testing to make our decision.

1. State H_A: 'The exercise programme reduces the time taken for patients to recover from orthopaedic surgery'. That is, the researcher claims that the independent variable (the treatment) has a 'real' or 'generalizable' effect on the dependent variable (time to recover).

2. State H_0: 'The exercise programme does not reduce the time taken for patients to recover from orthopaedic surgery'. That is, the statement claims that the independent variable has no effect on the dependent variable. The statement implies that the treated sample with $\bar{X} = 24$, and $n = 64$ is in fact a random sample from the population $\mu = 30$, $\sigma = 8$. Any difference between $\bar{X}$ and μ can be attributed to sampling error.

3. The decision level, α, is set before the results are analysed. The probability of α depends on how certain the investigator wants to be that the results show real differences. If he set $\alpha = 0.01$, then the probability of falsely rejecting a true H_0 is less than or equal to 0.01 (1/100). If he set $\alpha = 0.05$, then the probability of falsely rejecting a true H_0 is less than or equal to 0.05 or (1/20). That is, the smaller the α, the more confident the researcher is that the results support the alternative hypothesis. We also call α the level of significance. The smaller the α, the more significant the findings for a study, if we can reject H_0. In this case, say that the researcher sets $\alpha = 0.01$. (Note: by convention, α should not be greater than 0.05.)

4. Calculate the probability of H_0 being true. As stated above, H_0 implies that the sample with $\bar{X} = 24$ is a random sample from the population with $\mu = 30$, $\sigma = 8$. How probable is it that this statement is true? To calculate this probability, we must generate an appropriate sampling distribution. As we have seen in Chapter 17, the sampling distribution of the mean will enable us to calculate the probability of obtaining a sample mean of $\bar{X} = 24$ or more extreme from a population with known parameters. As shown in Figure 18.1, we can calculate the probability of drawing a sample mean of $\bar{X} = 24$ or less. Using the table of normal curves (Appendix A), as outlined previously, we find that the probability of randomly selecting a sample mean of $\bar{X} = 24$ (or less) is extremely small. In terms of our table, which only shows the exact probability of up to $z = 4.00$, we can see

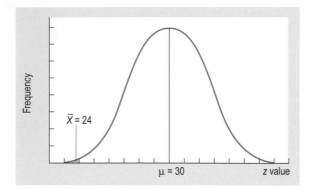

Figure 18.1 • Sampling distribution of means. Sample size = 64; population mean = 30; standard deviation = 8.

that the present probability is less than 0.00003. Therefore, the probability that H_0 is true is less than 0.00003.

5. Make a decision. We have set $\alpha = 0.01$. The calculated probability was less than 0.0001. Clearly, the calculated probability is far less than α. Therefore, the investigator can reject the statement that H_0 is true and accept H_A, that patients treated with the exercise programme recover earlier than the population of untreated patients.

Directional and non-directional hypotheses and corresponding critical values of statistics

In the previous example, H_A was directional in that we asserted that the difference between the mean of the treated sample and the population mean was expected to be in a particular direction. If we state that there was some effect due to the dependent variable, but do not specify which way, then H_A is called non-directional. In the previous example, if the investigator stated H_A as 'The exercise programme *changes* the time taken to recover following surgery' then H_A would have been non-directional.

In general, an alternative hypothesis is directional if it predicts a specific outcome concerning the direction of the findings by stating that one group mean will be higher or lower than the other(s). An alternative hypothesis is non-directional if it predicts a difference, without specifying which

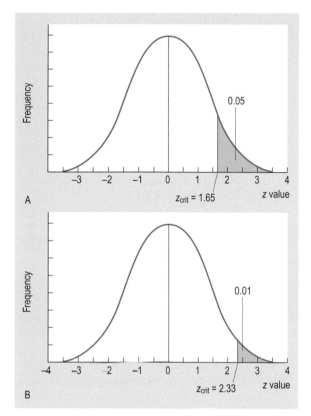

A

B

Figure 18.2 • Two examples of statistical decision making with directional (one-tail) hypothesis, H_A.

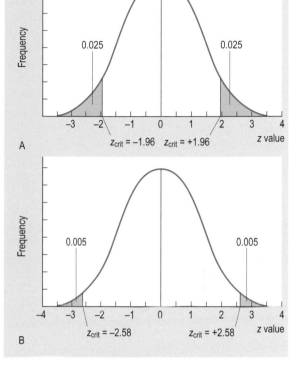

A

B

Figure 18.3 • Two examples of statistical decision making with non-directional (two-tail) hypothesis, H_A.

group mean is expected to be higher or lower than the others.

If we propose a directional H_A, it is understood that we have reasonable information on the basis of pilot studies or previously published research for predicting the direction of the outcome. The advantage of a directional H_A is that it increases the probability of rejecting H_0. However, the decision of the directionality of H_A must be decided before the data are collected and analysed.

Let us now examine the concept of the 'critical' value of a statistic. The critical value of a statistic is the value of the statistic which bounds the proportion of the sampling distribution specified by α. The critical value of the statistic is influenced by whether H_A is directional or non-directional.

Figures 18.2 and 18.3 represent the sampling distributions of the mean where n is large; that is, the sampling distribution for the statistic $\bar{X}$.

As we have seen in Chapter 17, these are the sampling distributions for $\bar{X}$ we would expect by the random selection of samples, as specified by H_0. Therefore, we can estimate from the distributions the probability of selecting any sample mean, $\bar{X}$, by chance alone. The α value (the level of significance) specifies the criterion for rejecting H_0. We can see that the critical value for the statistic (in this case z_{crit}) cuts off an area of the distribution corresponding to α ($p = 0.05$ or $p = 0.01$).

In Figure 18.2, we can see that $z_{crit} = 1.65$ (for $\alpha = 0.05$) and $z_{crit} = 2.33$ (for $\alpha = 0.01$). (These values are obtained from Appendix A.) Therefore, for any sample mean, $\bar{X}$, where the transformed (z) value is greater than or equal to z_{crit}, we will reject H_0 (that the sample mean was a random sample). However, if the absolute value of the transformed statistic is less than z_{crit}, then we must retain H_0. Note that when $\alpha = 0.01$, the z_{crit} is greater than when $\alpha = 0.05$. Clearly, the higher the level of significance set for rejecting H_0, the greater the absolute critical value of the statistic. Figure 18.2 shows statistical decision making with a directional H_A, where the probabilities associated with only one of the tails of the distribution are used.

Figure 18.3 shows the critical values for z with a non-directional H_A. Here, the probabilities associated with α (0.05 or 0.01) are divided between the two tails of the distribution. That is, where $\alpha = 0.05$, half (0.025) goes into each tail, and where $\alpha = 0.01$, half (0.005) also goes into each tail. This changes the values of z_{crit}, which becomes ± 1.96 or ± 2.58, respectively, as shown in Figure 18.3. Here, we reject H_0 if the calculated transformed z value of $\bar{X}$ falls beyond the values of z_{crit}. When we compare the values of z_{crit} for the one-tail and two-tail decisions, we find that the critical values are greater for the two-tail decisions. This implies that it is more difficult to reject H_0 if we are making two-tail decisions on the basis of a non-directional HA.

Decision rules

In general, Figures 18.2 and 18.3 illustrate the decision rules for statistical decision making for hypotheses concerning sample means. These rules are:

$|z_{obt}| \geq |z_{crit}|$; reject H_0
$|z_{obt}| < |z_{crit}|$; retain H_0

The same decision rules hold for the t distributions associated with the sampling distribution of the mean when n (the sample size) is small (see Ch. 17).

$|t_{obt}| \geq |t_{crit}|$; reject H_0
$|t_{obt}| < |t_{crit}|$; retain H_0

z_{obt} and t_{obt} refer to the calculated value of the statistic, based on the data:

$$z_{obt} = \frac{\bar{X} - \mu}{s_{\bar{x}}}$$

$$t_{obt} = \frac{\bar{X} - \mu}{s_{\bar{x}}}$$

z_{crit} and t_{crit} are the critical values of the statistic obtained from the tables in Appendices A and B. As we have seen, the values of these depend on α and the directionality of H_A. $|\ |$ is the symbol for modulus, implying that we should look at the absolute value of a statistic. Of course, the sign is important when considering if $\bar{X}$ is greater or smaller than μ. However we can ignore the sign ($+$ or $-$) when making statistical decisions. In effect, the greater z_{obt} or t_{obt}, the more deviant or improbable the particular sample mean, $\bar{X}$, is under the sampling distribution specified by H_0.

Statistical decisions with single sample means

The following examples illustrate the use of statistical decision making concerning a single sample mean, $\bar{X}$. Such decisions are relevant when our data consist of a single sample and we are to decide if the $\bar{X}$ of the sample is significantly different to a given population, with a mean of μ.

A statistical test is a procedure appropriate for making decisions concerning the significance of the data. The z test and the t test are procedures appropriate for making decisions concerning the probability that sample means reflect population differences. (As shown in Ch. 19, there is a variety of statistical tests available for hypothesis testing.)

Example 1

A researcher hypothesizes that males now weigh more than in previous years. To investigate this hypothesis he randomly selects 100 adult males and records their weights. The measurements for the sample have a mean of $\bar{X} = 70\,kg$. In a census taken several years ago, the mean weight of males was $\mu = 68\,kg$, with a standard deviation of $8\,kg$.

1. Directional H_A: males are heavier. That is, $\bar{X} = 70$ is not a random sample from population $\mu = 68$.
2. H_0: males are not heavier. That is, $\bar{X} = 70$ is a random sample from population $\mu = 68$.
3. Decision level: $\alpha = 0.01$.
4. Calculate probability of H_0 being true. Here, $\alpha = 0.01$, one-tail. We can find from the tables

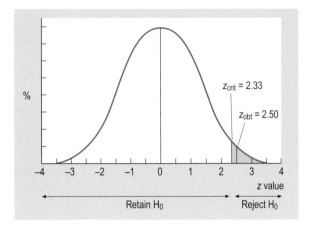

Figure 18.4 • Hypothesis testing: directional.

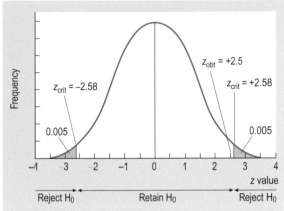

Figure 18.5 • Hypothesis testing: non-directional.

(Appendix A) z_{crit}, the z score which cuts off an area of 0.01 of the total curve. $z_{crit} = +2.33$ ($\alpha = 0.01$; one tail).

Calculating the z score (z_{obt}) representing the probability of the sample being drawn from the population under H_0 ($\mu = 68$), we use the formula:

$$z_{obt} = \frac{\bar{X} - \mu}{s_{\bar{x}}}$$

where $s_{\bar{x}} = s/\sqrt{n}$

$$z_{obt} = \frac{70 - 68}{8/\sqrt{100}}$$
$$= 2.5$$

Here, $z_{crit} = 2.33$

5. The decision rule is that if:

$|z_{obt}| \geq |z_{crit}|$; reject H_0
$|z_{obt}| < |z_{crit}|$; retain H_0

2.5 > 2.33, so the z_{obt} falls into the area of rejection, as shown in Figure 18.4. Therefore, the researcher can reject H_0, and accept H_A at a 0.01 level of significance. That is, the results of the investigation indicate that the mean weight of males has increased (consistent with the predictions of the research hypothesis). We conclude that the results are statistically significant at $p \leq 0.01$.

Example 2

A researcher hypothesized that men today have different weights (either more or less) than in previous years (assume the same information as for Example 1).

1. Non-directional H_A: males are of different weight, that is $\bar{X} - 70$ is not a random sample from population $\mu = 68$.
2. H_0: males are not different, that is $\bar{X}$ is a random sample from population $\mu = 68$.
3. Decision level: $\alpha = 0.01$.
4. Calculate the probability of H_0 being true. Here, $\alpha = 0.01$ (two-tail); the value of $z_{crit} = 2.58$ (from Appendix A); the value of $z_{obt} = 2.5$ (as calculated in Example 1).
5. Decision: applying the decision rule as outlined in Example 1:

$|z_{obt}| < |z_{crit}|$; as 2.5 < 2.58

z_{obt} falls into the area of acceptance, as shown in Figure 18.5. Therefore, the researcher must retain the H_0, and conclude that the study did not support H_A at a 0.01 level of significance. The investigation has not provided evidence that the mean weight of males has increased. The results are reported as not being statistically significant.

Example 3

The previous two examples involved sample sizes of $n > 30$. However, as we saw in Chapter 17, if

$n < 30$, the distribution of sample means is not a normal, but a t distribution. This point must be taken into account when we calculate the probability of H_0 being true. That is, for small samples, we use the t test to evaluate the significance of our data.

Assume exactly the same information as in Example 1, except that sample size is $n = 16$.

1. Directional H_A: as in Example 1.
2. H_0: as in Example 1.
3. $\alpha = 0.01$, one tail.
4. We can find from the t table (Appendix B) the value for t_{crit}. To look up t_{crit} we must have the following information:
   (a) α, the level of significance (0.05 or 0.01)
   (b) direction of H_A (directional or non-directional)
   (c) the degrees of freedom (df).
   In this instance:
   (a) $\alpha = 0.01$
   (b) H_A is directional, therefore we must look up a one-tail probability
   (c) df $= n - 1 = 16 - 1 = 15$
   Looking up the appropriate value for t; $t_{crit} = 2.602$. Calculating the t score (t_{obt}) representing the probability of the sample being drawn from the population under H_0, we use the formula:

$$t_{obt} = \frac{\bar{X} - \mu}{s_{\bar{x}}}$$
$$= \frac{70 - 68}{8/\sqrt{16}}$$
$$= 1.0$$

5. As we stated earlier, the decision rule is identical to that of the z test:

$$|z_{obt}| \geq |z_{crit}|; \text{ reject } H_0$$
$$|z_{obt}| < |z_{crit}|; \text{ retain } H_0$$

Here, $1.0 < 2.602$, such that t_{obt} falls into the area of retention (Fig. 18.6). Therefore, we must retain H_0 at a 0.01 level of significance. Clearly, when $n = 16$, the investigation did not show a significant weight increase for the males.

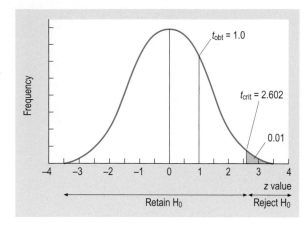

Figure 18.6 • Hypothesis testing: directional.

Conclusion

The above examples demonstrate the following points about statistical decision making:

- We are more likely to reject H_0 if we use a one-tail test (directional H_A) than a two-tail test (non-directional H_A). In effect, we are using the prediction of which way the differences will go to increase the probability of rejecting H_0 and therefore accepting H_A. Examples 1 and 2 demonstrate this point; in Example 1 we rejected H_0 with a directional H_A, while we retained H_0 in Example 2, with exactly the same data.
- The larger the sample size, n, the more likely we are to reject H_0 for a given set of data. Comparing Examples 1 and 3 demonstrates this; although μ, σ, and $\bar{X}$ were the same, where n was small we had to retain H_0. Also, when n is small, ($n < 30$), we must use the t test to analyse the significance of our sample mean being different.
- The more demanding the decision level (that is, if α is small), the less likely we are to reject H_0. To illustrate this point, repeat Example 2, but set $\alpha = 0.05$. Here, $z_{crit} = 1.96$ so that z_{obt} is greater than z_{crit}. Therefore, we can reject H_0, and accept H_A at a 0.05 level of significance. That is, with exactly the same data, we have rejected or accepted H_0, depending on the level of significance, α.

Errors in inference

When we say our results are statistically significant, we are making the inference that the results for

Table 18.2 Decision outcomes		
Reality	**Decision: reject H_0**	**Decision: retain H_0**
H_0 correct (no difference or effect)	'False alarm' Type I error	Correct decision
H_0 incorrect (real difference or effect)	Correct decision	'Miss' Type II error

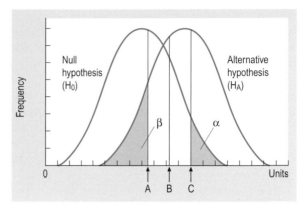

Figure 18.7 • Change of decision level to increase β and decrease α. As the decision criterion is moved from A to B to C, the relative frequency of Type I and Type II errors alters.

our sample are true for the population. It should be evident from the previous discussion that statistical decision making can result in incorrect decisions. There are two main types of inferential error: Type I and Type II.

A Type I error occurs when we mistakenly reject H_0; that is, when we claim that our experimental hypothesis was supported when it is, in fact, false. The probability of a Type I error occurring is less than or equal to α. For instance, in the previous Example 1 we set $\alpha = 0.01$. The probability of making a Type I error is less than or equal to 0.01; the chances are equal to or less than 1/100 that our decision in rejecting H_0 was mistaken. Therefore, the smaller α, the less the chance of making a Type I error. We can set α as low as possible, but by convention it must be less than or equal to 0.05.

A Type II error occurs when we mistakenly retain H_0; that is, when we falsely conclude that the experimental hypothesis was not supported by our data. The probability of a Type II error occurring is denoted by β (beta). In Example 3 we retained H_0, perhaps falsely. If n was larger, we might well have rejected H_0, as in Example 1. Type I errors represent a 'false alarm' and Type II errors represent a 'miss'. Table 18.2 illustrates this.

Table 18.2 illustrates that, if we reject H_0, we are making either a correct decision or a Type I error. If we retain H_0, we are making either a correct decision or a Type II error. While we cannot, in principle, eliminate these from scientific decision making, we can take steps to minimize their occurrence.

We minimize the occurrence of Type I error by setting an acceptable level for α. In scientific research, editors of most scientific journals require

that α should be set at 0.05 or less. This convention helps to reduce false alarms to a rate of less than 1/20. Replication of the findings by other independent investigators provides important evidence that the original decision to reject H_0 was correct.

How do we minimize the probability of Type II error?

1. Increase the sample size, n.
2. Reduce the variability of measurements ($s_{\bar{x}}$, either by increasing accuracy (Ch. 12) or by using samples that are not highly variable for the measurement producing the data).
3. Use a directional H_A, on the basis of previous evidence about the nature of the effect.
4. Set a less demanding α, Type I error rate. There is a relationship between α and β, such that the smaller α, the greater β. This relationship is illustrated in Figure 18.7. Figure 18.7 shows that, as α decreases, β increases. Inevitably, as we decrease the Type I error rate, we increase the probability of Type II error. This is the reason why we do not normally set α lower than $p = 0.01$. Although a significance level such as $\alpha = 0.001$ would reduce 'false alarms' it would also increase the probability of a 'miss'.

Summary

The problem addressed in the previous two chapters was that, although our hypotheses are general statements concerning populations, the evidence for verifying or supporting our hypotheses is based on sample data. We solve this problem through the use of inferential statistics.

It was argued in this chapter that, once the sample data have been collected and summarized, the investigator must analyse the findings to demonstrate their statistical significance. Significant results for an investigation mean that differences or changes demonstrated were real, rather than just the outcome of random sampling error.

The general steps in using tests of significance were explained, and several illustrative examples using the z and t tests for single sample designs were presented. A critical value is set for the statistic (in this case z_{crit}, t_{crit}) as specified by α. If the magnitude of the obtained value of the statistic (z_{obt}, t_{obt}) exceeds the critical value, H_0 is rejected. In this case, the investigator concludes that the data supported the differences predicted by the alternative hypothesis (at the level of significance specified by α). However, if the obtained value of the statistic is calculated to be less than the critical value, then the investigator must conclude that the data did not support the hypothesis. It was noted that following these steps does not guarantee the absolute truth of decisions made about the rejection or acceptance of the alternative hypotheses, but rather specifies the probability of the decisions being correct.

Two types of erroneous decisions were specified, Type I and Type II errors. A Type I error involves falsely concluding that differences or changes found in a study were real, that is, concluding that the data supported a hypothesis which is, in fact, false. A Type II error involves falsely concluding that no differences or changes exist, that is, concluding that the data did not support a hypothesis which is, in fact, true. It was demonstrated that the probability of these errors depends on factors such as the size of n, the directionality of H_A and the variability of the data.

The procedures of hypothesis testing and error were related to the logic of clinical decision making. The probabilities (α and β) of making Type I and Type II errors are interrelated. In this way, both researchers and clinicians must take into account the implications of possible error when setting levels of significance for interpreting the data.

Self-assessment

Explain the meaning of the following terms:

alternative hypothesis
critical value of a statistic
decision rule
directional or non-directional alternative hypothesis
null hypothesis
one-tail or two-tail test of significance
region of acceptance
region of rejection
significance (level of)
Type I and Type II error
z test or t test

True or false

1. The alternative hypothesis states that there is an effect or difference in the results.
2. If the probability of H_0 being true is greater than β, we can reject H_0.
3. Sampling distributions are used to enable the calculation of H_0 being true.
4. The critical value of a statistic is the value which cuts off the region for the rejection of H_0.
5. If the critical value of a statistic is less than the obtained or calculated value, we can reject H_0.
6. α is a probability, usually set at 0.01 or 0.05.
7. The t test requires that the sampling distribution of t should be normally distributed.
8. Hypothesis testing involves choosing between two mutually exclusive hypotheses, H_0 and H_A.
9. If α is set at 0.01 instead of 0.05, then the probability of making a Type I error decreases.
10. If we retain H_0, then we must conclude that the investigation did not produce significant results.
11. If n is greater than 30, the t test is more appropriate than the z test.
12. If results are statistically significant, the independent variable must have had a very large effect.
13. A directional H_A should be used when there is theoretical justification for the existence of a directional effect in the data.
14. When the results are statistically significant, they are unlikely to reflect sampling error.

15. It is impossible to prove the truth of H_A when using sample data as opposed to population data.
16. If we reject H_0 then we are in a position to accept H_A.
17. If α decreases (is made more stringent), then β increases.
18. If H_0 is true and we reject it, we have made a Type I error.
19. If H_0 is false and we reject it, we have made a Type II error.
20. If H_0 is false, and we fail to reject it, we have made a Type II error.

Multiple choice

1. Hypothesis testing involves:
   a deciding between two mutually exclusive hypotheses, H_0 and H_A
   b deciding if the investigation was internally and externally valid
   c deciding if the differences between groups was large or small
   d none of the above.
2. An α level of 0.01 indicates that:
   a the probability of falsely rejecting H_0 is limited to 0.05
   b the probability of Type II error is 0.01
   c the probability of a correct decision is 0.01
   d none of the above.
3. If α is changed from 0.01 to 0.001:
   a the probability of making a Type II error decreases
   b the probability of a Type I error increases
   c the error probabilities stay the same
   d the probability of a Type I error decreases.
4. If we reject the null hypothesis, we might be making:
   a a Type II error
   b a Type I error
   c a correct decision
   d a or c
   e b or c.
5. Statistical tests are used:
   a only when the investigation involves a true experimental design
   b to increase the internal validity of experiments
   c to establish the probability of the outcome of an investigation being due to chance alone
   d a and b.

6. The outcome of a statistical analysis is found to be $p = 0.02$. This means that:
   a the alternative hypothesis was directional
   b we can reject H_0 at $\alpha = 0.05$
   c we must conclude that H_A must be true
   d a and c.
7. When the results of an experiment are non-significant, the proper conclusion is:
   a the experiment fails to show a real effect for the independent variable
   b chance alone is at work
   c to accept H_0
   d to accept H_A.
8. It is important to know the possible errors (Type I or Type II) we might make when rejecting or failing to reject H_0:
   a to minimize these errors when designing the experiment
   b to be aware of the fallacy of accepting H_0
   c to maximize the probability of making a correct decision by proper design
   d all of the above.
9. An α level of 0.05 indicates that:
   a if H_0 is true, the probability of falsely rejecting it is limited to 0.05
   b 95% of the time chance is operating
   c the probability of a Type II error is 0.05
   d the probability of a correct decision is 0.05.
10. A directional alternative hypothesis asserts that:
   a the independent variable has no effect on the dependent variable
   b a random effect is responsible for the differences between conditions
   c the independent variable does not have an effect
   d there are differences in the data in a given direction.
11. If α is changed from 0.05 to 0.01:
   a the probability of a Type II error decreases
   b the probability of a Type I error increases
   c the error probabilities stay the same
   d the probability of Type II error increases.
12. If the null hypothesis is retained, you may be making:
   a a correct decision about the data
   b a Type I error
   c a Type II error
   d a or c
   e a or b.

13. When the results are statistically significant, this means:
    a the obtained probability is equal to or less than α
    b the independent variable has had a large effect
    c we can reject H_0
    d all of the above
    e a and c.

14. β refers to:
    a the probability of making a Type I error
    b the probability of $(1 - \alpha)$
    c the inverse of the probability of sampling error
    d the probability of making a Type II error.

15. Setting $\alpha = 0.0001$ would reduce the probability of Type I error. However, it would:
    a increase Type II error probability
    b increase the standard error of variance
    c reduce external validity
    d all of the above.

16. We retain H_0 if:
    a $|t_{obt}| \le |t_{crit}|$
    b $|t_{obt}| > |t_{crit}|$
    c $|t_{obt}| < |t_{crit}|$
    d none of the above.

17. If α is changed from 0.01 to 0.001:
    a the probability of a Type II error decreases
    b the probability of a Type I error increases
    c the error probabilities stay the same
    d none of the above.

A researcher believes that the average age of unemployed people has changed. To test this hypothesis, the ages of 150 randomly selected unemployed people are determined (A). The mean age is 23.5 years. A complete census taken a few years before showed a mean age of 22.4 years, with a standard deviation of 7.6 (B).

Questions 18–22 refer to these data.

18. The alternative hypothesis should be:
    a $\bar{X}_A = \bar{X}_B$
    b $\mu_A = \mu_B$
    c $\mu_A \ne \mu_B$
    d $\bar{X}_A \ne \bar{X}_B$

19. The z_{crit} where $\alpha = 0.01$ is:
    a $+2.58$
    b $+1.64$
    c $+2.33$
    d -1.64

20. The obtained value of the appropriate statistic for testing H_0 is:
    a 2.88
    b 2.35
    c 1.84
    d 1.77

21. What do you decide, using $\alpha = 0.01$?
    a retain H_0
    b reject H_0
    c it is not possible to decide
    d a and b.

22. Therefore, the researcher should conclude that:
    a unemployed persons are getting older on average
    b there is no evidence supporting the hypothesis that the average age of unemployed people has changed
    c too many young people are unemployed
    d b and c.

23. When the results are not statistically significant, this means that:
    a the experimental hypothesis was not supported by the data at a given level of probability
    b the null hypothesis was retained at a given level of probability
    c the alternative hypothesis must have been directional
    d the investigation was internally valid
    e a and b.

24. If $\alpha = 0.05$ and the probability of the statistic calculated from the data is $p = 0.02$, then:
    a we should retain H_0
    b we should reject H_A
    c we should reject H_0 at $\alpha = 0.05$
    d we should restate H_0 so that the findings will become significant at the 0.05 level.

Chapter Nineteen

19

Selection and use of statistical tests

Introduction

In the previous chapter, we examined the logic of hypothesis testing and the use of z and t tests for testing hypotheses about single sample means. There are numerous statistical tests available which are used in a conceptually similar fashion to analyse the statistical significance of the data. That is, all statistical tests involve setting up the relevant hypotheses, H_0 and H_A, and then, on the basis of the appropriate inferential statistics, computing the probability of the sample statistics obtained occurring by chance alone. We are not going to attempt to examine all statistical tests in this introductory book. These are described in various statistics text books or in data analysis manuals. Rather, in this chapter we will examine the criteria used for selecting tests appropriate for the analysis of the data obtained in specific investigations. To illustrate the use of statistical tests we will examine the use of the chi-square test (χ^2). This is a statistical test commonly employed to analyse nominally scaled data. Finally, we will briefly examine the uses of the Statistical Package for Social Sciences (SPSS) for data analysis in general.

The aims of this chapter are to:

1. Discuss the criteria by which a statistical test is selected for analysing the data for a specific study.

2. Demonstrate the use of the χ^2 test for analysing nominal scale data.
3. Explain how statistical packages are used for quantitative data analysis.

The relationship between descriptive and inferential statistics

As we have seen in the previous chapters, statistics may be classified as descriptive or inferential. Descriptive statistics are concerned with issues such as 'What is the average length of hospitalization of a group of patients?' Inferential statistics are used to address issues such as whether the differences in average lengths of hospitalization of patients in two groups are statistically significantly different. Thus, descriptive statistics describe aspects of the data such as the frequencies of scores, the average or the range of values for samples, whereas when using inferential statistics, one attempts to infer whether differences between groups or relationships between variables represent persistent and reproducible trends in the populations.

In Section 5 we saw that the selection of appropriate descriptive statistics depends on the characteristics of the data being described. For example, in a variable such as incomes of patients, the best statistics to represent the typical income would be the mean and/or the median. If you had a millionaire in the group of patients, the mean would give a distorted impression of the central tendency. In this situation the median would be most appropriate. The mode is most commonly used when the data being described are categorical. For example, if in a questionnaire respondents were asked to indicate their sex and 65 said they were male and 35 female, then 'male' is the modal response. It is quite unusual to use the mode only with data that are not nominal. As a rule, the scale of measurement used to obtain the data and its distribution determine which descriptive statistics are selected.

In the same way, the appropriate inferential statistics are determined by the characteristics

of the data being analysed. For example, where the mean is the appropriate descriptive statistic, the inferential statistics will determine if the differences between the means are statistically significant. In the case of ordinal data, the appropriate inferential statistics will make it possible to decide if either the medians or the rank orders are significantly different. With nominal data, the appropriate inferential statistic will decide if proportions of cases falling into specific categories are significantly different.

Thus, when the data have been adequately described, the appropriate inferential statistic will follow logically. However, when selecting an appropriate statistical test, the design of the investigation must also be taken into account.

Selection of the appropriate inferential test

Before addressing the issue of the selection of the appropriate inferential statistical test, it is useful to reiterate the reason why a statistical test should be employed.

In many studies, inferential statistical tests are not required. For example, if a health care needs-assessment survey is conducted in a particular community, using a full population, the investigator might not be overly concerned with generalizing the results to other communities, or with demonstrating that certain relationships between variables are reliable. It may be enough to be able to say, for example, that '35% of the respondents indicated that they were dissatisfied with the existing level of medical services'. In this instance, descriptive statistics are all that the investigator requires since the complete population was studied. If, however, the investigator wishes to argue that certain differences between groups or that certain correlations between variables for a sample are generalizable to the population, then inferential statistical tests are necessary.

The inferential statistic provides the investigator with a means of determining how reproducible the obtained results are, by enabling access to a probability. The probability associated with the value of an inferential statistic informs the investigator of the likelihood that the results obtained were due to chance factors, or if they are significant at a given level of probability.

Please note that we are not going to examine all of the numerous statistical tests available for decision making. Rather, the aim of this chapter is to examine the criteria used for selecting tests appropriate for the analysis of data obtained in investigations. To illustrate the use of statistical tests we will look at the χ^2 test, commonly employed for analysing nominal data. We examine the interpretation of findings which do not reach statistical significance and the relationship between statistical and clinical significance. In Chapter 20 we will consider some of the personal and social values implicit in making decisions concerning the actual adoption and use of treatments and diagnostic tests in clinical settings.

There is a variety of statistical tests, some of which are named in Table 19.1. The selection of the appropriate statistical test is determined by the following considerations:

1. The scale of measurement used to obtain the data (nominal, ordinal, interval, or ratio).
2. The number of groups used in an investigation (one or more).
3. Whether the measurements were obtained from independent subjects or from related samples, such as those involving repeated measurements of the same subjects.
4. The assumptions involved in using a statistical test, such as the distribution of the scores or the minimum required sample size.

Table 19.1 offers a sample of statistical tests in order to illustrate how statistical tests are selected for analysing data. Several points are worth noting.

1. It can be seen that appropriate tests are selected on the basis of the four criteria outlined above. When we have determined these four criteria for a given investigation, the cell containing the appropriate test can be readily selected. We might need additional criteria for deciding between two tests within a cell. For instance, we saw in the previous section that, if $n < 30$, we use the t test rather than the z test.
2. The tests appropriate for analysing ordinal and nominal data are called non-parametric or distribution-free. The tests for analysing interval or ratio data are called parametric tests. The parametric tests (for example, z, t or F) require that certain assumptions (such as normality and equal variance) be valid for the populations from which the samples were drawn. The non-parametric tests (e.g. χ^2, Mann–Whitney U) require few, if any, assumptions about the underlying population distributions.
3. Even before the data are collected, an investigator should have a good idea of which statistical test is appropriate for analysing the data. Sometimes, however, the distribution of the data is such that the test that was initially selected is found to be inappropriate.

Let us look at some examples to illustrate how statistical tests are selected.

An investigator wishes to evaluate the effectiveness of a new treatment in contrast to a conventionally used treatment. Assume that the outcome (dependent variable) is measured on a five-point

Table 19.1 Selection of tests of significance

Scale	Two groups		Three or more groups	
	Independent	Dependent	Independent	Dependent
Nominal	χ^2 test	McNemar's test	χ^2 test	Cochran's Q test
Ordinal	Mann–Whitney U test	Sign test	Kruskal–Wallis H test	Friedman two-way analysis of variance
Interval or ratio	t test (independent groups)	t test (dependent groups)	ANOVA (F) (independent groups)	ANOVA (F) (dependent groups)

ordinal scale. Each subject is assigned to one of the two treatment groups. Which test would the investigator use to analyse the significance of sample data when:

1. the measurement was ordinal?
2. there were two groups (new treatment, conventional treatment)?
3. subjects were independently assigned to a specific group?

By inspection of Table 19.1 the investigator would select the Mann–Whitney U test to analyse the significance of the data.

If we change the above example by stating that the dependent variable was measured on an interval scale, the appropriate test would now be a t test (for independent groups). Let us say that three groups were used (by the inclusion of a placebo group) by the investigator. Now, if the outcome measurement remained ordinal, the appropriate test for analysing the data is the Kruskal–Wallis H test. If, however, the outcome measures were interval, it follows from Table 19.1 that the appropriate test for analysing the results would be ANOVA (analysis of variance).

Finally, say that in the original example each of the subjects was treated with both the new and old treatments. Now, the data would have been obtained from the repeated measurement of the same subjects, and the appropriate statistical test would be the Sign test (ordinal, two groups, dependent).

Table 19.1 does not include all the available statistical tests and their uses. In fact, mathematical statisticians can generate inferential tests appropriate for a whole variety of designs. The basic idea is to use probability theory to generate appropriate sampling distributions in terms of which the probability of H_0 being true can be calculated, and the statistical significance of the findings evaluated.

Rather than examining all the tests and their underlying assumptions, we will look at the use of the χ^2 test in some detail. As well as being a very useful test for analysing nominal data, it (along with the z and t) illustrates how statistical tests are carried out to test hypotheses.

The χ^2 test

As shown in Table 19.1, χ^2 (chi-square) is appropriate for statistical analysis when:

1. variables were measured on a nominal scale
2. measurements were of independent subjects.

The χ^2 test is appropriate for deciding if proportions of cases falling into categories are different at a given level of significance.

The statistic, χ^2, is given by the formula:

$$\chi^2 = \sum \frac{(f_o - f_e)^2}{f_e}$$

where f_o = observed frequency for a given category and f_e = expected frequency for a given category, assuming H_0 was true.

The sampling distribution for χ^2 is a family of curves, which, like t, vary with degrees of freedom. The use of this inferential statistic is best illustrated by an example.

Suppose that an investigator is interested in finding out whether there is a difference in the relative frequency of different kinds of treatments currently offered to extremely depressed patients. A random sample of 150 patients is selected from a population of patients in Australia, and the type of treatment offered to them is determined from their medical records, as shown in Table 19.2.

The entries in each cell represent the frequency with which patients were given the various treatments. Thus, 45 patients were offered psychotherapy, 40 drugs and 65 electroconvulsive therapy. The χ^2 is the appropriate test for analysing these data. Let us follow the steps involved in hypothesis testing, as outlined in Chapter 18.

1. H_A: there is a difference in the population proportions for the three treatments. H_A is non-directional when we use χ^2.

Table 19.2 Treatments offered

Psychotherapy	Drugs	Electroconvulsive therapy
$n = 45$	$n = 40$	$n = 65$

2. H_0: there is no difference in the population proportions of the three treatments. The frequencies shown in each cell in the table occurred through random sampling from a population where there is an equal frequency of the three treatments.
3. Decision level, α: say the investigator sets a significance level of 0.05 for rejecting H_A ($\alpha = 0.05$).
4. Calculation of the statistic: x^2_{obt} is the value of x^2 calculated from the data obtained. To calculate x^2_{obt}, we must determine f_e for each cell (f_o is, of course, determined by the data). If the null hypothesis is true, then our expectation is that the frequencies in each cell should be the same. In this case, $n = 150$, so that f_e should be 150/3 = 50, given that there are three cells. Let us show this in tabular form (Table 19.3).

We can now calculate x^2_{obt}, by calculating $(f_o - f_e)^2/f_e$ for each cell, and then summing the values.

$$x^2_{obt} = \sum \frac{(f_o - f_e)^2}{f_e}$$
$$= \frac{(45 - 50)^2}{50} + \frac{(40 - 50)^2}{50} + \frac{(65 - 50)^2}{50}$$
$$= 0.5 + 2.0 + 4.5$$
$$= 7.0$$

The greater the discrepancy between f_e and f_o, the greater the calculated value of the chi-square statistic (x^2_{obt}). The direction of the difference is of no account as the difference between f_e and f_o is squared.

5. Making decisions concerning H_0: the decision rule for x^2 is similar to that of the z and t tests, as shown in the previous chapter:

$$x^2_{obt} \geq x^2_{crit}; \text{ reject } H_0$$
$$x^2_{obt} < x^2_{crit}; \text{ retain } H_0$$

Here, x^2_{crit} is the critical value of the statistic x^2, which cuts off a proportion of the sampling

distribution equal to α. The value of x^2_{crit} is obtained from the tables in Appendix C. To look up this statistic, we need to know:

(a) α, which was set at 0.05 for this example
(b) the degrees of freedom, df.

Note that with x^2 the degrees of freedom with one variable is $k - 1$, where k stands for the number of categories or groups. In this instance, we have $k = 3$ (three treatments) so that df = 3 - 1 = 2. Now we can look up the tables in Appendix C. In this case, $\alpha = 0.05$ and df = 2, therefore $x^2_{crit} = 5.99$.

Here, since $x^2_{obt} > x^2_{crit}$ we can reject H_0 at a 0.05 level of significance. The investigator is in a position to accept H_A (that the three treatments are offered at different frequencies to depressed patients). Clearly, electroconvulsive therapy is given most frequently for the condition (in this hypothetical example).

x^2 and contingency tables

In the previous example of x^2 we had clear expectations of the expected frequencies (f_e) and were dealing with only one variable. The x^2 test is also relevant for analysing nominal data where f_e is not known, and where we are interested in the effects of more than one variable. Thus, x^2 is a statistical test appropriate for deciding whether two variables are significantly related.

For example, an investigator compares the effectiveness of drug therapy with coronary artery surgery in males 55–60 years old, suffering from coronary heart disease. A sample of 40 patients consenting to the investigation is selected from this population, and randomly divided into the two treatment groups (drugs only or coronary artery surgery). The treatment outcome is measured in terms of survival over 5 years. The outcome of this hypothetical study is shown in Table 19.4.

Table 19.4 is called a contingency table. A contingency table is a two-way table showing the relationship between two or more variables. Note that the levels of the variables have been classified into mutually exclusive categories ('drugs or surgery' for the independent variable, and 'dead or alive' for the dependent variable, in this instance). The cells

Table 19.3 Treatments; f_e is shown in parentheses

Psychotherapy	Drugs	Electroconvulsive therapy
45	40	65
(50)	(50)	(50)

Table 19.4 Contingency table showing obtained frequencies for a hypothetical study comparing survival after treatments

	Drugs	Surgery	Row marginal
Dead	11	8	**19**
Alive	9	12	**21**
Column marginal	**20**	**20**	**n = 40**

Table 19.5 General format for 2 × 2 contingency table

A	B	j
C	D	k
l	m	n

Table 19.6 Sample calculation of chi-squared

	f_o	f_e	$(f_o - f_e)^2$	$(f_o - f_e)^2/f_e$
A	11	9.5	2.25	0.236
B	8	9.5	2.25	0.236
C	9	10.5	2.25	0.214
D	12	10.5	2.25	0.214
n	40			$\chi^2 = 0.90$

in the contingency table show the frequency of cases falling into each joint category (for example, 11 people who had 'drugs only' died during the 5 years). The row and column marginal scores are the sums of the frequencies. The row and column marginals necessarily add up to n, the sample size ($n = 40$ for this example).

Table 19.4 is called a two-by-two (2 × 2) contingency table. Depending on the number of categories (or levels) in each of the two variables, we might have 3 × 2 tables, 3 × 3 tables, etc. Let us now turn to analysing the data.

1. H_A: there is a difference in the proportion of patients surviving for 5 years following the two types of treatment.
2. H_0: there is no difference in the frequency of survival rates; any difference between observed and expected frequencies in the sample is due to chance.
3. Decision level: $\alpha = 0.05$.
4. Calculation of the statistic χ^2_{obt}

$$\chi^2_{obt} = \sum \frac{(f_o - f_e)^2}{f_e}$$

To make our explanation of the calculation easier, let us label the cells and the marginal values, as shown in Table 19.5. We calculate χ^2_{obt} by calculating f_e for each of the cells and then substituting this value into the equation for χ^2_{obt}. In order to calculate the expected frequencies, f_e, for each of the cells, we use the formula:

$$\frac{\text{Row total} \times \text{column total}}{n}$$

Substituting into the above formula for each of the cells:

$$A: f_e = \frac{j \times l}{n}, \quad B: f_e = \frac{j \times m}{n},$$

$$C: f_e = \frac{k \times l}{n}, \quad D: \frac{k \times m}{n}$$

Now f_o are the observed frequencies as in the data, summarized in contingency Table 19.5. Substituting the values for f_e and f_o for each cell is shown in Table 19.6.

5. Making decisions concerning H_0: the degrees of freedom for a contingency table are calculated by the following formula:

$$df = (r - 1)(c - 1)$$

where r = the number of rows and c = the number of columns. In this instance, given a 2 × 2 contingency table:

$$df = (2 - 1)(2 - 1) = 1$$

Now we can look up χ^2_{crit}, for $\alpha = 0.05$ and df = 1. From Appendix C, $\chi^2_{crit} = 3.84$. Therefore, since $\chi^2_{obt} < \chi^2_{crit}$ we must retain H_0: there is no statistically significant difference in the frequencies of survival over 5 years following the two kinds of treatments. Our data show that either there is no difference in the outcomes of the two treatments or we made a Type II error.

The χ^2 test can be used to analyse the statistical significance of nominal data arising from experimental or non-experimental investigations. This non-parametric test can be used provided that two simple assumptions are met:

1. Each subject has provided only one entry into the χ^2 table; that is, each of the entries is independent.
2. The expected frequency (f_e) in each cell is at least five. Therefore, if the sample size is too small, χ^2 may not be used.

If either of these assumptions is violated, the use of χ^2 is inappropriate for statistical decision making. Assumption 2 is particularly important when the degrees of freedom is one (df = 1) for a contingency table.

Statistical packages

We have been looking at a few simple examples of establishing the statistical significance of the results. These calculations were presented only for teaching purposes. Some older applied statistics text books are crammed with complicated formulae for calculating dozens of different inferential statistics. Researchers now use statistical packages which have made statistical analysis simpler and more accessible to all researchers. The following steps are followed when using statistical packages:

Select a statistical package

There are many packages on the market, including Statistical Package for Social Sciences ('SPSS'), 'STATISTICA', 'Statsview' or various spreadsheets with useful statistical functions. Each program has its strengths and weaknesses and some researchers have formed strong attachment to specific programs. If you are a beginner, you should be guided by your thesis supervisor or your workplace mentor about the availability of packages.

Training

It is useful to learn how to use a package before you begin data analysis. Depending on your aptitude and experience, training sessions take 1 or 2 days. With more complex scientific packages such as 'STATISTICA' it might require long-term usage before one feels like an expert user.

Encode the raw data

Using all packages we begin by encoding the data. You have to be clear about issues such as which are your independent or dependent variables or the scaling of the data (continuous/discontinuous). That is, designs and measurement procedures used in your research project influence the encoding process (e.g. Schwartz & Polgar 2003, Ch. 1).

Identifying the statistical analysis required

Some degree of statistical knowledge is required beyond that covered in this book to enable you confidently to select and interpret the appropriate statistical analyses. Keep in mind that our book is introductory; it is expected that you will complete a more advanced statistics subject. For more complex analyses it might be useful to seek expert help.

Printout

You will select the appropriate statistical analysis from the 'menu' and print out the results of the analysis.

Interpretation

Finally you will need to interpret the 'printout' in relation to your research questions and/or hypotheses.

Let us look at a simple example. Say we are interested in the benefits of exercise for improving mobility in nursing home residents. A sample of 24 ($n = 24$) residents with reduced mobility are selected and give informed consent to participate. The participants are randomly assigned to either of two groups: 'E', which involves them undertaking an exercise programme suitable for improving mobility in elderly patients, and 'C', which involves undertaking alternative activities of equal duration. The outcome or dependent variable is measured as the distance in metres safely walked by the residents unassisted at the completion of the exercise and control programmes. The research hypothesis here is: exercise improves mobility in nursing home residents. We will look at a set of created data to illustrate hypothesis testing using a statistical package (SPSS).

Let us follow the steps for analysing the data:

1. Assume that the SPSS package is readily available in your workplace and you are informed by your computing expert or supervisor.
2. You have had some training. Even if no formal training is available, self-help books such as *SPSS: Analysis Without Anguish. Version 11.0 for Windows* (Coates & Steed 2003) are very useful.
3. After accessing the spreadsheet for the program, we encode the data in the two columns representing 'E' and 'C'. We inform the program that the data are 'continuous' (ratio-scale data).
4. We refer to Table 19.1 to identify the required statistical analysis. Here we have:
   - two groups
   - independent groups
   - ratio-scale data.

   Therefore, we select the independent *t* test for analysing the data from the 'menu' of inferential tests available.
5. Printouts: Tables 19.7 and 19.8 for SPSS are based on printouts presented in Coates & Steed (2003, p.73). We changed the original example which contains additional information: the interested reader might wish to examine it further in Coakes & Steed (2003).

Table 19.7 shows key descriptive statistics:

- n refers to the sample size for each group
- mean ($\bar{X}$) for each group
- standard deviation (s) for each group
- standard error mean ($s_{\bar{x}}$) for each group. You will recall from Chapter 17 that $s_{\bar{x}} = s/\sqrt{n}$. Here, for the control group 'C' the standard error mean = $2.864 /\sqrt{11} = 0.863$, as shown in the printout.

The group mean for the exercise group does in fact indicate a better overall performance. However, we are justified in concluding that exercise in general produces improved mobility in nursing home residents. To answer this question we must look at the results of the *t* test, as shown in Table 19.8.

The following information was presented:

- The *t* obtained was −0.695, the minus sign simply reflecting that the mean for the exercise group was less than the mean for the control group. A *t* value of 0.695 is quite 'small' in relation to the critical values for *t* shown in Appendix B.
- 'df' refers to degrees of freedom. For the control group's *t* test, df = $n_1 + n_2 - 2$ (Schwartz & Polgar 2003). Here, df = $11 + 11 - 2 = 20$, as shown in Table 19.8.
- 'Sig. (2-tailed)' refers to the probability of a difference between the means being obtained by chance, i.e. p (H_0 is true) (see Ch.18). The decision rule is that we reject H_0 if $p \leqslant 0.05$. Here the calculated probability is 0.495 and therefore we retain H_0. We conclude that the results were not statistically significant.
- The 'mean difference' refers to the difference between the two sample means; that is, $8 - 9 = -1$, as shown in Table 19.8.
- 'Standard error difference' refers to the standard error of the distribution of sample means. We will

Table 19.7	Printout for descriptive statistics			
Treatment	n	Mean	Standard deviation	Standard error mean
Control (C)	11	8.00	2.864	0.863
Exercise (E)	11	9.00	3.821	1.152

Table 19.8	*t* test for equality of means					95% confidence interval of the difference	
Treatment	t	df	Sig. (2-tailed)	Mean difference	Standard error difference	Lower	Upper
Control (C)	−0.695	20	0.495	−1.00	1.440	−4.003	2.003
Exercise (E)	−0.695	18.539	0.496	−1.00	1.440	−4.018	2.013

not discuss this statistic in detail. However, as shown in Chapter 17, the standard error enables us to calculate a 95% confidence interval; in this case for $\bar{X}_C - \bar{X}_E$.

- The lower and upper limits show that the true (i.e. population) difference ($\mu_C - \mu_E$) probably ($p = 0.95$) falls between -4.003 and 2.003. This is a wide range for a confidence interval and therefore indicates that residents who exercise might be able to walk either four extra metres or, for that matter, two metres less than those who don't exercise. Of course, any other difference between the two limits is possible. Clearly, such results are far too variable to attribute any clinical benefits to the exercise programme.

Summary

There are a variety of statistical tests available for analysing the significance of the obtained data. The statistical test appropriate for analysing a given set of data is selected on the basis of:

1. the scaling of the data
2. the dependence/independence of the measurements
3. the number of groups being studied
4. specific requirements for using a statistical test.

Generally, parametric and non-parametric statistical tests were distinguished on the grounds of the scaling of the data and the assumptions underlying the sampling distributions.

None of the individual statistical tests was discussed in detail, except the χ^2 test, which was presented as an example. Together with the discussion on the z and t tests in Chapter 18, the χ^2 test illustrates the principle that theoretical sampling distributions can be generated, and the probability of obtaining specific outcomes can be calculated. If the obtained value of the inferential statistic is greater than or equal to the critical value, the null hypothesis can be rejected at the level of significance specified by the Type I error rate (α). This is the case regardless of which particular statistical test is being used.

The retention of H_0 might reflect a correct decision, or a Type II error. Sample size is a factor which contributes to Type II error rate, as shown in both Chapters 18 and 20.

Self-assessment

Explain the meaning of the following terms:

chi-square
contingency table
expected frequency
non-parametric test
observed frequency
parametric test

True or false

1. Inferential statistics are used to decide if differences obtained in sample data are persistent, 'real' trends.
2. The selection of descriptive and inferential statistics is independent of the scaling of the data.
3. Inferential statistics must be used regardless of the nature and aims of an investigation.
4. Parametric tests are used to analyse the significance of interval or ratio data.
5. The use of non-parametric tests depends on the normal distribution of the underlying population.
6. Each statistical test entails the use of sampling distributions for calculating the probability of the obtained sample outcomes.
7. It is impossible to select an appropriate statistical test before the data are collected.
8. The number of groups being compared in an investigation influences the selection of the appropriate statistical test.
9. A basic assumption for using t is that the samples were drawn from a normally distributed population. A basic assumption of χ^2 is that the scores in each cell are independent.
10. When using χ^2, the closer the observed frequency for each cell is to the expected frequency, the higher the probability of rejecting H_0.
11. In order to reject the null hypothesis, $\chi^2_{obt} > \chi^2_{crit}$.
12. The χ^2 sampling distribution is a family of curves, the distribution of which varies with the degrees of freedom.
13. The χ^2 test is appropriate for testing hypotheses about proportions.
14. Each entry in a χ^2 table is a frequency.
15. The value of f_e is looked up in the appropriate χ^2 table.
16. If the f_e and f_o values are the same for each cell, χ^2_{obt} will not be statistically significant.

17. The decision level, α, is generally set at 0.05 or 0.01 with χ^2.
18. If we use sample data to calculate the values of f_e, then we use contingency tables for calculating χ^2_{obt}.
19. A 2×2 contingency table shows the relationship between two variables.
20. 'rc' stands for the degrees of freedom for a 2×2 contingency table.

Multiple choice

1. In a study, three independent samples are compared and the dependent variable is measured on a ratio scale. A statistical test appropriate for analysing these findings is:
   a χ^2
   b Mann–Whitney U
   c t
   d ANOVA (analysis of variance).
2. In a study, two independent samples are compared and the dependent variable is measured on an ordinal scale. A statistical test appropriate for analysing these findings is:
   a χ^2
   b Mann–Whitney U
   c t
   d Wilcoxon.
3. Which of the following is a 'non-parametric' test?
   a ANOVA (analysis of variance)
   b t
   c z
   d Kruskal–Wallis H.
4. Which of the following is a 'parametric' test?
   a Median test
   b McNemar's test
   c z
   d Cochran's Q.
5. Which of the following tests is appropriate for analysing data where three or more groups were used?
   a z
   b t
   c χ^2
   d Sign test.
6. The larger the discrepancy between f_o and f_e for each cell in a contingency table:
   a the more likely it is that the results will not be significant

b the more likely it is that H_0 will be rejected
c the more likely it is that the population proportions are the same
d the more likely it is that the population proportions are different
e a and c
f b and d.
7. For any given level of significance, χ^2_{crit}:
   a increases with increases in sample size
   b decreases with increases in degrees of freedom
   c increases with increases in degrees of freedom
   d decreases with increases in sample size.
8. A contingency table:
   a always involves two degrees of freedom
   b always involves two dependent frequencies
   c always involves two variables
   d all of the above
   e a and b.
9. Entries into the cells of a contingency table should be:
   a frequencies
   b means
   c percentages
   d degrees of freedom.
10. The degrees of freedom for a contingency table:
    a equal $n - 1$
    b equal $rc - 1$
    c cannot be determined if $r = c$
    d equal $(r - 1)(c - 1)$.
11. χ^2 should not be used with a 2×2 contingency table if:
    a df > 1
    b f_e is below 5 in any cell
    c f_o is below 5 in any cell
    d $f_e = f_o$
    e b and c.

An investigator is interested in determining whether there is a relationship between gender and susceptibility to a substance known to trigger an allergic response. 'Susceptibility' is measured as yes or no.

Questions 12–15 refer to this example. The raw data are presented in the contingency table below.

	Not susceptible	Susceptible	Total
Female	90	110	200
Male	60	140	200
Total	150	250	400

12. The value of χ^2_{obt} is:
    a 2.50
    b 8.09
    c 9.60
    d 11.05
13. The value of df is:
    a 2
    b 1
    c 3
    d need more information.
14. Using $\alpha = 0.05$, χ^2_{crit} is:
    a 3.841
    b 5.412
    c 2.706
    d −3.841
15. Using $\alpha = 0.05$, what is your conclusion?
    a Accept H_0: there is no relationship between gender and susceptibility.
    b Reject H_0: there is a significant relationship between gender and susceptibility.
    c Fail to reject H_0: the study does not show a significant relationship between gender and susceptibility.
    d Fail to reject H_0: this study shows a significant relationship between gender and susceptibility.
16. In selecting an appropriate statistical test:
    a z should be used as it is most powerful
    b t should be used as it takes the sample size into account
    c the choice depends on the design of the study
    d χ^2 should be avoided.
17. The χ^2 test requires that:
    a data be measured on a nominal scale
    b data conform to a normal distribution
    c expected frequencies are equal in all cells
    d all of the above occur.

The following information should be used in answering questions 18–25. Aerobics classes are conducted by the student union of a tertiary institution; although there are equal numbers of male and female students enrolled at the institution, it is observed that far more female than male students attend. A test is performed to see whether the proportion of the two sexes at the class is representative of the proportion of the two sexes enrolled at the institution as a whole. Of the 50 students who attend the classes, 10 are male. A χ^2 is conducted on these data.

18. What type of χ^2 will be conducted?
    a one-way
    b two-way
    c contingency analysis
    d parametric.
19. How many cells will there be in the χ^2 table?
    a 1
    b 2
    c 3
    d 4
20. What is the expected frequency of male students at the aerobic classes?
    a 10
    b 40
    c 25
    d 8
21. What is the obtained value of χ^2?
    a 4.5
    b 2.5
    c 18.0
    d 9.0
22. What are the degrees of freedom?
    a 1
    b 2
    c 49
    d 48
23. If α is set at 0.01, what is the critical value of χ^2?
    a 0.0201
    b 4.605
    c 9.210
    d 6.635
24. What statistical decision should be made on the basis of these data?
    a Reject null hypothesis.
    b Retain null hypothesis.
    c Increase α.
    d Increase size of sample.

25. What conclusion can be drawn on the basis of these data?

    a Overall, the tendency for more females than males to attend the classes is not statistically significant.

    b There is a statistically significant tendency for more females than males to attend the classes ($\alpha = 0.01$).

    c The aerobics classes should have their format changed to attract more male students.

    d There is a statistically significant trend ($\alpha = 0.01$) for differential attendance by the two sexes, but it is impossible to state the direction of this trend.

The following information should be used in answering questions 26–31. In a test of the effectiveness of phenothiazine in treating schizophrenia, 60 patients are randomly assigned to receive either the drug or a placebo; after 2 weeks of daily treatment each patient is assessed by the chief psychiatrist as 'improved' or 'not improved'. A 2×2 table is constructed to indicate improved number of patients falling into each category:

Assessment	Treatment	
	Phenothiazine	Placebo
Improved	20	10
Not improved	10	20

26. The degrees of freedom in this table are:

    a 1

    b 2

    c 3

    d 4

27. The obtained χ^2 is:

    a 1.33

    b 13.5

    c 8.71

    d 6.67

28. With α set at 0.05, the critical value of χ^2 is:

    a 3.841

    b 5.991

    c 6.635

    d 0.013

29. The correct statistical decision in this case is to:

    a reject H_0

    b retain H_0

    c decrease α

    d increase α.

30. The appropriate conclusion to be drawn from these data is:

    a Patients receiving the active drug are not significantly more likely to get an 'improved' rating than those receiving the placebo.

    b Those receiving the active drug are significantly more likely to be rated as 'improved' ($\alpha = 0.05$).

    c The drug cures schizophrenia.

    d The improvements cannot be due to the drug, as some people received the drug and did not improve.

31. Following the publication of this study, it is revealed that the psychiatrist who did the ratings of improvement was also the person who had assigned the patients to phenothiazine or placebo groups. What type of problem could have invalidated these findings?

    a Rosenthal effects.

    b Placebo effects.

    c Instrumentation effects.

    d All of the above.

Chapter Twenty

20

The interpretation of research evidence

Introduction

When researchers have demonstrated statistical significance within a study, what have they actually established? Statistical significance suggests that it is likely that there is a similar effect or phenomenon in the population from which the study sample has been drawn. However, it is not correct to assume that statistical significance necessarily implies clinical importance or usefulness. We must also establish the *clinical* or *practical significance* of our results following the step of demonstrating statistical significance.

The aims of this chapter are to discuss the following:

1. Effect size, that is, how large the relationships or differences observed in the data are.
2. The relationship between effect size and statistical and clinical significance.
3. The determinants of statistical power.
4. Basic principles of clinical decision making.

Effect size

In a clinical intervention study, the effect size is the size of the effects that can be attributed to the intervention. The term *effect size* is also used more broadly in statistics to refer to the size of the phenomenon under study. For example, if we were studying gender effects on longevity, a measure of effect size could be the difference in mean longevity between males and females. In a correlational study, the effect size could be represented by the size of the correlation between the selected variables under study. There are many measures or indicators of effect size selected on the basis of the scaling of the outcome or dependent variable (Sackett et al 2000).

The concept of effect size can be illustrated by results from two student research projects supervised by the authors.

Study 1: Test–retest reliability of a force measurement machine

In the first study, the student was concerned with demonstrating the test–retest reliability of a device designed to measure maximum voluntary forces being produced by patients' leg muscles under two conditions (flexion and extension). Twenty one patients took part and the reliability of the measurement process was tested by calculating the Pearson correlation between the readings obtained from the machine in question during two trials separated by an hour for each patient. The results are shown in Table 20.1. Both results reach the 0.01 level of significance.

The student was ecstatic when the computer data analysis program informed that the correlations were statistically significant at the 0.01 level (indicating that there was less than a 1 in 100 chance that the correlations were illusory or actually zero). We were somewhat less ecstatic because, in fact, the results indicated that approximately 69% ($1 - 0.56^2$) and 71% ($1 - 0.54^2$) of the variation was not shared between the measurements of the first and second trial. In other words, the measures were 'all over the place', despite statistical significance being reached. Thus, far from being an endorsement of the measurement process, these results were somewhat of a condemnation. This is a classic example of the need for careful interpretation of effect size in conjunction with statistical significance.

Study 2: A comparative study of improvement in two treatment groups

The second project was a comparative study of two groups: one group suffering from suspected repetition strain injuries (RSI) induced by computer keyboard input and a group of 'normals'. An Activities of Daily Living (ADL) assessment scale was used and yielded a 'disability' index of between 0 and 50. There were 60 people in each group. The results are shown in Table 20.2.

The appropriate statistic for analysing these data happens to be the independent groups t test, although this is not important for understanding this example. The t value for these data was significant at the 0.05 level. Does this finding indicate that the difference is clinically meaningful or significant? There are two steps in interpreting the clinical significance of the results.

First, we calculate the effect size. For interval or ratio-scaled data the effect size 'd' is defined as:

$$d = \frac{\mu_1 - \mu_2}{\sigma}$$

where $\mu_1 - \mu_2$ refers to the difference between the population means and σ, the population standard deviation.

Since we rarely have access to population data we use sample statistics for estimating population differences. The formula becomes:

$$d = \frac{\bar{X}_1 - \bar{X}_2}{s_1}$$

Table 20.1 Pearson correlations between trials 1 and 2	
Flexion	**Extension**
0.56	0.54

Table 20.2 Mean ADL disability scores		
	RSI group	**Normals**
Mean	33.2	30.4
Standard deviation	1.6	1.2

where $\bar{X}_1 - \bar{X}_2$ indicates the difference between the sample means and s_1 refers to the standard deviation of the 'normal' or 'control' group. Therefore, for the above example, substituting into the equation yields:

$$d = \frac{30.4 - 33.2}{1.2}$$
$$= -2.33$$

In other words, the average ADL score of the people with suspected RSI was 2.33 standard deviations under the mean of the distribution of 'normal' scores. The meaning of d can be interpreted by using z scores. The greater the value of d, the larger the effect size.

Second, we need to consider the clinical implications of the evidence. It might be that the difference of 2.8 units of ADL scores is important and clinically meaningful. However, if one inspects the means, the differences are slight, notwithstanding the statistical significance of the results. This example further illustrates the problems of interpretation that may arise from focusing on the level of statistical significance and not on the effect sizes shown by the data.

When we say that the findings are clinically significant we mean that the effect is sufficiently large to influence clinical practices. It is the health workers rather than statisticians who need to set the standards for each health and illness determinant or treatment outcome. After all, even relatively small changes can be of enormous value in the prevention and treatment of illnesses. There are many statistics currently in use for determining effect size. The selection, calculation and interpretation of various measures of effect are beyond our introductory book, but interested readers can refer to Sackett et al (2000).

How to interpret null (non-significant) results

As we discussed in previous chapters, the researcher will sometimes analyse data that show no relationships or differences according to the chosen statistical test and criteria. In other words,

the researcher cannot reject the null hypothesis. There are several reasons why the researcher may obtain a null result.

1. The trend or difference that the researcher originally hypothesized is incorrect.
2. The sample included in the analysis is unrepresentative, so the effect does not show up, although it exists in the wider population.
3. There are insufficient cases in the sample to detect the trend; this is especially a problem if the trends are subtle (i.e. the effect size is small).
4. The measurements chosen have very high or inherent random variability.

Therefore, if the researcher obtains a null result, one or more of the above explanations may be appropriate. There are, however, steps that can be taken to minimize the chance of missing real effects. In order to understand these measures, it is necessary again to invoke the table illustrating the possible outcomes of a statistical decision (as shown in Table 20.3).

There are four possible outcomes. On the basis of the statistical evidence you may: (i) correctly conclude there is an effect when there is indeed an effect; (ii) decide that there is an effect when there is not (this is a false alarm or Type I error); (iii) decide that there is not an effect when there really is (this is a miss or Type II error); or (iv) correctly decide there is not an effect when indeed there is not. The probability that researchers derive from their statistical tables is in fact the probability of making a false alarm or Type I error. This value does not tell us, however, how many times we will fail to identify a real effect. The probability of missing a real effect (or making a Type II error) is affected by the size of the actual effect and the number of cases included in our study. If you have large effects and large samples, the number of misses will be small. To detect a small effect size larger samples are needed.

Table 20.3 Statistical decision outcomes		
Reality	**Decision: effect**	**Decision: no effect**
Effect	Correct	'Miss' Type II error
No effect	'False alarm' Type I error	Correct

Table 20.4 The relationship between effect size, sample size and decision making

Effect size	Sample size	
	Large	*Small*
High	Both statistical and clinical significance are likely to be demonstrated	Statistical significance might not be demonstrated, but clinical significance would be indicated
Low	Statistical significance would be likely, but the results might not indicate clinically applicable outcomes	Neither statistical nor clinical significance is likely. Statistically significant results might result in Type I error

Statistical power analysis

In statistical analysis we need to know how likely a miss is to occur. We can do this by calculating the statistical power of a design. The statistical power for a given effect size is defined as 1 – probability of a miss (Type II error or β). Thus, if the power of a particular analysis is 0.95, for a given effect size we will correctly detect the existence of the effect 95 times out of 100. Power is an important concept in the interpretation of null results. For example, if a researcher compared the improvements of two groups of only five patients under different treatment circumstances, the power of the analysis would almost certainly be low, say 0.1. Thus 9 times out of 10, even with an effect really present, the researcher would be unable to detect it.

It is essential to be careful in the interpretation of null results where they are used to demonstrate a lack of superiority of one treatment method over another, especially when there is a low number of cases. This may be purely a function of low statistical power rather than the equivalence of the two treatments. Unfortunately the calculation of statistical power is complicated and beyond the scope of this text. However, there are technical texts, such as Cohen (1988), that are available to look up the power of various analyses. There are also statistical programs that perform the same function. The best defence against low statistical power is a good-sized sample. Before quantitative research projects are approved by funding bodies or ethics committees, there is the requirement that sufficient data will be collected to identify real effects.

Effect size is a key determinant of both statistical and clinical significance. We are more likely to detect a significant pattern or trend in our sample data when a factor has a strong influence on health or illness outcomes. A very powerful treatment such as the use of antibiotics for bacterial infections could be demonstrated even in a small sample. Table 20.4 shows the association between effect size and sample size for determining statistical and clinical significance for the results of research and evaluation projects. The most useful results for clear decision making occur when both effect size and sample size are large. Where the effect size is large but the results are not statistically significant, it might be useful to replicate the study with a larger sample size. Unfortunately, in real research it might be difficult to obtain a large sample and the effect size, we discover, might be disappointingly small. It is for this reason that researchers make the best use of previous research and, if possible, complete pilot studies. The evidence from previous research and the results of pilot studies enable us to conduct power analyses for estimating the minimum sample size for detecting an effect if it is really there.

Table 20.5 shows how evidence for statistical and clinical significance can be combined to interpret the findings of a study. A clear positive outcome is when there is strong evidence for both clinical and statistical significance. In this case we are confident that the information obtained is clinically useful and generalizable to the population.

Table 20.5 How to interpret findings

Clinical significance	Statistical significance	
	Yes	**No**
Yes	Clear: strong evidence for treatment effect	Inconclusive: need for further research (e.g. with larger samples)
No	Inconclusive: suggests findings might not be meaningful – need further research	Clear: strong evidence for lack of a treatment effect

Acknowledgement: We are grateful to Dr. Paul O'Halloran (La Trobe University) for this table.

Another clear finding, provided that the sample size was adequate, is the lack of clear treatment effect. Such negative findings can be very useful in eliminating false hypotheses or ineffectual treatments.

Clinical decision making

The decisions confronting a clinician making a diagnosis on the basis of uncertain information are similar to the scientist's hypothesis testing procedure. As a hypothetical example, assume that a clinician wishes to decide whether a patient has heart disease on the basis of the cholesterol concentration in a sample of the patient's blood. Previous research of patients with heart disease and 'normals' has shown that, indeed, heart patients tend to have a higher level of cholesterol than normals.

When the frequency distributions of cholesterol concentrations of a large group of heart patients and a group of normals are graphed, they appear as shown in Figure 20.1. You will note that, if patients present with a cholesterol concentration between 1.0 and 2.4 mg/cc, it is not possible to determine with complete certainty whether they are normal or have heart disease, due to the overlap of the normal and heart disease groups in the cholesterol distribution.

Therefore, the clinician, like the scientist, has to make a decision under uncertainty: to diagnose pathology (that is, reject the null hypothesis) or normality (that is, retain the null hypothesis). The

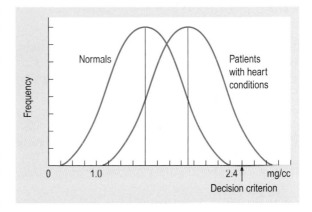

Figure 20.1 • Decision criterion: risk of Type II error (miss).

Table 20.6 Clinical decision outcomes

Reality	Decision: pathology	Decision: no pathology
No pathology	'False alarm' Type I error	Correct decision
Pathology	Correct decision	'Miss' Type II error

clinician risks the same errors as the scientist, as shown in Table 20.6.

The relative frequency of the type of errors made by the clinician can be altered by moving the point above which the clinician will decide that pathology is indicated (that is, the decision criterion). For example, if clinicians did not

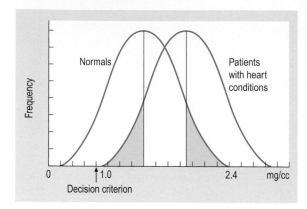

Figure 20.2 • Decision criterion: risk of Type I error (false alarm).

bother their colleagues or patients with false alarms (Type I errors), they might shift the decision criterion to 2.5 mg/cc (Fig. 20.1). Any patient presenting with a cholesterol level below 2.5 mg/cc would be considered normal. In this particular case, with a decision point of 2.5 mg/cc, no 'false alarms' would occur. However, a huge number of people with real pathology would be missed (Type II errors).

If clinicians value the sanctity of human life (and their bank balance after a successful malpractice suit) they will probably adjust the decision criterion to the point shown in Figure 20.2. In this case, there would be no misses but lots of false alarms.

Thus, most clinicians are rewarded for adopting a conservative decision rule, where misses are minimized, by receiving lots of false alarms. Unfortunately, this generates a lot of useless, expensive and sometimes even dangerous clinical interventions.

Summary

In the interpretation of a statistical test, the researcher calculates the statistical value and then compares this value against the appropriate table to determine the probability level. If the probability is below a certain value (0.05 is a commonly chosen value), the researcher has established the statistical significance of the analysis in question.

The researcher must then interpret the implications of the results by determining the actual size of the effects observed. If these are small, the results may be statistically significant but clinically unimportant. Statistical significance does not imply clinical importance.

A null result (indicating no effects) must be carefully interpreted. It is possible that the researcher has missed an effect because of its small size and/or insufficient cases in the analysis. The statistical analysis measures the chance of correctly detecting a real effect of a given size. Thus, a null result may be a function of low statistical power, rather than there being no real effect. It is necessary to carry out a statistical power analysis *before* undertaking a research project.

There are several criteria, beyond statistical significance, which need to be considered before making decisions concerning the clinical relevance of investigations. The most important criterion is a large and consistent effect size. In addition to effect size, the determination of clinical significance is influenced by values and economic limitations concerning the administration of health care in a given community.

Self-assessment

Explain the meaning of the following terms:

clinical significance
effect size
null result
power analysis
social significance
statistical significance

True or false

1. If the effect size is small, clinical significance will be large.
2. In order to establish statistical significance, clinical significance must first be established.
3. In order to establish clinical significance, statistical significance must first be established.
4. The effect size in an analysis is directly measured by the size of the p value associated with the statistic.

5. High inherent variability in measures will promote the detection of effects within data.
6. If a statistical analysis has high power, this means that β will be low.
7. A 'miss' is a correct rejection of the null hypothesis.
8. If a statistical analysis has low power, the null hypothesis will be accepted more frequently.
9. Power = $1 - \beta$ (Type II error).
10. It is more difficult to detect small effects in data where the statistical power is high.

Multiple choice

1. If $\beta = 0.80$ and $\alpha = 0.1$, the power of an analysis equals:
   a 0.9
   b 0.7
   c 0.2
   d 0.65
2. In a study, there was a 1% difference in improvement of systolic blood pressure for two groups of patients receiving different treatments. This was statistically significant at $p = 0.05$. The results probably demonstrate:
   a clinical and statistical significance for the difference
   b clinical significance only
   c statistical significance only
   d neither clinical nor statistical significance.
3. A study of the relationship between family income and probability of occurrence of nutritionally related disorders demonstrated a correlation of 0.8 with $p < 0.001$. The results probably demonstrate:
   a clinical and statistical significance of the relationship
   b clinical significance only
   c statistical significance only
   d neither clinical nor statistical significance.
4. If the effect size in a study is large, the results are likely to have:
   a clinical and statistical significance for the difference

   b clinical significance only
   c statistical significance only
   d neither clinical nor statistical significance.
5. If the power of the statistical analysis of a study is high there will be:
   a fewer misses
   b fewer correct rejections
   c fewer correct acceptances
   d more misses.
6. The effect of large sample sizes in a study upon statistical power is generally to:
   a increase it
   b decrease it
   c not affect it.
7. In a study, the effect of larger sample sizes upon clinical significance is generally to:
   a increase it
   b decrease it
   c not affect it.
8. In a study, the effect of a larger sample size upon obtained statistical significance as measured by p is generally to:
   a increase it
   b decrease it
   c not affect it.
9. If a null result is obtained in an experimental clinical study, the clinical significance of any observed differences between treatment groups:
   a cannot be supported
   b can be supported if it is big
   c can be supported if it is small
   d should be determined by power analysis.
10. If a power analysis is not performed, is it sensible to accept a null result from a study at face value?
   a Yes
   b No.

Section Six

Discussion, questions and answers

Inferential statistical tests arise from the desire of clinical researchers to generalize from the data they have collected in a sample to the population from which the sample has been drawn. 'Is what I have found in my sample a true representation of the population (and hence other samples)?' is the basic question to be answered through the use of inferential statistical tests.

Inferential statistical tests all have the same basic format. The data are processed using the appropriate calculation procedure (often with the support of a computer program) and the value of the statistic is calculated. This value obtained is then compared with a table of known values in order to interpret the outcome of the statistical test. This is very much like the application of clinical tests where, in order to interpret the value of the test result, it is compared with a known standard. As with the clinician, the clinical researcher needs to know which test to choose in which circumstance. It would not be appropriate to try to measure the weight of a patient by giving her an X-ray. Similarly, it is not appropriate to use a χ^2 test when the t test is required. It is beyond the scope of an introductory text to have an extended discussion of the various types of statistical tests and when they might be used (although it should be noted that there are many fewer statistical than clinical tests). However, it is essential that the student understands the basic use of inferential tests.

Consider the following analysis using χ^2. This statistic is designed to test the relationship between variables with nominal or categorical scales (i.e. the values are categories).

The clinical researcher is using the χ^2 test to examine the relationship between length of stay in hospital and the rate of unplanned readmissions. These data are described more fully in Section 5. The goal is to determine whether there is a statistically significant association between the two variables. The raw data appear in Table D20.1.

As demonstrated in Section 5, we could use the Pearson correlation to analyse these data. However, to illustrate the use of χ^2 we will recode the data to categorical data and use this technique. The data will be recoded using the averages for each variable to convert the data from ratio data to categorical data. For example, all those cases (hospitals) with a mean length of stay of 13.6 days or greater will be considered as having an 'above-average' length of stay. Those cases (hospitals) with a stay below 13.6 days will be considered as having a 'below-average' length of stay. The same procedure will be followed for readmission rates of 4.47 or greater. These are the respective means for the two variables shown in Table D20.1. The recoded data appear as Table D20.2.

From these data we can construct a contingency table which shows the relationship between

Table D20.1 Average lengths of stay and readmission rates per 100 patients for patients with fractured neck of femur at 30 hospitals

Hospital	Average length of stay (days)	Unplanned readmission rates per 100 patients	Hospital	Average length of stay (days)	Unplanned readmission rates per 100 patients
1	11.100	7.800	16	13.200	4.500
2	11.200	6.500	17	13.200	5.500
3	11.200	4.300	18	13.300	4.100
4	11.200	5.500	19	13.700	3.200
5	11.700	5.100	20	13.900	3.400
6	12.100	5.200	21	14.100	3.500
7	12.100	5.000	22	14.200	3.400
8	12.100	4.900	23	14.200	6.000
9	12.300	4.800	24	14.900	4.400
10	12.400	3.400	25	15.300	3.300
11	12.400	5.000	26	15.400	4.200
12	12.500	4.300	27	15.400	4.300
13	13.100	3.900	28	15.500	4.100
14	13.100	3.300	29	16.300	3.200
15	13.200	4.700	30	22.400	3.300

the two newly coded variables. We do this by counting the number of times the 30 cases fall into the appropriate categories.

As can be seen from Table D20.3, only one hospital with an above-average length of stay had an above-average readmission rate, while 11 hospitals with above-average lengths of stay had below-average readmission rates.

These data can be subjected to χ^2 analysis. If these calculations are performed, we obtain a χ^2 value of 9.98, df = 1, $p < 0.01$. In other words there is a statistically significant association between length of stay and readmission rates for the 30 hospitals. This confirms the analysis conducted in Section 5.

Questions

1. From Table D20.1, how many hospitals have a below-average length of stay, if the average length of stay is 13.6 days? How many have an above-average length of stay? Why is it not 15 above and below?

2. From Table D20.3, why is there one degree of freedom in this analysis?

3. On the basis of this analysis, what would you conclude about the relationship between average length of stay in hospital and unplanned readmission rates for patients with fractured neck of femur at the 30 hospitals?

4. To what other groups of patients could these findings be generalized?

Table D20.2 Recoded average lengths of stay and readmission rates per 100 patients for patients with fractured neck of femur at 30 hospitals

Hospital	Average length of stay (days)	Unplanned readmission rates per 100 patients	Hospital	Average length of stay (days)	Unplanned readmission rates per 100 patients
1	Below average	Above average	16	Below average	Above average
2	Below average	Above average	17	Below average	Above average
3	Below average	Below average	18	Below average	Below average
4	Below average	Above average	19	Above average	Below average
5	Below average	Above average	20	Above average	Below average
6	Below average	Above average	21	Above average	Below average
7	Below average	Above average	22	Above average	Below average
8	Below average	Above average	23	Above average	Above average
9	Below average	Above average	24	Above average	Below average
10	Below average	Below average	25	Above average	Below average
11	Below average	Above average	26	Above average	Below average
12	Below average	Below average	27	Above average	Below average
13	Below average	Below average	28	Above average	Below average
14	Below average	Below average	29	Above average	Below average
15	Below average	Above average	30	Above average	Below average

Table D20.3 Contingency table of relationship between average length of stay and readmission rates at 30 hospitals for patients with fractured neck of femur

| Length of stay | Unplanned readmission rate | |
	Above average	Below average
Above average	1	11
Below average	12	6

Answers

1. In this sample, 18 hospitals have a below-average length of stay. Twelve hospitals have an above-average length of stay. Although that is how the median is defined, i.e. the score above which and below which half of the cases fall, the mean does not always fall at the exact half-way point of the sample.

2. The number of degrees of freedom in a contingency table is calculated by the formula:

   df = (number of rows − 1) ×
       (number of columns − 1)
   = (2 − 1) × (2 − 1)
   = 1

3. There is a moderately sized statistical association between average length of stay in hospital and unplanned readmission rates. That is, those hospitals with shorter lengths of stay for patients with a fractured neck of femur tend to have higher unplanned readmission rates.

4. It is difficult to say. The current data include patients with one condition only, i.e. fractured neck of femur. These patients may be atypical of other acute/surgical patients; they are likely to be older and perhaps more debilitated. These analyses would need to be extended to other types of patients before the results could be generalized. The country in which the study has been performed also needs to be considered, as procedures and incentives may vary considerably from one country to the next.

Section **Seven**

Dissemination and critical evaluation of research

Having completed the analysis and interpretation of our data, we are now ready to communicate our results to the community of health scientists and professionals. Depending on the context in which our research was carried out, this entails the writing up of a report, a thesis or a 'paper' for a health sciences journal. The most common way of communicating research findings by established researchers is first to report the results at a professional conference and then to write a more formal paper for a relevant journal.

Each journal has its particular set of rules and requirements for how research projects should be written up for publication. In general, at least for quantitative research, the format for presenting our research follows the sequential stages of the research process outlined in the present book. This general format is outlined in Chapter 22, which includes a detailed discussion of the specific sections of a research paper and outlines some 'stylistic' considerations required by journal editors.

It is an ethical requirement that we report our results in an accurate and honest fashion. Before a paper is published in a reputable journal, it is critically evaluated by experts in the area (called referees) for errors or problems. However, sometimes problems remain unidentified. Ultimately, it is our task as health professionals to read important publications in a critical fashion. We owe it to our patients and clients to be cautious and critical concerning recent developments in theories and practices. However, being critical does not imply the adoption of a cynical or derogatory approach towards the work of other health researchers. We are aware that ethical and economic constraints, and the complex nature of the subject matter, as discussed in Section 2, make it difficult to ensure the external and internal validity of research projects.

The critical evaluation of a paper is not like judging a dog show; we do not simply award or subtract points for the strengths and weaknesses of a research project. Rather, if the information is relevant to advancing the effectiveness of our practices, we have a stake in the project (even as readers). In this way, we take an active role in trying to 'repair' the problems which might cloud or invalidate the evidence.

In Chapter 23, we outline some of the criteria which we generally apply to evaluate specific sections of a research paper. We also discuss the implications of finding serious problems with the design, data collection and analysis and interpretations of a research project.

In effect, a single research project is rarely sufficient either to verify or falsify a theory, or to demonstrate the effectiveness of a treatment programme convincingly. Rather, we need to evaluate and summarize the literature as a whole, that is, conduct a literature review. Conflicting findings or gaps in the knowledge for a given area of health care identified in our literature review provide the impetus for further research, as outlined in Section 2. In this way research is a circular process.

Chapter Twenty One

Qualitative data analysis

Introduction

Qualitative data are collected through techniques such as in-depth interviews, focus groups, participant observation and narratives spoken and written by the participants and researchers involved in the study. Qualitative data analysis refers to the processes by which researchers organize the information collected and analyse the meanings of what was said and done by the participants. In qualitative data analysis we bring our values, experiences and social understanding into analysing and constructing the meaning of what our respondents were telling us about their lives. At the same time, qualitative data analysis is principled; there are various explicit and shared strategies for summarizing and making sense of the data and checking the accuracy of our interpretation.

The aims of this chapter are to:

1. Describe the process of interpreting qualitative research data.
2. Describe the basic procedures involved in conducting content analysis, thematic analysis and semiotic analysis.
3. Discuss the comparative advantages and disadvantages of using different types of qualitative analyses.
4. Explain basic strategies for ensuring the accuracy of interpretations.

Understanding meaning in everyday life

Understanding people involves discovering the contents of people's minds – their beliefs, desires, intentions. There is nothing remarkable or supernatural being implied by this, simply that we infer mental contents by listening to and observing what people say and do, taking into account the social settings in which these actions occur.

For instance, one person says to another: 'Would you like to come in for a coffee?' What are the intentions of the speaker? Does he or she simply want to prepare the dark beverage and consume it in silence? Or should we look for 'hidden' or 'latent' meanings in order to understand the speaker's true intentions? Consider these two everyday scenarios (Polgar & Swerissen 2000):

1. You have been given a lift by a work mate who had to go out of his way to drive you home. Although you are tired, it seems the right thing to offer the driver refreshments. However, your intention is to be polite and acknowledge the colleague's effort; in fact you are hoping that the invitation will be refused. The 'hidden message' here is: 'Thank you and goodbye!' The worst-case outcome is that the colleague is too insensitive to read your intentions and stays around gossiping until midnight. Bad luck!

2. The British film 'Brassed Off' (1996) has a scene where a young woman is escorted home after a date by a young man. A dialogue was (approximately) as follows:
   She: Come up for a cup of coffee.
   He: I don't drink coffee.
   She: That's alright; I don't have any.

The above dialogue shows the nuances in the everyday use of language. Just as we sometimes misunderstand meanings and intentions in everyday life, we can also misinterpret the data produced by qualitative data collection. To avoid error we need to cross-check the accuracy of our interpretation.

Coding qualitative data

Qualitative data analysis frequently involves analysis of verbatim transcripts of dialogues and narratives. A common point of departure for analysing the transcript data is to develop a coding system. A coding system is to organize the data into specific classes or categories. There are two fundamental approaches to coding: predetermined and emerging with thematic analysis.

Predetermined coding

Predetermined coding uses predetermined categories to organize and analyse the transcripts.

For example, you might be conducting a survey to determine how clients experienced a rehabilitation programme at your workplace. Say that you conducted 20 in-depth interviews and produced a 100-page transcript representing what people said in these interviews. Considering your research aims, you might code the statements into three categories:

1. Satisfaction with the rehabilitation programme.
2. Dissatisfaction with the rehabilitation programme.
3. Neutral statements.

At the simplest level, analysing the first two categories would enable us to understand the reasons why the clients found the rehabilitation programmes to be satisfactory or unsatisfactory. This information could be useful for improving the programme. In most studies the coding system would be a good deal more elaborate.

Coding and thematic analysis

An alternative approach to using predetermined codes is to develop a coding system that identifies common themes as they emerge from the text. Different qualitative researchers advocate different approaches to coding but it typically involves the following steps. The researchers first study their materials, in this case transcripts, and develop a close familiarity with the material. During this process, all the concepts, themes and ideas are noted to form major categories. Often, the researcher will then attach a label and/or number to each category and record their positions in the transcript. Coding is an iterative process (we retrace our steps), with the researcher coding and recoding as the scheme develops. The researchers, having developed the codes and coded the transcripts, then attempt to interpret their meanings in the context in which they appeared. The reporting of this process typically involves 'thick' or detailed description of the categories and their context, with liberal use of examples from the original transcripts.

Content analysis

Content analysis allows the quantification of units of meaning occurring in a text or a number of texts. Content analysis can be seen as a blending of quantitative and qualitative methods. The recognition and coding of meaning are qualitative, while the counting of the meaningful 'chunks' is quantitative. The 'meaningful chunks' can be words, sentences or paragraphs, that is, the units of language that were coded by the researchers from the narratives and dialogues.

For example, in an unpublished study one of the authors was interested in how leading newspapers were representing the use of stem cells in medical research. The following research questions were asked:

1. How extensive was the newspaper coverage of the medical use of stem cells?
2. What was the attitude of the newspapers (positive, negative or neutral) to the use of stem cells?

In relation to question 1, the data were collected by identifying relevant newspaper articles published on the topic and measuring the length of the columns. They were quantified by counting the number of articles published per month across the selected time interval. The data relevant to question 2 were obtained by identifying statements supportive or critical of using stem cells or simply 'neutral' descriptions of the nature and possible uses of stem cells. The column lengths for each of the three categories were measured and the percentages devoted to each were graphed across the months. Therefore, the content analysis provided evidence for the level of interest and changing attitudes of the media towards the use of stem cells. This evidence was relevant to understanding the cultural context in which government policy for using stem cells was being formulated.

The discussion of content analysis provides a good opportunity for raising the issue of computer-assisted data analysis. As the texts are often transcribed using personal computers the text is available in electronic form. This means that the text can be fed into a software package to assist with its analysis. For example, say that the data representing the contents of a hundred newspaper articles were transcribed into a software package. We could now introduce our codes and identify the segments of the whole text which use the relevant words/phrases/sentences. The segments can then be retrieved, examined or modified (cut and paste) on screen. Also, various frequency counts can be readily performed using software tools.

A detailed discussion for selecting and using computer packages is beyond the scope of the present book. Interested readers might find Liamputtong Rice & Ezzy (1999, pp 202–210) a useful introduction to selecting and using currently available software packages for expediting and improving qualitative data analysis in general (not only for content analysis). Liamputtong Rice & Ezzy have discussed the ambivalent attitude among qualitative researchers to computer-assisted data analysis. A key objection has been the distancing of the researcher from the creativity and surprising insights afforded by the more hands-on approaches. Another objection is that meanings of words and sentences sometimes do not follow dictionary definitions but rather have to be understood in the general context. The true meaning of certain subtle and ambiguous communications can be missed in crude and electronically conducted data analyses.

Content analysis is a technique that combines elements of both qualitative and quantitative approaches. We interpret the meaning of the text for developing our coding strategy for organizing or 'chunking' the text and then we use statistics to describe the quantities of text devoted to a specific point of view. Content analysis can be used to test hypotheses, for example hypotheses addressing media perspectives on embryonic stem cell research.

Thematic analysis, verstehen and grounded theory

Counting and hypothesis testing is not the essence of the qualitative approach. What we are trying to do is to see things from the perspectives of our informants and to explain their actions from their points of view. The German word *verstehen* is often used in phenomenological research to express the notion of 'putting ourselves in someone else's shoes' or attaining a strong empathy with their situation. Empathy with other people might seem quite simple, just something we do as human beings. It is worthwhile remembering, however, that sometimes we misunderstand how people feel or think, even when they are our close friends or family. In the same way, we might misunderstand the points of view of persons who are very different to us in age, gender, education, language and culture. Yet, it is essential to understand the points of views of the people to whom we offer health services. So how does 'verstehen' arise through qualitative health research?

First, as we described earlier, our data collection must use a technique (in-depth interviews, written materials, focus groups, etc.) which enables our respondents to express their point of view. Second, we can adopt a theoretical framework for explaining our understanding of the respondents' experiences. The key point, in the context of *grounded theory*, is that our explanations or theories must emerge inductively from the information provided by our informants. The theory is constructed gradually as more evidence is provided by additional informants. Third, the data are often analysed by coding and thematic analysis as we outlined earlier in this chapter.

A theme is a grouping of ideas or meanings which emerge consistently in the text. The themes emerging from the data illuminate the experiences of the informants and enable us to understand their points of view (verstehen). Let us consider an example of thematic analysis.

In a study titled 'The plight of rural parents caring for adult children with HIV', Fred McGinn (1996) studied the experiences of parents caring for their adult children with acquired immuno-deficiency syndrome/human immuno-deficiency virus (AIDS/HIV). In-depth interviews were conducted with eight mothers and two fathers from rural families involved in this task. The interview transcripts were analysed using a thematic analysis/grounded theory approach (Miles & Huberman 1984).

McGinn extracted three major themes:

1. *Physical and mental problems related to HIV/AIDS*. Here the parents discussed their experiences of their children's problems and the emotional consequences of physical decline and death, e.g:

   'He would fall over, so I would sit him in the wheelchair. And then from within a week in November he went from not being able to sit in the wheelchair to not getting out of bed. And he went from eating little bits of food along with taking a liquid nutrition to just liquid nutrition . . . and then he got to where he wouldn't swallow the liquid nutrition and he subsisted on just water and juices and Pepsi . . . and then in the end he even refused them: he wouldn't take anything . . . He just wasted away.'

2. *Stigma associated with having AIDS*. Because of the mode of transmission of AIDS and superstitious fears of contacting the condition, many of the parents found themselves socially isolated at such a very difficult time of their lives, e.g:

   'That Sunday, I never will forget. I asked him, 'Do you want anybody to know?' And I don't remember if he said no, but his head . . . he almost shook it off. No way did he want anybody to know what the real problem was. But I want you to know that that was a terrible, stressful time. People who came, who normally would be support for me . . . weren't. It was a real traumatic experience.'

3. *Health care*. This theme summarizes the difficulties of accessing necessary health services in rural settings. Even though there were serious deficiencies in health services, one mother reported:

   'As for the hospital, I couldn't have asked for a better hospital. There may have been *nurses who refused to work with him, I don't know, but the nurses that did come in were great . . . They even hugged and kissed him goodbye whenever he got well and left. They didn't act like they didn't want to be around him and I appreciated that. I think that's important.'*

These three themes enable us to understand and empathize with the parents of these very sick young people. Also, they were the bases for recommending improvements in rural health care which directly address the needs of AIDS sufferers and their families in non-metropolitan environments.

Also, we must note that McGinn's paper reported the experiences of people in the mid-1990s, living in rural Canada. With improvements in the treatment and prevention of AIDS and a decrease in the stigma attached to the condition, the experiences of families caring for sufferers have improved. Because of differences and changes in practices and the cultural context, it is always important to note the time at and place in which interpretive research was carried out.

Interpretation and social context

As we have seen, qualitative data analysis is a systematic way of interpreting texts. There are many areas of study (e.g. history, politics, theology) where the interpretation of texts is an essential part of the research process. What these diverse disciplines have in common with qualitative health research is the recognition that the meaning of language and texts must be interpreted in a cultural context.

An example is *hermeneutics*, which is a method that was originally used to analyse the meaning of religious texts. Consider the meaning of the term 'god'. When the Romans spoke of Augustus Caesar as a 'god', they were referring to him as a hero who was immortal in the history of Rome. The use of the term 'god' by a polytheistic is quite different to meanings in the context of contemporary Judaeo–Christian or Muslim traditions.

The meaning of the term must be interpreted in the context of the religious tradition (polytheistic, monotheistic) and the position of the speaker (believer, non-believer).

An important issue in reading texts is that they might have implicit (in addition to explicit) meanings. Semiotics is a method of textual interpretation which seeks to uncover the hidden, omitted meanings implicit in a text. In order to do this, we must adopt a theoretical framework in terms of which we can 'deconstruct' a text. The theoretical framework reflects our understanding of the culture within which the text was produced. You have probably read the book *Animal Farm* by George Orwell. There are several levels at which one can read this story; for example:

- A fairy tale about the imaginary lives of farm animals where animals have human traits and concerns.
- A morality tale in Aesop's style about how power corrupts and leads to betrayal.
- A critique of Stalinism and a retelling of the bloody history of the Bolshevik revolution and its social consequences in the Soviet Union.

In order to identify Orwell's book as a political critique, one needs to understand the historical/cultural context in which the author worked and lived.

To illustrate these points, we will examine a letter to the editor in a Melbourne newspaper by a woman writer who was apparently concerned about the physical and mental health of young men:

They're just asking for it.

Since the weather improved, it seems that young men all over the place are discarding their shirts and going about half-naked. I worry for them. Do they have any idea of what a provocative and inviting image they put across?

To my mind, they would be doing themselves a far greater service if they would just compromise a little and get dressed properly. It might not seem fair, and it might be less comfortable, but at least then there wouldn't any longer be the danger of urge-driven women raping young men because of the confusing visual signals they so often put across.

(In Polgar & Swerissen 2000).

Let us analyse the text consistent with a procedure outlined in Daly et al (1997). First, let us analyse the explicit content of the letter.

1. *Tone*. Serious and condescending as that used by authority figures such as teachers and magistrates; '. . . now, see here young man, this is for your own benefit . . .' type of communication.
2. *Language*. Moralistic (e.g. 'dressed properly', 'going about half-naked') and calling for responsibility ('compromising a little'). Also the language is alarmist, predicting that men non-compliant to a dress code will be assaulted.
3. *The aim*. The explicit aim of the letter is to warn young men of the dire consequences of dressing immodestly and thereby inviting attention by 'urge-driven women'.
4. *Repetition of ideas*. The main idea seems to be that a scantily dressed man is sexually provocative to women. Another notion is that women are struggling to control powerful sexual urges. It is implied that men should accept responsibility for suppressing these urges in women. If men dress immodestly then they have to accept the consequences.
5. *Themes*. The first basic explicit theme is the importance of men taking responsibility in projecting a safe, chaste image. The second is the power and danger of women's sexual urges which can explode into assault when provoked by scantily dressed males. An underlying theme which you might have detected is one of 'blaming the victim'; if men are assaulted it is their fault, they should have been more careful.
6. *Oppositional elements*. If men ignore the letter writer's message and move towards the choice of scanty dress then they are putting themselves at risk. That is, modest dress means safety while immodest dress means assault. Another dichotomy is gender: women are sexually powerful and dangerous; men are presented as naive victims lacking any defined sexuality. In different ways the overt themes emerging from the text are demeaning of both males and females.

You may have different views about how best to interpret the text. As Daly and her colleagues (1997, p. 183) noted: 'Let us now make some basic semiotic moves across the data'. Let us interrogate the 'data' further using the six points suggested by Daly et al (1997).

- Is the content of the letter preposterous? Are there scantily dressed male construction workers being dragged into alleys by out-of-control schoolgirls? Are there gangs of libidinous females cruising our streets with evil purposes on their minds? Preposterous! The incidence of assault by women is, to all intents and purposes, very low, regardless of how men choose to dress. Therefore, the letter is unsound or it may be a parody.
- In order to understand the meaning of the letter, we play a language game as follows: read 'male' for 'female' in the text. The story now reads quite differently; in fact it resembles a more usual story told to women concerning their responsibility for ensuring that men don't assault them.
- One might propose that the latent agenda for the letter was to ridicule the notion that victims are in some way responsible for the violence of the perpetrator.
- The apparent hero of the explicit story was the author, the caring woman dispensing advice to young men to keep themselves safe by dressing in a chaste fashion. In the implicit story the villains are people who blame women for contributing to violence simply by the clothes they wear.
- What is missing from the original story? Or what was introduced? The writer introduced the notion of female sexuality as an urge that could transform at the slightest provocation into violence. If this notion is ludicrous for females, the question is, how can it be tenable for males? You might ask that if the true intention of the author was to denounce myths of male sexuality then why didn't she say so directly? This is like asking why George Orwell wrote a fairy tale with talking farm animals rather than a direct denouncement of totalitarianism and Stalinist terror. It is a question of how we use language; we use metaphors, parables, hyperboles and so on for expressing ourselves in an interesting, colourful fashion. Semiotics is one of the ways for interpreting the meanings that might be hidden or camouflaged in the original narrative.
- A basic principle for semiotic analysis is selecting a theoretical framework in terms of which we can deconstruct the original narrative and identify its hidden, repressed or mystifying elements. The key to the previous analysis was that the basic idea underpinning the argument (that immodestly dressed males are in danger of being assaulted by out-of-control women) was false and absurd.

Our interpretation of the meaning is that the text is a parody of the victim-blaming discourses in patriarchal societies. By adopting a feminist theoretical framework we are in a position to identify the hidden meaning of the text and infer the intentions of the author.

- There is always the possibility that we have misinterpreted the text and misrepresented the intentions of the author. What if she was genuinely concerned about the welfare of young men? The fact of the matter is that there are no absolute guarantees. It might be that, regardless of his well-known interest in political affairs, George Orwell was simply intending to create a children's story when he wrote *Animal Farm*.

In the next part of this chapter we will outline some strategies for ensuring validity and reliability for qualitative research.

The accuracy of qualitative data analysis

How can we be sure that the themes we identified in a text accurately reflect the actual views of the participants? Also, how do we know that similar themes would emerge from the reports of other people who had similar experiences to our sample?

There are a number of qualitative researchers who ensure that the collection and interpretation of their evidence are carried out in a methodologically rigorous fashion. The following represent some of the key methodological criteria for conducting qualitative research (Lincoln & Guba 1985):

1. *Data saturation*. This refers to ensuring that we have collected sufficient data from our respondents. Saturation occurs when the themes and ideas emerging from the text become repetitive and we are confident that the inclusion of new participants or further engagement with current participants will not lead to novel themes or interpretations.
2. *Credibility*. Checking if the interpretation of the evidence is judged as accurate by both the research participants and also independent clinicians or scholars. In other words, does your interpretation make sense and if not, why not?
3. *Auditability*. This refers to each of the steps of the research process being clearly described, so that an independent scholar can critique the research

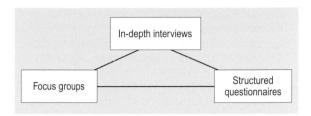

Figure 21.1 • Triangulation using different approaches to data collection.

process from its beginning to the analysis and interpretation of the data. The auditor confirms or rejects the researcher's methodology.

4. *Triangulation*. This strategy involves the use of multiple independent methods for collecting data and checking if the themes and interpretations emerging from these different methods are consistent and matching. For example, in order to evaluate client satisfaction with a health service you might use three different data collection strategies (Fig. 21.1). It is useful (but not essential) to use three different data collection methods. The researcher might, if appropriate, use both qualitative (e.g. in-depth interviews) and quantitative (e.g. structured questionnaires) methods for data collection. These are called 'mixed' designs (see also Chs 1 and 9).

As you can see, the methodological concerns in qualitative research are parallel to those of quantitative research (i.e. reliability and validity). However, because of the differences in the way the two types of research are conducted, the terminology for describing the methodological principles is somewhat different.

Summary

There are different approaches to analysing qualitative data depending on the theoretical framework and data collection strategies adopted by the researchers. However, as we saw in this chapter, there are several common aspects to qualitative data analysis:

- 'Immersion' in the data; reading and re-reading the texts to develop a sense of what it is that respondents are trying to say.

- Developing a coding system and identifying the themes emerging from the text.
- Using these themes as a basis for insight, empathy (verstehen) with the experiences, emotions and thinking of the respondents.
- Interpreting and theorizing the respondents' experiences in the context of cultural or historical settings.
- Ensuring the accuracy of the interpretations by cross-checking themes and explanations with other sources of data, other researchers' interpretations of the data, and the respondents.

Self-assessment

Explain the meaning of the following terms:

auditability
coding
coding and thematic analysis
content analysis
credibility
data saturation
grounded theory
hermeneutics
predetermined coding categories
semiotics
theme
theoretical framework
triangulation
verstehen

True or false

1. Hermeneutics refers to understanding meanings in their cultural contexts.
2. Quantitative data analysis is a far more subjective process than qualitative analysis.
3. Qualitative data analysis is a systematic way of 'reading' another person's mental states.
4. In the context of qualitative data analysis, the term 'text' refers to the transcripts of in-depth interviews, focus groups, etc.
5. Predetermined coding is based on categories of meaning emerging as the texts are analysed.
6. When coding and thematic analysis are carried out together, it is essential to maintain the first coding system chosen to avoid thematic confusion.
7. Content analysis often employs statistical analyses of the data.

8. A basic objection to computer-assisted coding and analysis is that this technique might obscure more subtle meanings communicated by the respondents.
9. 'Verstehen' is a German word referring to the precise dictionary definitions of the words used in a text.
10. A fundamental objective of qualitative data analysis is to enable the researcher to see health-related events from the perspectives of the respondents.
11. A theme is a specific idea which reflects the unique experiences of only one respondent.
12. Hermeneutics is a form of religious practice requiring withdrawal from everyday life.
13. Semiotics requires the adoption of a theoretical framework for identifying hidden meanings in a text.
14. The results of a qualitative study represent experiences which are useless unless they are true for all times and places.
15. 'Auditability' refers to the clarity of the methodology employed in conducting a qualitative research project.
16. 'Data saturation' addresses an issue analogous to external validity in quantitative research.
17. The results of quantitative and qualitative research cannot be compared with each other.
18. As there are no absolute guarantees for the truth of our interpretation of other people's experiences, all qualitative research lacks credibility.
19. Qualitative analyses produce evidence relevant for constructing social theories, but have no relevance to evidence-based health care.
20. In conducting evidence-based health care, we should combine the results of qualitative and quantitative research to identify the best practice for our clients.

Multiple choice

1. Which of the following statements is *not* an aspect of 'intepretivist' approaches?
   a Society exists as the result of meaningful social interactions.
   b It is the actors themselves who are best able to define social situations.
   c A society is defined by the sum of the total behaviours of individuals constituting a population.

d Data collection requires a degree of empathy with the way in which people experience their social situation.

2. Themes are:

 a the planning process used by the researcher

 b organized around interview data

 c the result of the research question

 d ideas represented in a pattern.

3. A qualitative researcher could develop codes for interview data:

 a after conducting all of the interviews

 b before collecting data

 c both before and during data collection

 d all of the above.

4. Latent content of themes in qualitative data refers to:

 a the hidden or underlying themes

 b the second level of data collection

 c what was not said directly in the data

 d both *a* and *c*.

5. Which of the following statements is true in coding data?

 a Words, concepts and themes are selected.

 b The researcher must wait until all data are collected before establishing codes.

 c Concepts are weighted as far more important than themes

 d The researcher must be trained in using a qualitative computer program.

6. In a qualitative study of public perceptions of people with mental illness, you intend to identify the social significance of being perceived as mentally ill. You are well aware that most of your respondents will attempt to *appear* caring and tolerant, even when they hold strong prejudices against people with mental illness. A useful approach for analysing the data in relation to the above question is called:

 a grounded theory

 b semiotic analysis

 c content analysis

 d typological categorization.

7. The term 'grounded theory' refers to:

 a any sociological theory that is based on empirical evidence

 b any theory, sociological or otherwise, that is based on empirical evidence

 c a systematic way of formulating theories which are the sources for empirically testable hypotheses

 d generating and testing interpretive theories during the course of data collection.

8. Generally, an interpretive theory aims to explain:

 a the social causes of human action

 b the experiences of people in the context of their cultural settings

 c why people do what they do

 d the factors which interact in a society for generating human personality.

9. The process of interpreting texts (such as the Bible) in the cultural contexts in which they were written is called:

 a hermeneutics

 b content analysis

 c semiotics

 d discourse analysis.

10. The term 'data saturation' as used in qualitative research is most closely related to what in quantitative research?

 a Sample size.

 b Validity of the evidence.

 c Reliability of the evidence.

 d 'Scaling' of the data (nominal, ordinal, etc.)

11. The term 'triangulation' as used in qualitative research is most closely related to what in quantitative research?

 a Reliability.

 b Validity.

 c Hypothesis testing.

 d Descriptive data analysis.

12. Which of the following is *not* a traditional approach to qualitative research?

 a Ethnomethodology.

 b Grounded theory.

 c Phrenology.

 d Phenomenology.

Chapter Twenty Two

22

Presentation of health science research

Introduction

Knowledge in the health sciences is the sum of the individual efforts of investigators working all over the world. Professional journals in science and health care provide the dominant medium for disseminating information about the outcome of specific investigations. Investigators must report their procedures and results in an accurate and complete fashion. In this chapter, we outline the format and style generally followed for presenting the results of empirical investigations.

The specific aims of this chapter are to:

1. Describe the conventional way in which quantitative research is presented for publication.
2. Discuss the style or language used to describe research.
3. Outline briefly the way in which research papers are selected for publication.

The structure of research publications

The format of a professional publication reporting empirical research reflects the stages of the

Table 22.1 Format of research publications and the research process

Publication format	Research process
Title	
Abstract	
Introduction	Research planning

Method:
  Subjects
  Apparatus
  Procedure
	Design
	
	Measurement

Results	Descriptive statistics Inferential statistics
Discussion	Interpretation of the data
References	
Appendices	

research process discussed in this book. Table 21.1 represents the relationship between the stages of research and the commonly used publication format. This format is generally used to report quantitative empirical research, although you will find that some variations on this theme are adopted by some professional journals. This format is not necessarily followed for certain types of scholarly communications, such as for qualitative research, theoretical papers or literature reviews. In the subsections following, we examine in detail each of the components of a research report shown in Table 21.1.

Title and abstract

The *title* is a descriptive sentence stating the exact topic of the report. Many titles of research reports take one of the following two forms:

- *y* as a function of *x*
- the effect of *x* upon *y*.

In causal research, such as experiments, *y* refers to the dependent variable being measured

and *x* refers to the independent variable being manipulated. For example:

- The incidence of alcoholism in health professionals as a function of work-related stress.
- The effect of major tranquillizers on the cognitive functioning of persons with schizophrenia.

For descriptive or qualitative research the title should inform the reader about the groups being studied and the characteristics being reported, for example: 'The attitudes of physicians to the professional functions of podiatrists'. In general, titles should be concise and informative, enabling a prospective reader to identify the nature of the investigation. Immediately below the title should appear the name(s) of the investigator(s) and affiliation.

The *abstract* is a short (not more than 250 words) description of the entire report. The purpose of this section is to provide the reader with a general overview of the communication. It should provide enough details to enable the reader to decide whether or not the article is of interest. This section can be difficult to write because of its precise nature. When writing an abstract you should include:

1. A brief statement about previous findings which led you to conduct your own research.
2. The hypothesis and/or aim of your research.
3. Methods, including subjects, apparatus and procedure.
4. A short description of what you found and how you interpreted your results.
5. What you concluded.

In some journals, this section may appear at the end of the manuscript in the form of a summary. For our purposes, however, we will treat this section as an abstract.

The title and the abstract together are important and should contain key words that enable the efficient retrieval of the information.

Introduction

The introduction is equivalent to the planning stages of research, discussed in Section 2. A good introduction will set the stage for the hypotheses being tested. It should do this by discussing the theoretical background of the problem under consideration and evaluating the relevant research done previously. The introduction thus serves as a link between the past and the present.

Generally, all aspects of the literature cannot be covered in a relatively brief research paper, therefore the review of past research is done with a bias towards only those aspects of the problem which are of direct relevance to your report. In this way the hypotheses being tested can be derived in a logical manner. For this reason, a good introduction starts out by making a few general statements about the field of research, leading logically to a narrow and specific set of statements which represent the aims or hypotheses. The final paragraph of the introduction should state the precise aims or the hypotheses being investigated.

Method

The purpose of the method section is to inform the reader of how the investigation was carried out. It is important to remember that the method section should contain enough detail to enable another researcher to replicate your investigation. (Of course, replications may not be feasible for a unique event, such as a case study of a specific individual.) Conventionally, three subsections are used: subjects, apparatus and procedure.

- *Subjects*. Three questions must be answered concerning the subjects: who were they, how many were there and how were they selected? Specific information must be given concerning the subjects, as results may vary from one sample to another.
- *Apparatus*. A description of all equipment, including questionnaires, etc., used in the research must be provided. If it is commercially available, provide the reader with the manufacturer's name and the commercial identification of the equipment. Alternatively, if the equipment was privately made, provide the reader with enough information to allow replication. Measurements and perhaps a diagram will be necessary.
- *Procedure*. Once again, this section should provide enough information for other researchers to replicate the investigation. Details of how the research was carried out should include how subjects were assigned to groups, how many subjects per group, the experimental procedure and a description of how the data were collected.

In a sense, the method section should read like a cookbook. The 'subjects' subsection describes the ingredients. The 'apparatus' subsection describes the equipment necessary for baking (note we did not say 'cooking' the experiment) and, finally, the 'procedure' subsection describes how the ingredients were mixed to produce the final outcome: the results section.

Results

The results section presents the findings of the investigation and draws attention to points of interest. Raw data and statistical calculations are not presented in this section. Rather, we use the principles of descriptive and inferential statistics to present the summarized and analysed data: graphs, tables and the outcomes of statistical tests are presented in this section. It is essential that all the findings are presented and that the graphs and tables are correctly identified.

Discussion

The discussion section restates the aim(s) of the investigation and discusses your results with reference to the aims or experimental hypothesis stated in the introduction. Did you find what you expected? How do the present results relate to previous research?

It is important to remember that one experiment in isolation cannot make or break a theory or establish the effectiveness of a practice. Thus, the discussion should connect the findings with similar studies and especially with the theory underlying such studies. If unexpected results were obtained, possible reasons for the outcome (such as faulty design and controls) should be discussed. By this, the discussion will point the way to further problems which remain to be solved. Unconstructive, negative or unimportant criticism should be avoided, so that the report does not end with long discussions of possible reasons for the outcome. Brief, concise discussion is more appropriate.

In the conclusion, which is usually the last paragraph of the discussion section, the main findings are summarized and suggestions made for further research. For example, you may have demonstrated certain phenomena which may have implications for explaining broader concepts which can be empirically tested. You are therefore taking your findings and generalizing them to phenomena not directly tested in the present research.

References and appendices

It is expected that all the literature discussed in the paper is listed in the references section. This enables your reader to evaluate your sources. You should refer to appropriate style manuals for information on how references should be listed. Sufficient information must be provided for an interested reader to be able to identify and retrieve the sources. In addition, a report may include labelled appendices. These might include a full description of questionnaires or other measuring instruments, raw data or statistical calculations if required.

The style of research publications

It is essential that you read research publications in your professional area to gain a 'feel' for the appropriate style of writing. In general, the following points should be kept in mind when writing reports:

1. Avoid long phrases or complicated sentences. Short, simple sentences are far more easily understood by your reader. In other words, try not to posture but to communicate.
2. Use quotations sparingly; put ideas in your own words. Quotations are only used when it is necessary to convey precisely the ideas of another researcher, for instance while conducting a critique of a paper.
3. Use past tense when writing your research report.
4. Use an objective style, avoiding personal pronouns wherever possible.
5. Make sure you are writing to your audience; if the material is specialized or difficult, explain it clearly.
6. Make sure that you are concise and clear; do not introduce issues and concepts which are not strictly relevant to reporting your investigation.

Raising interesting but superfluous issues might distract and confuse your reader.

In general, you should aim to improve your report writing and your ability to communicate your findings and ideas by seeking constructive criticism from your colleagues and supervisors.

The publication process

The formal knowledge representing the empirical and professional basis for your professional practice is in large part stored in journals, books and conference reports. Journals are published by appropriate professional associations, government departments or private companies. Having completed a research project, how does one publish it in a professional journal? After all, the value of research is negligible if it is not made public.

In general, the prospective author will:

1. Select a professional or scientific journal appropriate for the material.
2. Present the research report in a format required by the journal.
3. Send the completed manuscript to the journal's editor.

The editor is generally a person of high standing in a given scientific or professional area. If the article is judged as being appropriate for the journal, the editor will send the article to two or more referees and, on the basis of the referees' reports, publish or reject the manuscript. Sometimes the referees recommend certain additions or changes which have to be made by the author before the manuscript is judged to be publishable.

Therefore, when you read research publications in refereed journals, you can be confident that the articles have been scrutinized by experts. However, as shown in the next subsection, this does not necessarily guarantee the truth of either the evidence or the conclusions.

Ethics of presenting research

The health science researcher has an obligation to publish honest and accurate results that would not harm those people who participated in the research.

Most ethics committees in health care institutions and universities have the twin objectives of not only advancing knowledge for the common good but also preventing harm to those participating in the research. This is particularly so in the situation where the participants may have a diminished capacity to consent freely to their involvement (e.g. children or people who are unconscious or seriously ill). It is crucial to maintain the dignity and confidentiality of participants in health research.

Therefore, in the process of ethical evaluation of health science research, the researcher can expect to be closely questioned on these issues. If the researcher cannot convince the ethics committee that the research will deliver knowledge for the common good and that it will not harm the participants, then the research will not usually proceed.

In research performed for a higher degree, many universities will not accept a thesis without an accompanying ethical clearance from the relevant ethics committee. Most hospitals and universities have strict ethical procedures that must be followed before any research work is commenced by their staff. Most, if not all, health research grant bodies require an ethical clearance before they will release the funds to successful applicants. Many journals also require certification from the researcher that the work complies with ethical principles. It is likely that this trend towards tightening of procedures will continue.

The ultimate unethical act is to manufacture data. Broad & Wade (1982), in their book *Betrayers of the Truth*, describe this problem. It would seem to be a growing problem that may be associated with the 'publish or perish' requirements placed upon health science researchers by granting bodies and employers.

In the health sciences, it is not only the participants in research who may be harmed or assisted by the research. If an erroneous research finding is widely applied, it may harm many thousands of people. Ethics are therefore not simply concerned with whether the researcher has good intentions and treats the research participants well; there is also the issue of competence. Poorly designed research is unethical in that it may bring great harm to others. Thus, the ethical researcher must also be a competent researcher.

Summary

In this chapter we outlined the general format followed by researchers for publishing their results. The format is related to the logical steps of planning, conducting and interpreting research. The style involves clarity, accuracy and sufficient completeness for colleagues to understand or replicate the research project. Research is published in journals, which are generally edited by persons of high standing in the field. Every effort is made by editors to ensure the validity of the research published in their journals. The individual researcher is also ethically bound to report findings in an unbiased and truthful fashion.

Although the format and style outlined in this chapter might seem rather arduous, poor presentation may destroy the intrinsic value of a research project.

Self-assessment

Explain the meaning of the following terms:

abstract
apparatus
discussion
method
plagiarism
procedure
refereed journal
subjects

True or false

1. As a rule, the title of a research investigation should not contain more than seven words.
2. Generally, the research hypothesis should be presented in the introduction.
3. A research report should contain sufficient information so that the investigation can be replicated.

4. The results section should contain all computational details for each statistic.

5. The abstract should normally contain the key tables of the results.

6. The design of an investigation influences the content of the method section.

7. All the names and addresses of your subjects must be published to enable replication of your investigation.

8. Quotations should be used sparingly in a research report.

9. A research report should be written in the past tense.

10. The outcomes of statistical analyses are reported in the results section.

11. Scientists do not normally report the results of their investigations, in case their work is stolen or misrepresented.

12. Calculations are best presented in appendices.

13. The 'referees' are hired by the investigator in order to convince the editor that an investigation should be published.

14. The role of an editor for a scientific journal is to censor research publications for pornographic, blasphemous or politically undesirable material.

15. Good research is unique and cannot be replicated.

16. A researcher should report data even if it is inconsistent with the researcher's original preconceptions.

17. Scientific and professional journals are important for disseminating and storing knowledge.

18. Fortunately, there have been no major scandals concerning scientists publishing fabricated data.

19. Provided that the results are statistically significant, there is no need to present descriptive statistics.

Multiple choice

1. Scientific journals:
   a only publish empirical evidence
   b depend on the services of referees to comment on the validity of the research project
   c publish only true knowledge
   d b and c.

2. The literature review is normally found in which section of a research report?
   a Abstract.
   b Introduction.

c Discussion.
d References.

3. A literature review for a research report should:
   a contain a detailed review of all previously published reports
   b contain a selective review of evidence pertinent to the current research project
   c be at least 5000 words
   d a and c
   e b and c.

4. Which of the following is most inadequate as a title for a research report?
   a The effects of the twentieth century culture on being human: an empirical evaluation of personal functioning in declining cultures.
   b Electrical stimulation of the limbic system: effects on emotion and memory.
   c A survey of the incidence of mental illness in the London metropolitan area.
   d Popularity, friendship selection and specific peer interaction among children.

5. The methods section of a research report:
   a informs the reader of the purpose of an investigation
   b informs the reader about the state of methodological advances in the subject area
   c informs the reader as to how the investigation was carried out
   d informs the reader as to how the hypothesis or aim of the investigation was formulated.

6. When writing a scientific report one should:
   a make sure the introduction contains 250 words or less
   b use personal pronouns as much as possible
   c try to impress the readers by one's level of general knowledge
   d use the past tense.

7. In which part of a research report are the descriptive and inferential statistics normally reported?
   a Abstract.
   b Results.
   c Discussion.
   d Appendices.

8. In writing a discussion, one should:
   a relate the results to findings reported in previous publications
   b establish if the results of the investigation supported the hypothesis

c neither *a* nor *b*

d both *a* and *b*.

9. Which of the following statements is true?

  a The discussion section should relate present findings to previous research.

  b The literature review should be conducted in a special appendix labelled 'references'.

  c The results section should contain only tables and graphs, but not any verbal descriptions of the data.

  d All the above statements are true.

  e None of the above statements are true.

10. Which of the following statements is false?

  a The abstract should be a brief summary of the research.

  b It is unethical to fabricate data.

  c A refereed journal is one in which experts independently evaluate a research report before it is published.

  d A well-designed research project need not have a procedure section.

Chapter Twenty Three

Critical evaluation of published research

CHAPTER CONTENTS

Introduction

By the time a research report is published in a refereed journal, it has been critically scrutinized by several experts and, usually, changes have been made to the initial text by the author(s) to respond to the referees' comments. Nevertheless, even this thorough evaluation procedure doesn't necessarily guarantee the validity of the design or the conclusions presented in a published paper. Ultimately, you as a health professional must be responsible for judging the validity and relevance of published material to your own clinical activities. The evidence-based practice movement focuses on the ways in which practitioners can incorporate better procedures into their practice based upon well-founded research and evaluation evidence. The systematic review processes employed by bodies such as the Cochrane and Campbell Collaborations are intended to assist clinicians in the selection of interventions that are well proven (Ch. 24).

The proper attitude to take with published material, including systematic reviews, is hard-nosed scepticism, notwithstanding the authority of the source. This attitude is based on our understanding of the uncertain and provisional nature of scientific and professional knowledge. In addition, health researchers deal with the investigation of complex phenomena, where it is often impossible for ethical reasons to exercise the desired levels of control or to collect crucial information required to arrive at definitive conclusions. The aim of critical evaluation is to identify the strengths and weaknesses of a research publication, so as to ensure that patients receive assessment and treatment based on the best available evidence.

The aim of this chapter is to demonstrate how select concepts in research design, analysis and measurement can be applied to the critical evaluation of published research. The chapter is organized around the evaluation of specific sections of research publications.

The specific aims of this chapter are to:

1. Examine the criteria used for the critical evaluation of a research paper.
2. Discuss the implications of identifying problems in design and analysis in a given publication.
3. Outline briefly strategies for summarizing and analysing evidence from a set of papers.
4. Discuss the implications of critical evaluation of research for health care practices.

Critical evaluation of the introduction

The introduction of a paper essentially reflects the planning of the research. Inadequacies in this section might signal that the research project was erroneously conceived or poorly planned. The following issues are essential for evaluating this section.

Adequacy of the literature review

The literature review must be sufficiently complete so as to reflect the current state of knowledge in the area. Key papers should not be omitted, particularly when their results could have direct relevance to the research hypotheses or aims. Researchers must be unbiased in presenting evidence that is unfavourable to their personal points of view. This is why we now have systematic review procedures, such as those utilized by the Cochrane Collaboration, so as to avoid inappropriate and biased exclusion or inclusion of work that supports or challenges a point of view favoured by the researcher or other researchers who hold contrary opinions. Poor review of the literature could lead to the unfortunate situation of repeating research or making mistakes that could have been avoided if the previous work's findings had been incorporated into formulation of the research design.

Clearly defined aims or hypotheses

As stated in Chapter 2, the aims or hypotheses of the research should be clearly stated. If this clarity in expression of the aims is lacking, then the rest of the paper will be compromised. In a quantitative research project, it is usual to see a statement of the hypotheses as well as the research aims. All research, whether qualitative or quantitative, should have a clear and recognizable statement of aim(s).

Selection of an appropriate research strategy

In formulating the aims of the investigation, the researcher must have taken into account the appropriate research strategy. For instance, if the demonstration of causal effects is required, a survey may be inappropriate for satisfying the aims of the research. If the purpose of the study is to explore the personal interpretations and meanings of participants then a qualitative strategy will be best. Some researchers now advocate mixed designs where multiple studies are performed to examine different perspectives of the same issues. Thus in a study of views concerning health practices, a focus group discussion may also be accompanied by a structured questionnaire even within the same study sample, so that the findings from each may be used to inform the total understanding of the research issue(s) under study.

Selection of appropriate variables/ information to be collected

In a quantitative study, if the selection of the variables is inappropriate to the aims or questions being investigated, then the investigation will not produce useful results. Similarly, in a qualitative study, the information to be collected must be appropriate to the research aims and questions.

Critical evaluation of the methods section

A well-documented methods section is a necessary condition for understanding, evaluating and perhaps replicating a research project. In general, the critical evaluation of this section will allow a judgment of the validity of the investigation to be made.

Research subjects/participants

This section shows if the study participants were representative of the intended target group or population and the adequacy of the sampling model used.

Sampling model used

In Chapter 3, we outlined a number of sampling models that can be employed to optimize the representativeness of a study sample. If the sampling model is inappropriate, then the sample might be unrepresentative, raising questions concerning the external validity of the research findings. In qualitative research, although the participant sampling method may be less formal than in a quantitative study, the issue of participant representativeness is still pertinent in terms of being able to apply the results more broadly.

Sample size/number of participants

Use of a small sample is not necessarily a fatal flaw of an investigation, if the sample is representative. However, given a highly variable, heterogeneous population, a small sample will not be adequate to ensure representativeness (Ch. 3). Also, a small sample size could decrease the power of the statistical analysis in a quantitative study (Ch. 20). As discussed in the qualitative sampling section of this text, unlike in quantitative sampling procedures, there is not widespread agreement among qualitative researchers as to the issue of how many participants are needed in such studies.

Description of the study participants

A clear description of key participant characteristics (for example age, sex, type and severity of their condition) should be provided. When necessary and possible, demographic information concerning the population from which the participants have been drawn should be provided. If not, the reader cannot adequately judge the representativeness of the sample.

Instruments/apparatus/tools

The validity and reliability of observations and/or measurements are fundamental characteristics of good research. In this section, the investigator must demonstrate the adequacy of the tools used for the data collection.

Validity and reliability

The investigator should use standardized tools, or establish the validity and reliability of new tools used. A lack of proven validity and reliability will raise questions about the adequacy of the research findings.

Description of tools

A full description of the structure and use of novel tools should be presented so that they can be replicated by independent parties.

Procedure

A full description of how the investigation was carried out is required for both replication and for the evaluation of its internal and external validity. This requirement applies to both qualitative and quantitative studies.

Adequacy of the design

It was stated previously that a good design should minimize alternative conflicting interpretations of the data collected. For quantitative research aimed at studying causal relationships, poor design will result in uncontrolled influences by extraneous variables, muddying the identification of causal effects. In Section 3, we looked at a variety of threats to internal validity which must be considered when critically evaluating an investigation.

In a qualitative study the theoretical approach taken in the study design or approach should be clearly stated.

Control groups

In quantitative research a common way of controlling for extraneous effects is the use of control groups (such as placebo, no treatment, conventional treatment). If control groups are not employed, then the internal validity of the investigation might be questioned. Also, if placebo or untreated groups are not present, the size of the effect due to the treatments might be difficult to estimate.

Subject assignment

When using an experimental design, care must be taken in the assignment of subjects so as to avoid significant initial differences between treatment groups. Even when quasi-experimental or natural comparison strategies are used, care must be taken to establish the equivalence of the groups.

Treatment parameters

It is important to describe all the treatments given to the different groups. If the treatments differ in intensity, or the administering personnel take different approaches, the internal validity of the project is threatened. The adherence of the study in the delivery of the intervention to the intended intervention is sometimes called *treatment fidelity*.

Rosenthal and Hawthorne effects

Whenever possible, intervention studies should use double- or single-blind procedures. If the participants, researchers or observers are aware of the aims and predicted outcomes of the investigation, then the validity of the investigation will be threatened through bias and expectancy effects. In qualitative research, it is very important that the research findings are not unduly influenced by the personal positions of the researchers in a way that obscures the meanings and interpretations of the research participants. Of course, the position of the researcher in any study, whether qualitative or quantitative, will to some extent influence the findings but this needs to be kept to a minimum.

Settings

The setting in which a study is carried out has implications for external (ecological) validity. An adequate description of the setting is necessary for evaluating the generalizability of the findings. The context of the investigation may have important effects on the study outcomes. Research conducted in the investigator's lab or office may yield different results to the same work conducted in the field.

Times of treatments and observations

In intervention studies the sequence of any treatments and observations must be clearly indicated, so that issues such as series and confounding effects can be detected. Identification of variability in treatment and observation times can influence the internal validity of experimental, quasi-experimental or $n = 1$ designs, resulting in, for instance, internal validity problems.

Critical evaluation of the results

The results should represent a sound and, where appropriate, statistically correct summary and analysis of the data. Inadequacies in this section could indicate that inferences drawn by the investigator were erroneous.

Tables and graphs

Data should be correctly tabulated or drawn and adequately labelled for interpretation. Complete summaries of all the relevant findings should be presented.

Selection of statistics

Where appropriate both descriptive and inferential statistics must be selected according to specific rules. The selection of inappropriate statistics could distort the findings and lead to inappropriate inferences.

Calculation of statistics

Clearly, both descriptive and inferential statistics must be correctly calculated. The use of computers generally ensures this, although some attention must be paid to gross errors when evaluating the data presented.

Methods of qualitative analysis

The methods chosen must complement the theoretical approach taken in the study and be performed according to the specified protocols.

Critical evaluation of the discussion

In the discussion, investigators draw inferences from the information or data they have collected in relation to the initial aims, questions, and/or hypotheses of the investigation. Unless the inferences are correctly made, the conclusions drawn might lead to useless and dangerous treatments being offered to clients.

Drawing correct inferences from the collected information/data

The inferences from the collected information or data must take into account the limitations of the study and the analytical methods used to analyse them. In the quantitative domain we have seen, for instance in Chapter 16, that correlations do not necessarily imply causation, or that a lack of significance in the statistical analysis could imply a Type II error or incorrect missing of a real trend or finding (see Ch. 20). In the qualitative domain, the findings must follow reasonably from the information collected in the investigation according to the paradigm used.

Logically correct interpretations of the findings

Interpretations of the findings must follow from the information collected, without extraneous evidence being introduced. For instance, if the investigation used a single-participant design, the conclusions should not claim that a procedure is generally useful for the entire population.

Research protocol deviations

In interpreting the data or information collected in a study, the investigator must indicate, and take into account, unexpected deviations from the intended research protocols. For instance, in a quantitative study a placebo/active treatment code might be broken, or 'contamination' between control and experimental groups might be discovered.

In a qualitative study, it could be that participants have conversed with each other about the research prior to one of the participants completing participation. If such deviations are discovered by investigators they are obliged to report these, so that the implications for the results might be taken into account.

Generalization from the findings

Strictly speaking, the data obtained from a given sample are generalizable only to the population from which the participants were drawn. This point is sometimes ignored by investigators and the findings are generalized to subjects or situations which were not considered in the original sampling plan. Qualitative researchers may vary in their willingness to claim generalizability of their findings outside the actual research participants but this must also be systematically considered.

Statistical and clinical significance

As was explained in Chapter 22, in quantitative studies, obtaining statistical significance does not necessarily imply that the results of an investigation are clinically applicable or useful. In deciding on clinical significance, factors such as the size of the effect, side effects and cost-effectiveness, as well as value judgments concerning outcome, must be considered.

Theoretical significance

It is necessary to relate the results of an investigation to previous relevant findings that have been identified in the literature review. Unless the results are logically related to the literature, the theoretical significance of the investigation remains unclear. The processes involved in comparing the findings of a set of related papers are introduced in the next subsection.

Table 23.1 summarizes some of the potential problems, and their implications, which might emerge in the context-critical evaluation of an investigation. A point which must be kept in mind is that, even where an investigation is flawed, useful knowledge might be drawn from it. The aim of critical analysis is not to discredit or tear down published work, but to ensure that the reader

Table 23.1 Checklist for evaluating published research

Problems which might be identified	Possible implications in a research article
1. Inadequate literature review	Misrepresentation of the conceptual basis for the research
2. Vague aims or hypotheses	Research might lack direction; interpretation of evidence might be ambiguous
3. Inappropriate research strategy	Findings might not be relevant to the problem being investigated
4. Inappropriate variables selected	Measurements might not be related to concepts being investigated
5. Inadequate sampling method	Sample might be biased; investigation could lack external validity
6. Inadequate sample size	Sample might be biased; statistical analysis might lack power
7. Inadequate description of sample	Application of findings to specific groups or individuals might be difficult
8. Instruments lack validity or reliability	Findings might represent measurement errors
9. Inadequate design	Investigation might lack internal validity; i.e. outcomes might be due to uncontrolled extraneous variables
10. Lack of adequate control groups	Investigation might lack internal validity; size of the effect difficult to estimate
11. Biased subject assignment	Investigation might lack internal validity
12. Variations or lack of control of treatment parameters	Investigation might lack internal validity
13. Observer bias not controlled (Rosenthal effects)	Investigation might lack internal and external validity
14. Subject expectations not controlled (Hawthorne effects)	Investigation might lack internal and external validity
15. Research carried out in inappropriate setting	Investigation might lack ecological validity
16. Confounding of times at which observations and treatments are carried out	Possible series effects; investigation might lack internal validity
17. Inadequate presentation of descriptive statistics	The nature of the empirical findings might not be comprehensible
18. Inappropriate statistics used to describe and/or analyse data	Distortion of the decision process; false inferences might be drawn
19. Erroneous calculation of statistics	False inferences might be drawn
20. Drawing incorrect inferences from the data analysis (e.g. Type II error)	False conclusions might be made concerning the outcome of an investigation
21. Protocol deviations	Investigation might lack external or internal validity
22. Over-generalization of findings	External validity might be threatened
23. Confusing statistical and clinical significance	Treatments lacking clinical usefulness might be encouraged
24. Findings not logically related to previous research findings	Theoretical significance of the investigation remains doubtful

understands its implications and limitations with respect to theory and practice.

Summary

The critical evaluation of published material at a level of detail suggested by this chapter can be a time-consuming, even pedantic, task. One undertakes such detailed analysis only when professional communications are of key importance, for example, when writing a formal literature review or when evaluating current evidence for adopting a new intervention or approach. Nevertheless, it is a necessary process for an in-depth understanding of the empirical and theoretical basis of your clinical practice.

Even when some problems are identified with a given research report, it is nevertheless likely that the report will provide some useful additional knowledge. Given the problems of generalization, an individual research project is usually insufficient for firmly deciding upon the truth of a hypothesis or the usefulness of a clinical intervention. Rather, as we will see in Chapter 24, the reader needs to scrutinize the range of relevant research and summarize the evidence using qualitative and quantitative review methods. In this way, individual research results can be evaluated in the context of the research area. Disagreements or controversies are ultimately useful for generating hypotheses for guiding new research and for advancing theory and practice.

Self-assessment

Explain the meaning of the following terms:

critical evaluation
protocol deviation

True or false

1. Critical analysis of a publication aims to identify the internal and external validity of the investigation.
2. If an investigation is published in a reputable journal by established investigators then the validity of the investigation can be taken for granted.
3. Random assignment of subjects to treatment groups ensures that the investigation uncovers causal effects.
4. The outcome of an investigation can be useful even with a small sample size.
5. If an investigation produces statistically significant results, its design must have been adequate.
6. Obtaining statistical significance in an investigation is a condition for the demonstration of the clinical significance of a quantitative study.
7. The replication of an investigation demonstrates the internal validity of the original investigation.
8. Without adequate controls the size of an effect might be difficult to estimate.
9. If a study is internally valid, the investigator is justified in generalizing the results to any other population.
10. Provided that the outcomes are statistically significant, it doesn't matter which statistical tests were chosen to analyse the data.
11. If the design of an investigation is inadequate, none of the empirical findings are of scientific or clinical use.
12. Controversies in an area of science usually reflect the presence of fraudulently published evidence.
13. One of the problems with using human subjects for research is the expectations of the subjects concerning the purpose of the investigation.
14. Even poorly planned research can provide some useful results.
15. The application of the scientific method ensures the validity of a researcher's conclusions.
16. Disagreements among researchers in an area are useful for generating new hypotheses.

Multiple choice

1. The aim of the critical analysis of a publication is to:
   a identify the relevance of the results for clinical practice
   b identify the internal and external validity of the investigation
   c identify and attack incompetent researchers in one's area of interest
   d a and b.

2. If the internal validity of a study is adequate, then:
   a   the results will be statistically significant
   b   the results will be clinically useful
   c   the investigation may demonstrate causal effects
   d   a and b.

3. Say that an investigation has generated some interesting findings. However, you find that the investigators selected an inappropriate statistical test to analyse their findings. You should:
   a   regretfully discard the study as useless
   b   re-analyse the data from the descriptive statistics provided
   c   write to the investigators for their raw data, and re-analyse yourself
   d   b or c.

4. The reason one should evaluate the 'literature' as a whole is to:
   a   identify general patterns of findings in the area
   b   condense results from related papers into a single statistic
   c   identify and attempt to explain controversies in the area
   d   all of the above.

5. In judging the clinical significance of a well-designed investigation one should consider:
   a   the cost-effectiveness of the interventions
   b   the size of the therapeutic effects
   c   the possible undesirable side effects of the treatment
   d   all of the above.

An investigation was carried out in order to show that 'prepared childbirth' was an effective method for reducing pain during delivery. Ninety women attending a large hospital constituted the sample. Sixty of the women chose to participate in childbirth preparation, based on the Lamaze method, provided by trained instructors working at the hospital. This method encourages 'natural' (drug-free) childbirth through teaching physical and mental strategies for coping with pain or discomfort occurring during childbirth. The other 30 women chose not to attend the childbirth preparation programme. The level of pain experienced was assessed on the McGill Pain Questionnaire, which has been shown to be a valid and reliable interval scale for pain. It was administered following the childbirth. In addition the number of women seeking analgesia during childbirth was recorded as a measure of levels of discomfort experienced. The results for the investigation are as shown in the table below.

Questions 6–14 refer to the above investigation.

6. The strategy for the investigation is best described as:
   a   an experiment
   b   a quasi-experiment
   c   a correlational study
   d   an $n = 90$ design.

7. One of the problems with the above investigation was that:
   a   the subjects could not be randomly assigned to treatment groups
   b   the dependent variable was irrelevant to the aims
   c   basic ethical issues were not considered
   d   the instructors teaching the Lamaze method were incompetent.

8. From the information given above, it is clear that the investigators controlled for:
   a   Hawthorne effects
   b   Rosenthal effects
   c   subject assignment
   d   none of the above.

Groups	Mean pain scores	Number given medication
Women with no training ($n = 30$)	38	24
Women with childbirth preparation ($n = 60$)	32	49
	(The difference was statistically significant at $\alpha = 0.05$)	(The difference was not statistically significant at $\alpha = 0.05$)

9. If you wanted to calculate the proportion of women with no training who had greater McGill pain scores than women with childbirth preparation, then the required statistics are:
   a the distribution of t for $n = 98$
   b the normal distribution
   c the indices for reliability and validity
   d the standard deviations for the two groups.

10. Which of the following statistical tests is most appropriate for analysing the significance of the data for the McGill pain scores?
   a Mann–Whitney U
   b Sign test
   c z test for two means
   d χ^2 test.

11. Which of the following statistical tests is most appropriate for analysing the significance of the data for women requiring medication?
   a Mann–Whitney U
   b Sign test
   c t test for two means
   d χ^2 test.

12. The lack of statistical significance for the data on medication implies that:
   a the power for the test may have been too low

   b equal sample sizes should have been used
   c training has no effect
   d both a and c.

13. The outcome of this investigation can be generalized to:
   a women having children and undergoing Lamaze training
   b women having children without Lamaze training
   c women who choose the type of childbirth they undergo
   d none of the above groups.

14. Considering the evidence provided, one concludes that:
   a prepared childbirth is a waste of time
   b there is evidence that Lamaze preparation at this hospital results in statistically significant reductions in pain during delivery
   c women undergoing childbirth find Lamaze preparation useless at this hospital
   d a and c.

Chapter Twenty Four

24

Synthesis of research evidence

Introduction

The research papers published in scientific and professional peer-reviewed journals contain the basic information currently available for understanding the causes and consequences of health problems. Each research publication contributes to the overall knowledge regarding a health problem. However, given the problems of generalization, an individual research project is usually insufficient for firmly deciding the truth of a hypothesis or the efficacy of a clinical intervention. In order to understand the progress of a research programme (Ch. 1) we need to compare, contrast and synthesize the results of related research papers. Consistent results across diverse research reports are the most appropriate bases for justifying the delivery of health services.

The term literature refers to the set of publications containing the network of theories, hypotheses, practices and evidence representing the current state of knowledge in a specific area of the health sciences. A literature review contains both the critical evaluation of the individual publications and the identification of emergent trends and patterns of evidence. The literature review is a synthesis of the available knowledge in an area and therefore constitutes the strongest foundations for initiating further advances in theory and practice.

The overall aim of this chapter is to outline the basic strategies used for synthesizing evidence and producing a literature review.

The specific aims of the chapter are to:

1. Identify the basic methodological principles relevant to writing a health sciences review.
2. Describe the process for conducting a systematic review.
3. Explain how to interpret the findings of a published meta-analysis.
4. Explain the uses and limitations of systematic reviews and meta-analyses.

Basic principles

The first thing to consider is that writing a literature review is a demanding intellectual challenge. The facts do not 'speak' for themselves. Rather, the evidence has to be extracted, critically evaluated, organized and synthesized into a logical, coherent representation of the current state of knowledge. For example, consider the review by Olanow (2004) tilted 'The scientific basis for the current treatment of Parkinson's disease'. This relatively brief 15-page review is based on only 75 references, although there are thousands of research papers, articles and reports available on the anatomy, physiology and treatment of Parkinson's disease. In writing the review, the author had to make a series of expert judgments regarding which were the nine key papers, containing the most salient, up-to-date information for understanding the medical treatment of Parkinson's disease.

Second, the outcome of the review process is influenced by the theoretical orientation and professional background of the reviewer. Olanow, a leading neurologist, provided an authoritative review written from a biomedical perspective. In contrast, a physiotherapist working in neurological rehabilitation might take a different conceptual approach to the causes and treatment of Parkinson's disease. He or she might place more emphasis on psychological and social factors as integral components of the etiology and treatment of Parkinson's disease.

Third, the selection, analysis, critique and synthesis of the materials is an active, interpretive process drawing on the personal experiences, interests and values of the reviewer. Even if their professional backgrounds were identical, there are no guarantees that two reviewers interpreting the evidence from the same set of publications will arrive at exactly the same conclusions. Depending on how these reviewers approached the subject matter, they might emphasize different aspects of the evidence or select different patterns in the data as being important, resulting in different syntheses. In Chapter 1, we discussed the post-positivist position that theories and preconceptions can influence our perceptions of what is happening in the world, and therefore shape the way in which we construct knowledge.

Last, the notion that we all have our experiences, opinions and prejudices does not imply that 'anything goes' when writing health sciences reviews. On the contrary, we need to apply the principles of scientific methodology to ensure that we provide an accurate overview of the literature. In other words, there are principles which we must follow in preparing a literature review.

As stated before, in preparing literature reviews and evaluating research findings, a multiplicity of papers must be considered, at least according to the following general steps:

1. Identify relevant literature; select key papers.
2. Critically evaluate key papers, as discussed in this section. You might decide to discard some papers if irreparable problems are discovered.
3. Identify general patterns of findings in the literature. Tabulate findings, where appropriate.
4. Identify crucial disagreements and controversies.
5. Propose valid explanations for the disagreements. Such explanations provide a theoretical framework for resolving controversies and proposing future research.
6. Provide a clear summary concerning the state of the literature, identifying progress, obstacles and further research.

Systematic reviews

There are several approaches to conducting health sciences reviews. For example, the previously mentioned review by Olanow (2004) can be classified as a 'narrative' review. This approach entails producing a 'story-like' overview of the state of current evidence and theories. Although reviewers adhere to the principles of science and logic in conducting a narrative review, there have been concerns about bias and lack of clarity. More recently, systematic reviews and meta-analyses have been introduced to enhance the rigour for combining and interpreting the state of the literature. Systematic reviews rely on the explicit use of the methodological principles discussed in previous chapters. In effect, systematic reviews follow the problem-solving approach as used for conducting empirical research (Schwartz & Polgar 2003, Ch. 14). Let us examine a published example (Polgar et al 2003) to illustrate the logic and principles underlying the conduct of systematic reviews.

Research questions

When conducting a systematic review, we are expected to formulate a clear research question which will be answered by the outcomes of the review. You might have read about the current research using embryonic or stem cells for reconstructing the brains of people suffering from neurological conditions such as stroke and Parkinson's disease. We were interested in reviewing the evidence for answering the research question 'How effective is reconstructive neurosurgery (i.e. the grafting of immature cells) for improving the signs and symptoms of Parkinson's disease?' (Polgar et al 2003).

Theoretical framework

Although this principle is not adhered to by all reviewers, it is very useful to specify the theoretical framework(s) which guides a specific review. The theoretical framework used for conducting the review was identified as the 'Repair Model'. This is a purely biomedical, quantitative view of neural reconstruction based on the notion that recovery is due to the replacement of dopaminergic cells damaged in Parkinson's disease. An explicit theoretical framework is essential for understanding a given area of health as a coherent research programme (Ch. 1).

Search strategy

The next step is to identify the relevant publications. For example, in Polgar et al (2003) we conducted the following search:

A search of MEDLINE (1994–2000 and 2000/01–2000/10) using the exploded terms fetal tissue transplantation, Parkinson's disease, human or fetal tissue transplants, Parkinson's disease, human, also using the author Kopyov was conducted. In conjunction with this search, abstracts from the American Society for Neural Transplantation and Repair conferences (1999; 2000) were hand searched for authors that may have been overlooked. The reference lists of key papers were searched to identify papers that might not have been identified through on-line search mechanisms. An additional electronic search was conducted using the following databases: Medline (1966–March Week 2, 2001), Embase (1994–April Week 1, 2001), CINAHL (1982–March Week 2, 2001).

The general point here is that reviewers must be diligent in identifying all the publications which constitute the literature in the area targeted for review. The search should include both 'electronic, on-line searches' and 'hand' searches of key journals for cross-checking if the relevant papers were identified by the search engines. It is essential to have a working knowledge of who the key researchers are in a particular field and what critical issues exist in a research programme before we can undertake a formal published review.

Selection of key papers

Depending on the area of health sciences being reviewed, literature searches might yield any number of publications, from one or two to many hundreds. Relying on the outcome of the search, the reviewers might restate the research questions and redefine the scope of the proposed systematic review. This will expand or restrict the number of studies for further searchers. In addition, explicit inclusion/exclusion criteria are used to identify the most relevant sources. For example, Polgar et al (2003) used the following criteria for including a study in a review. In order to be included in the review, a study had to:

- be published in a peer-reviewed journal
- have transplantation surgery performed after 1993, following consensus for optimal donor characteristics
- have grafted human or embryonic cells
- have followed 'best practice' stereotactic surgery procedures
- have followed standard post-surgical assessment protocols.

It would be tedious in the present context to explain the specific reasons for each of the above selection criteria; interested readers will find that they were justified in the original review. The point is that we must have explicit, objective criteria for including or excluding studies.

The key papers function as a sample of the best available information accessible in the literature. Parallel to empirical research, we use the evidence from key papers to draw inferences about the state of knowledge in the area under review. The use of diagnostic searches and explicit inclusion/exclusion criteria ensure that the 'sample' of papers produces a representative, rather than biased, sample of the overall knowledge.

Coding the research studies

When the process of selecting and collecting the publications is complete, we have the available evidence relevant to answering our research question. The information that we seek is embedded in the text of research publications. We need to extract the key information from the text of each of the papers selected for the review. We can approach the analysis of the meaning of this information in a way that is similar to qualitative data analysis (Ch. 21). Similarly to the predetermined codes used in content analysis, reviewers use the constant features of quantitative research for identifying the categories appropriate for analysing the key papers (Schwartz & Polgar 2003). These features include:

1. the design of the studies
2. the sampling strategies used and the sample characteristics
3. the ways in which the treatment or intervention was administered
4. the data collection strategy used (i.e. the measurement strategy)
5. the statistical and clinical significance of the results.

Other dimensions or features might also be coded or the above features can be modified according to the judgments of the authors. These aspects of the research process are often presented in a table form, as shown in Table 24.1. We used a hypothetical example rather than the previous published review.

To illustrate coding, consider a set of four hypothetical studies reporting on levels of diabetics' compliance to insulin administration. The results and key features of the hypothetical studies are tabulated in Table 24.1.

Table 24.1 represents how findings from several publications might be tabulated. Key information

Table 24.1 Compliance with insulin use by diabetics

Publication	Sample size	Average age of patients (years)	Method of measuring compliance	Percentage of patients compliant
Smith (2000)	50	55	Self-report	85
Jones (2001)	60	58	Self-report	82
Brown (2001)	50	59	Blood sugar level	40
Miller (2002)	55	56	Blood sugar level	35

about each study, as well as the outcomes, is presented in the table, enabling the emergence and demonstration of an overall pattern.

Interpretation of the evidence

The coding of the hypothetical studies enables the reviewer to answer the research question: 'How compliant are patients with diabetes with using insulin?' The hypothetical summarized evidence illustrates that sometimes no clear overall trends emerge from the tabulated findings.

In the simple hypothetical example shown in Table 24.1, the percentage of compliance reported by Smith (2000) and Jones (2001) is over twice that reported by Brown (2001) and Miller (2002). Clearly, there is an inconsistency in the literature. A possible explanation for this discrepancy might emerge by the inspection of Table 24.1. Neither differences in sample size nor the average ages of the patients provide an explanation for the difference. However, the method by which compliance was measured emerges as a plausible explanation. The investigators Smith and Jones relied on the patients' self-reports and might have overestimated compliance levels, in contrast to Brown and Miller, who used a more objective method and found poor levels of compliance. Of course, this explanation is not necessarily true, but is simply a hypothesis to guide future investigations of the problem. There are other possibilities which might account for the pattern of findings. It appears that more research is needed.

Meta-analysis

Dooley (1984) discussed the availability of two general types of strategies for summarizing research findings from multiple papers:

1. *Qualitative*. A qualitative review involves the selection of key features of related publications such as designs, subject characteristics or measures used in the studies. These features are presented in a table form, such that differences in the features of the research can be related to outcomes. The qualitative reviews identified by Dooley (1984) are related to the systematic reviews, as we discussed above.

2. *Quantitative*. A quantitative review calls for the condensation of the results from several papers into a single statistic. This statistic represents an overall or pooled effect size. These procedures are meta-analyses which are systematic procedures for summarizing the results published in a set of research papers.

Although many statistical procedures can be used for synthesizing data, meta-analysis also refers to an active area of statistics examining strategies most suitable for synthesizing published evidence. Statisticians have developed software packages such as 'Comprehensive Meta-Analysis' which expedite the computational difficulties entailed in synthesizing evidence from diverse studies (http://www.metaanalysis.com, info@metaanalysis.com).

Combining data from diverse studies

How are results synthesized? Let us look at a simple example for combining data. Say that you are interested in the average age of the participants in three related studies: A, B and C (Table 24.2).

Say we wish to calculate the average age for all the 230 participants in the three studies. Could we calculate the overall mean, $\bar{X}$, simply by adding up the three means and dividing by three? The answer is no, because there are different numbers of participants across the groups. We must give a weight to each of the statistics depending on 'n', the sample size for each study. The equation which we use is:

$$\bar{X} = \frac{(\bar{X}_A \times n_A) + (\bar{X}_B \times n_B) + (\bar{X}_C \times n_C)}{n_A + n_B + n_C}$$

$$= \frac{(40 \times 80) + (45 \times 50) + (60 \times 100)}{80 + 50 + 100}$$

$$= 49.8$$

Table 24.2 Participants' ages in three hypothetical studies

Study	Number of participants (n)	Average age ($\bar{X}$)
A	80	40
B	50	45
C	100	60

The point here is that, in order to calculate the correct overall statistics, we must give a weight to each study. In general, the weight assigned to a study represents the proportion of information the study contributes to the overall analysis. For the above calculation, weight was determined by the sample size used in each study. In general the weight assigned to a study represents the proportion of the information contributing to the calculation of the overall statistic.

Even the calculation of a simple statistic like 'average overall age' can be useful for understanding the state of a research programme. For instance, in Polgar et al (2003) we found that the mean age of Parkinson's disease sufferers was 56 years, with the mean overall duration of the illness being 13 years. These results indicated that the average age of onset of the disease was only about 43 years, indicating that experimental reconstructive neurosurgery has been offered to an unrepresentative sample of Parkinson's disease sufferers. Typically people with Parkinson's disease are in their late sixties or early seventies.

Of course we need to synthesize other clinically and theoretically relevant statistics appearing across the papers constituting a research programme, including the overall pooled standard deviation, the overall statistical significance, the overall effect size and the confidence intervals for the overall effect sizes. These analyses are best carried out using statistical software packages. You can check the Internet for further information regarding the logic of meta-analysis and currently available software packages.

Interpreting the results of a meta-analysis

There are different ways for conducting and reporting the results of meta-analyses which have become quite frequent in the health sciences literature. A typical way of presenting the results is shown in Figures 24.1 and 24.2, which show the hypothetical outcome of a computer-assisted meta-analysis (modified from www.metaanalysis. com). The graphics shown in these figures are referred to as 'forest plots'. A forest plot is a visual representation of the results of a meta-analysis.

Say that the printout showed the results of five randomized double-blind trials (see Ch. 5) aiming to demonstrate the effectiveness of a vaccine for influenza. In each of the studies volunteers were given either the vaccine (treated) or a placebo (control) injection. The following features of Figures 24.1 and 24.2 are important for interpreting the outcomes of a meta-analysis.

Studies

Following searching and critical analysis of the relevant literature, as discussed previously, the reviewer selected the five papers shown. If you look carefully at the sample sizes in each of the groups under Treated (odds) and Control (odds), you will find that the sample sizes are not equal. If they represent randomized trials, you might ask why the groups were unequal in the studies. Sometimes unequal groups represent people dropping out because of harmful side effects to the treatment.

Effect

The effect size was represented as an odds ratio (OR), which is a commonly used statistic for outcomes measured on a nominal scale. For this measure the outcome is: diagnosed with influenza following vaccination or placebo over, say, 6 months: 'yes' or 'no'. Looking at the first (English) study, the odds of 'yes' to 'no' are 30/530 for the treated group and 40/540 in the control group. The statistical software package computed an OR of 0.750, indicating a slight reduction in the odds of contracting influenza. Note that an $OR = 1$ means equal odds or no difference at all, while decreasing OR under 1.0 favours treatment. For example, an OR of 0.5 would indicate that the vaccination halved the odds for contracting influenza in the sample.

Confidence intervals

As we discussed in Chapter 17, a 95% confidence interval contains the true population parameter at $p = 0.95$. The lines produced from the 'squares' containing the sample OR represent the 95% confidence intervals. You can see in Figure 24.1 that all the confidence intervals for the five studies overlap with 1.0, indicating that we cannot infer that the studies favour the treatment.

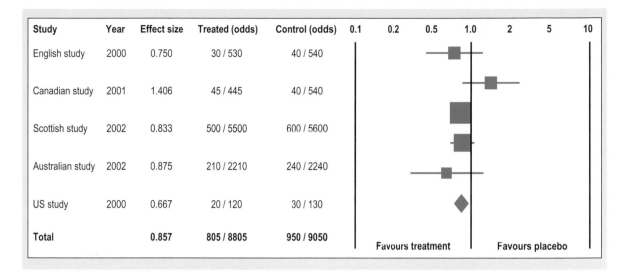

Figure 24.1 • Results of a hypothetical meta-analysis: negative findings.

Figure 24.2 • Results of a hypothetical meta-analysis: positive findings.

Weights and totals

When you look at the 'odds' columns in Figures 24.1 and 24.2, you can see that there is a variation in the sample sizes used in the hypothetical studies. For example, the 'Scottish' study included 12 200 participants, while the 'US' study included only 300 participants. These differences contribute to the relative 'weight' of the study represented graphically by the area of the 'squares' in the forest plots. Clearly, the larger the square, the greater the sample size. You will also note that the confidence intervals are wider with the smaller squares in comparison to the larger squares. As discussed in Chapter 20, the larger the sample size, the more 'power' we have for making accurate inferences.

The 'Totals' in Figures 24.1 and 24.2 refer to the overall statistics synthesized from the results of the five hypothetical studies. These statistics are represented by the diamond shapes on the forest plots. In Figure 24.1 the total OR was 0.857, indicating a very weak effect for the vaccination. The OR is close to one or equal 'odds' for having influenza. For the results shown in Figure 24.2, the total OR was 0.492. This represents a strong effect, indicating that the odds for contracting influenza would have been more than halved by the vaccination. Such results are suggestive of the clinical or practical significance of introducing the treatment.

Validity of systematic reviews

The interpretation of the results of published meta-analyses is far more difficult than indicated in the above example. Let us look at some of the sources of difficulties.

Sampling

The results reported in the papers selected for review generally represent a sample of the total information published in a field. This leads us to the first problem: studies that do not report statistically significant findings are often not submitted or accepted for publication. By not having access to these 'negative' findings, the selection of papers becomes biased towards those with reported 'positive' outcomes. Also, in published research papers where outcomes for multiple dependent variables are reported, only the statistically significant outcomes are reported, undermining attempts to synthesize the evidence accurately (Polgar et al 2003).

In addition, the exclusion/inclusion criteria used for selecting the studies can result in a sampling bias. Some practitioners of evidence-based medicine (e.g. Sackett et al 2000) are reluctant to include studies which have not adopted a randomized experimental design. While this approach has strong methodological justifications, valuable information can be lost by using highly selective inclusion criteria. Of course, the more information that is lost, the weaker the external validity of the review or meta-analysis in relation to the 'population' of research results constituting a research programme. The reduced external validity is a trade-off

for including only methodologically stronger studies in the review.

Extracting the data

Another source of error arises when extracting the data from an individual meta-analysis. Some authors report very clear, descriptive statistics but others report their results in an obscure, uninterpretable fashion. Also, some journals and authors only discuss the statistical significance of the results. Obscure and incomplete reporting of the evidence leads to errors in synthesizing overall statistics.

The state of the research programme

The validity of a systematic review or meta-analysis is limited by the methodological rigour and statistical accuracy of the studies selected for review. To put it bluntly, many health-related problems cannot be resolved and questions cannot be answered on the basis of the currently available evidence. An inconclusive systematic review or meta-analysis is not necessarily a waste of time. Although inconclusive attempts to synthesize data cannot be used to make valid clinical decisions, they provide strong evidence for gaps in knowledge and provide objective grounds for identifying further research required to advance the research programme (e.g. Polgar et al 2003). Until better evidence becomes available we simply provide the best practices suggested by tradition and experience.

The Cochrane Collaboration

Cochrane (1972), a Scottish medical practitioner, was one of the first influential practitioners in the modern era to advocate the systematic use of evidence to inform clinical practice.

In recognition of Cochrane's pioneering work, the Cochrane Collaboration, the Cochrane Library and the Cochrane Database of Systematic Reviews were established. The Cochrane Collaboration is now a large international venture with a series of special-interest groups commissioning and maintaining reviews on a wide range of topics. There are also detailed protocols that have been established for the conduct and presentation of Cochrane systematic reviews. Although the scope of the Cochrane database is very broad, much of it is quite focused on intervention research, i.e. what intervention approaches work best for specific health problems and populations. The database is now expanding into other areas but there is a strong intervention focus.

The Cochrane approach adheres to a hierarchy of evidence. There are five levels of evidence, with systematic reviews of multiple randomized controlled trials at the top, followed by single randomized controlled trials, evidence from trials without randomization but with pre–post, cohort or time series measurement, evidence from non-experimental studies and, at the bottom level, opinions of respected authorities. Many reviews, however, only focus on the top two levels of the evidence categories. Obviously, because of the intervention-oriented nature of many Cochrane reviews, qualitative research, case study and policy research do not yet figure prominently in this system.

The Cochrane Database of Systematic Reviews is available on a wide range of websites in different countries. Access arrangements for the reviews vary widely from country to country. In some countries some fees are payable, but in others, such as Australia, the government has taken out a national subscription so that access may be freely available. In order to access the database, we suggest that you use a search engine to search for 'Cochrane Collaboration' and follow the links or consult your librarian.

Evidence-based practice

Although the name of evidence-based medicine or evidence-based practice is relatively new, the idea of using research evidence to inform the design of clinical interventions is very old. Muir Gray (1997) provides a very good review of this approach. The quality movement in health care, at which commentators such as Donabedian (1990) have been at the forefront, has also been influential in promoting the need for the systematic use of evidence to promote the delivery of high-quality health care.

As Muir Gray (1997) notes, evidence-based practice has at its centre three linked ideas. These are how to find and appraise evidence, how to develop the capacity for evidence-based decision making and how to get research evidence implemented into practice. The finding and appraising of evidence draw heavily upon systems such as the Cochrane Collaboration approach where evidence is systematically collected and appraised according to pre-defined principles and protocols. However, the facilitation and implementation elements of evidence-based practice are important additions to the basic establishment of research evidence to support particular approaches in the provision of health services. The evidence-based practice movement is based upon the recognition that the mere existence of evidence for the effectiveness of particular interventions does not mean that it will necessarily be effectively implemented. This is the new element of evidence-based practice, the systematic implementation of programmes based upon sound research evidence.

Summary

We have seen in this chapter that the advancement of knowledge and practice depends not only on the results of individual research projects but also on the information provided by the synthesis of the results across the literature. Where the projects share the same clinical aims and theoretical frameworks, they are said to constitute a research programme. In this chapter we outlined the process of identifying and selecting publications which contain theoretically or practically relevant research findings. We argued that reviewing a research programme is an active, creative process which is influenced by our expectations and attitudes. While absolute objectivity is not a realistic requirement of a reviewer, there are basic rules to ensure that the review of the evidence is carried out with a minimal degree of bias.

A systematic review of the literature proceeds by identifying the basic components of research papers for organizing the evidence. We use these dimensions to identify patterns or trends which enable us to synthesize the information and answer the research questions. When studies are sufficiently similar, their results can be condensed into single statistics such as overall effect size. In this chapter, we examined how the results of meta-analyses are interpreted.

The relationships between the state of a research programme and practice are very complex. We examined hypothetical situations where there was a strong consistency in the research findings and clear trends emerging in the literature could be identified. In these cases, applying the results is relatively straightforward in that we can either adopt or reject the use of a treatment on the basis of the evidence. Systematic reviews and meta-analyses are essential means for identifying best practices available for our patients. However, even well-conceived reviews and meta-analyses can fail to identify clear trends or clinically meaningful effect sizes. When the evidence is inconclusive, we simply continue with traditional practices and identify further research required for resolving unanswered questions concerning improved efficacy. In this way research in the health sciences is a continuous process, producing better information for advancing theory and practice, as we discussed in Chapter 1 of this book.

Self-assessment

Explain the meaning of the following terms:

Cochrane Collaboration
combined or pooled results
evidence-based practice
exclusion criteria
extraction (of data)
forest plots
inclusion criteria
literature
literature review
meta-analysis
odds ratio
systematic review
weight (for a study)

True or false

1. The term 'literature' refers to the set of papers purposefully selected by a reviewer.

2. 'Trends' in the literature refer to consistent outcomes across a number of publications.

3. The conduct and outcomes of a carefully written review are not influenced by the theoretical positions of the reviewers.

4. The methodological principles relevant to conducting empirical research are not applicable to writing literature reviews.

5. Contemporary literature searches use both 'online' and traditional means for identifying relevant papers.

6. Explicitly stated inclusion and exclusion criteria ensure the objective selection of publications.

7. When conducting a systematic review, the 'population' is defined as the literature for an area of research.

8. Only studies employing randomized double-blind designs should be included in a systematic review.

9. Odds ratios are used to represent effect sizes for interval and ratio-scaled data.

10. An odds ratio of 0.95 indicates a large effect size.

11. An overall weighted mean is a useful statistic for synthesizing the results of studies using continuous outcome measures.

12. Inconsistent findings should not be included in a meta-analysis.

13. The results of a meta-analysis can be graphed as a forest plot.

14. The 'weight' of a study in a meta-analysis is inversely proportional to the sample size.

15. Confidence intervals are used to estimate the range for the probable true values of overall statistics.

16. The outcomes of systematic reviews and meta-analyses enable researchers and practitioners to make decisions based on overall evidence.

Multiple choice

1. Which of the following statements is true about systematic reviews?
   a Systematic reviews are the same as narrative reviews.
   b The 'system' referred to follows the problem-solving strategy of applied empirical research.
   c Systematic reviews are appropriate for synthesizing evidence from qualitative research.
   d Narrative reviews are preferable to systematic reviews for minimizing reviewers' bias in selecting key papers.
   e Systematic reviews are alternative strategies to meta-analyses for synthesizing evidence.

2. Which of the following statements is false regarding the use of meta-analyses?
   a Meta-analyses are statistical strategies for synthesizing evidence from several empirical studies.
   b Meta-analyses can provide significant outcomes even when the individual studies lacked statistical significance.
   c Meta-analyses are alternative strategies to systematic reviews for synthesizing evidence.
   d Using meta-analyses increases the statistical power for identifying therapeutically useful outcomes.
   e Meta-analyses are an important component of evidence-based health care.
3. Consider the forest plots shown in Figure 24.1 and 24.2. These figures indicate that:
   a the larger the sample size in a study, the greater the weight contributed to the overall results
   b the narrower the confidence interval, the larger the sample size in an individual study
   c the key outcome measure is the total or overall effect size for the studies included in the analysis
   d all of the above (a, b and c) are true
   e none of the above (a, b and c) are true.
4. Which of the following is problematic for conducting a meta-analysis?
   a 'Negative' findings are sometimes not reported in health sciences journals.
   b Some outcomes are measured on a nominal scale.
   c Not all published research involves randomized controlled designs.
   d The Cochrane Collaboration favours the use of narrative reviews for synthesizing evidence.
   e Differences such as samples, measurement strategies, etc. in each of the studies makes the synthesis of the evidence 'invalid'.
5. The best evidence for implementing a treatment based on a meta-analysis is:
   a a large overall effect size
   b very wide confidence intervals
   c large overall sample sizes
   d both a and b
   e none of the above.

Assume that you are working as a rehabilitation provider in your area of professional practice. Your supervisor asks you to review the relevant literature in order to decide if 'Rehabilitation A' or 'Rehabilitation B' should be implemented at your centre. Having identified and critically evaluated the relevant studies in the area, you find only two well-designed comparative experiments in which the outcomes were measured on the same standardized inventory. The outcomes were as follows:

The t values were calculated for an independent groups t test, with non-directional H_A. Questions 6–10 refer to the above information.

	Type of rehabilitation	$\bar{X}$	df	t	p
Experiment 1	A	50	10	2.0	>0.05
	B	30			
Experiment 2	A	45	58	2.8	<0.01
	B	30			

6. A standardized inventory was used to measure rehabilitation outcome, where $\mu = 40$ and $\sigma = 10$. What was the effect size for Experiment 1? (Hint: use σ for calculating effect size.)
   a 0.05
   b 0.2
   c 1.67
   d 2.0
   e 10.0
7. On the basis of the evidence provided, a plausible explanation for the results of Experiment 1 being non-significant is that:
   a the sample size was too small
   b the variability was too large
   c the effect size was very small
   d both a and b
   e all of the above (a, b and c).
8. The results of Experiment 1 indicate the importance for evaluating the _____ of a statistical analysis.
   a application
   b sampling error
   c variability
   d power
   e reproducibility.
9. Assume that the higher the scores on the inventory, the better the rehabilitation outcome. If the clinical significance of the results is set

at d (effect size) $\geqslant 1$, then the trends shown in Experiment 1 and Experiment 2 indicate that:

a both studies demonstrate clinical significance

b both studies demonstrate statistical significance

c Rehabilitation A should be implemented

d both *a* and *b*

e *a*, *b* and *c*.

10. Your supervisor is concerned that the literature did not demonstrate a clear trend, considering the different values for *p* in the two studies. If you are not in a position to carry out further research, you could test the hypothesis 'Rehabilitation A is superior to Rehabilitation B' by:

a using a different statistical test

b using your clinical knowledge

c applying narrative analysis

d using a computer model of the outcome

e carrying out a quantitative meta-analysis.

Consider the following two hypothetical scenarios representing research findings for randomized controlled trials (RCTs) evaluating the differences between the outcomes of two treatments, X and Y. Assume that an independent samples *t* test was used to analyse the data. A positive effect size represents outcomes in favour of treatment X.

Questions 11–13 are based on the information below:

Scenario A

Study	Effect size (d)	df	p
A	1.0	30	<0.01
B	1.0	30	<0.01
C	1.2	14	>0.05
D	1.2	14	>0.05

Scenario B

Study	Effect size (d)	df	p
A	0.2	80	>0.05
B	0.2	100	>0.05
C	−0.1	200	>0.05
D	−0.2	200	>0.05

11. Which of the following is correct for Scenario A?

a There was a large effect size.

b The results were consistently in favour of treatment X.

c The outcomes for the four studies were statistically significant.

d Both *a* and *b*.

e All of the above (*a*, *b* and *c*) are correct.

12. Which of the following is correct for Scenario B?

a There was a large effect size.

b The results were consistently in favour of treatment X.

c The outcomes for the four studies were not statistically significant.

d Both *a* and *b*.

e All of the above (*a*, *b* and *c*) are correct.

13. Which scenario demonstrates that treatment X is more effective than treatment Y?

a Scenario A, because all the studies provided statistically significant outcomes.

b Scenario B, because all the studies provided *p* values greater than 0.05.

c Scenario A, because the studies provided evidence for large and consistent effect sizes.

d Scenario B, because the studies provided evidence for large and consistent effect sizes.

e Scenario B, because the sample sizes in the studies were significantly larger than those in Scenario A.

14. A well-known project for constructing and disseminating the results of systematic reviews and meta-analyses online is called:

a the Cochrane Collaboration

b the Meta-Analyses Database (MAD)

c Medline

d CINAHL

e Embase.

Section **Seven**

Discussion, questions and answers

This question is based on a survey which was published in an Australian newspaper. Of course, such surveys do not represent research published in scientific journals, but they are important sources for public knowledge and/or attitudes towards health sciences issues. The survey questioned a sample of adults concerning their smoking habits. Only one of the questions asked is discussed here and the results are hypothetical.

Table D24.1 Survey characteristics

Sample	1000 voters
Coverage	Australia-wide
Method	Telephone
Question	Do you smoke? (Yes or No)

Table D24.2 Results

Percentage of replies to the question in two major cities		
	Melbourne	**Sydney**
Yes	24	18
No	76	82

Questions

The following questions involve the critical analysis of the above survey.

1. If we assume that cigarette smoking is now a 'stigmatized' behaviour, do you think the telephone survey produced valid answers?
2. A total of 180 people were interviewed in Melbourne and 220 in Sydney. If the population of Australia is 17 million and the populations of Melbourne and Sydney are 2.5 and 3.2 million respectively, do the samples appear to be quota samples?
3. Which categories of smokers may not have been reached by this survey? What implications might this have for the external validity of the survey?
4. A journalist commented on the results, saying: 'This difference is ironic, given that anti-smoking lobbyists have applauded Melbourne as a pacesetter for smoking law reform, such as tobacco tax-funded health promotion'.
   (a) Explain why this comment is inappropriate given the design of the survey.
   (b) What research design would be appropriate to show a causal effect on smoking due to health promotion on smoking? (Hint: see Ch. 6.)
5. Explain why the comment quoted in question 4 is inappropriate, given that the statistical significance of the results was not calculated.
6. Which statistical test should be used to analyse the significance of the results concerning

differences in smoking between the two cities? Justify your selection.

7. Setting $\alpha = 0.05$, calculate the statistic and decide if the results were significant (note that we gave the results in percentages).

8. Do you think the sample size ($n = 1000$) was adequate? Explain.

Answers

1. Although telephone interviews and mailed-out questionnaires are a relatively cost-efficient strategy for collecting data, we have problems validating the responses. This is particularly true for conditions and behaviours which are socially stigmatized: why should respondents disclose such information about themselves? In face-to-face interviews, we can explore issues, for example if the respondents have nicotine-stained fingers or smell of cigarettes, we may pursue the issue further to establish the accuracy of the replies.

2. Given that $n = 1000$, 18% of the respondents were from Melbourne and 22% from Sydney. For a quota sample, the expected samples would be:

Melbourne: $\dfrac{2.5}{17} \times 100 = 14.7\%$

and

Sydney: $\dfrac{3.2}{17} \times 100 = 18.8\%$

Assuming that the information used to calculate the above figures is correct, it seems that the sample included more respondents from Melbourne. This may reflect the different proportion of 'voters' in the two cities, or a rather poor quota sample.

3. People who are not on the electoral roll, such as persons under 18 years of age, and people who do not have or do not answer their telephones, would not have been contacted. In this way, the sample may not be representative of all the smokers in the city (e.g. young people, poor or itinerant people, people with unlisted telephone numbers). Therefore, the survey may not be externally valid if we generalize to all persons in Australia who smoke.

4. (a) The present survey did not tell us how rates of smoking have changed over a period of time.
   (b) We may use a quasi-experimental design and introduce the programme in one city, A, but not in the other equivalent city, B. If the

reduction is greater over time in A than in B, we may argue that this difference could reflect the causal effect of health promotion.

5. Although results for the samples show a difference between the two cities, this may simply reflect sampling error. We must establish the significance of the results before we can draw inferences ('ironic' or otherwise) about populations.

6. χ^2; nominal data and independent measurements or samples.

7. Convert the data into frequencies (see Ch. 19) before entering obtained values into a 2×2 contingency table (values rounded to closest whole number).

Table D24.3

	Melbourne	Sydney	Total
Smokers	43 (cell 1)	40 (cell 2)	83
Non-smokers	137 (cell 3)	180 (cell 4)	317
Total	180	220	400

Expected values (for calculation procedure, see Ch. 19):

f_e (cell 1) $= \dfrac{83 \times 180}{400} = 37.4$

f_e (cell 2) $= \dfrac{83 \times 220}{400} = 45.7$

f_e (cell 3) $= \dfrac{317 \times 180}{400} = 142.6$

f_e (cell 4) $= \dfrac{317 \times 220}{400} = 174.3$

$\chi^2_{obt} = \Sigma \dfrac{(f_o - f_e)^2}{f_e} = 1.96$

Table D24.4 Calculation of χ^2

Cell	f_o	f_e	$(f_o - f_e)^2$	$\dfrac{(f_o - f_e)^2}{f_o}$
1	43	37.4	31.36	0.84
2	40	45.7	32.49	0.71
3	137	142.6	31.36	0.22
4	180	174.3	32.49	0.19

Critical value of χ^2; $\alpha = 0.05$ where degrees of freedom (df) = 1 (Appendix C)

$\chi^2_{crit} = 3.84$

In this case we would retain H_0: there is no association between the variables 'city' (Melbourne or Sydney) and smoking (Yes or No). (For details of the decision-making process, refer to Ch. 19.) It is apparent that the results are not significant, therefore we are not justified in drawing any inferences concerning the different proportions of smokers in Melbourne and Sydney.

8. Although a sample size of $n = 1000$ appears quite large, this was an Australia-wide sample which was divided up to represent regions. It is possible that the null results obtained in question 7 are because there are no differences in smoking rates between the two cities, but there are other possibilities (see Ch. 20). Perhaps the sample size was inadequate and we made a Type II error in our decision. Replicating the study with larger sample sizes might enable us to show significant differences in smoking rates.

Section **Eight**

SECTION CONTENTS

Glossary of research terms

AB design A type of experimental design in which the participant is monitored during a baseline phase followed by an intervention phase.

ABAB design A type of experimental design in which the participant is monitored during a baseline phase followed by an intervention phase which, in turn, is followed by further baseline and intervention phases.

Abstract An abbreviated summary of a research report, generally found at the beginning of the report.

Acquiescent response mode A style of answering questions which results in the respondent choosing the middle category in a response scale.

Alternative hypothesis Sometimes also known as the experimental hypothesis. This is the hypothesis for which the researcher is trying to gain support in a statistical analysis, by rejecting the null hypothesis. The alternative hypothesis is represented by the symbol H_A or H_1.

Apparatus Any equipment or special facilities used in a research project.

Area sample A type of sampling procedure in which the units of the sample are where people live or work, rather than who they are. The researcher divides the target area into sections and then samples the sections.

Assignment The process in an experiment where the researcher allocates subjects to the various groups. Matching and random assignment are the two most common methods. The goal of assignment is to achieve identical groups.

Assignment errors A situation that arises in an experiment where the assignment or allocation of people to groups results in groups with different characteristics.

Authority An appeal to authority argument is based on the proposition that someone of high status knows best, not whether the argument is soundly based.

Bar graph A method of displaying data where the frequency of a particular category is reflected in the height of the bar in the graph.

Baseline A phase in an intervention study where the participant is receiving no intervention.

Bell-shaped curve This is the characteristic shape of the normal distribution.

Bias In a questionnaire, bias is introduced by inappropriately framed questions, such as leading questions.

Biased sample A biased sample is one that is not representative. It does not reflect the composition of the population to which the researcher is attempting to generalize.

Causal explanation An attempt to explain the occurrence of a particular phenomenon or event by identifying the cause(s).

Causality An event or factor (A) is generally argued to have caused another one (B) if the following conditions are met: (i) if (A) occurs then (B) occurs; (ii) if (A) does not occur then (B) does not occur; (iii) if (A) precedes (B) in time.

Central tendency The central tendency of a frequency distribution is the average, middle or most common score. Measures of central tendency include the mean, the median and the mode.

Chi-square (χ^2) A statistical test often used with categorical data. It is based on a comparison of the frequencies observed and the frequencies expected in the various categories.

Clinical significance The clinical significance of a research finding is the extent to which that finding is clinically meaningful.

Closed-response format A method of eliciting answers from people in a questionnaire in which the researcher provides fixed response categories, e.g. yes or no.

Coding A qualitative method of analysis of materials such as interviews where categories are formed and their interrelationships examined.

Complete observer A type of research strategy in which the researcher observes social interactions with no direct personal input; for example, observation via a one-way mirror or through the analysis of a video tape.

Complete participant A research strategy in which the researcher completely participates in the research setting in order to experience its characteristics.

Confidence interval The confidence interval of a sample statistic is the expected range in which the actual population value will be found, at a given level of confidence or probability.

Content validity The extent to which a test or assessment matches the real requirements of the situation, e.g. a living skills assessment would have high content validity if it measured cooking, self-care, etc.

Contingency table A method of presenting the relationship between two categorical variables in the form of a table.

Continuous data Data with values that do not fall into discrete categories, for example measures of temperature and mass.

Control In an experiment, the researcher attempts to control or eliminate the influence of extraneous variables so that any changes or differences may be attributed solely to the intervention.

Control group In an experiment, a control group is generally a non-treatment group which is compared with the experimental group to study the effects of the intervention.

Correlation coefficient A statistic designed to measure the size and direction of the association between two variables. The values vary between 0 and ± 1.

Correlational studies Studies that are concerned with investigating the associations between variables.

Critical theory In qualitative research, critical theory explains how personal meanings and actions are influenced by the person's social environment.

Critical value of a statistic The value of the statistic (obtained from appropriate tables) that the calculated value for a given result must exceed, in order to attain statistical significance.

Curvilinear correlation coefficient A measure of association between variables designed to investigate curved rather than straight-line relationships.

Data The information collected by a researcher.

Deduction A process where a general principle is applied to a particular case to explain it, e.g. all humans die; this is a human, therefore he/she will die.

Descriptive statistics Statistics designed to describe characteristics of a sample. For example, the most common or typical value or the extent of variation among such values.

Determinism The view that all events are caused by other events.

Directional hypothesis A directional hypothesis is one that asserts that differences between groups in the data will occur in a particular direction. For example, the hypothesis 'smokers die younger than non-smokers' is a directional hypothesis.

Discontinuous data Sometimes termed discrete data; variables that have discrete categories, for example male versus female.

Discussion A section of a research report in which the research findings are discussed.

Dispersion Sometimes known as variability: the extent to which scores in a group of scores vary. This may be measured by statistics such as the standard deviation, variance, range and semi-interquartile range.

Ecological validity The extent to which the results of a study may be generalized to the real world.

Effect size The amount of change created by an intervention, especially in an experimental study.

Empathy In qualitative research, the ability to understand the perspectives of others.

Epidemiology The study of the distribution and determinants of disease within a community.

Ethics A project is ethical to the extent that its design and execution conform to a set of standards or conventions guiding research.

Ethnography A descriptive qualitative study, often of an individual or situation, usually written from the perspective of the participant(s) in the first person.

Ethnomethodology A qualitative approach to research which involves the study of social processes associated with the ways in which people perceive, describe and explain the world.

Expected frequency In the analysis of categorical data, the expected frequency is the one that would be expected in a particular category, under certain theoretical conditions. The expected frequency of women in a sample of 100 people would be 50, if equal proportions of sexes were assumed.

Experiment A research design involving the random allocation of subjects to groups and the application of different interventions to these groups. A non-intervention control group is often employed in an experimental design. The aim of an experiment is to be able to conclude validly that differences in outcomes for the groups were caused by the different interventions.

External validity The extent to which the results of the study may be generalized to the population.

Extreme response mode A method of responding to questions in which the respondent chooses the most extreme available response categories.

Factorial design A type of research design in which combinations of several independent variables are manipulated concurrently. A 2×2 factorial design involves the manipulation of two independent variables, each with two levels.

False negative The situation that occurs when a diagnostic test indicates that the person being assessed does not have a disease when he/she actually does.

False positive The situation that occurs when a diagnostic test indicates that the person being assessed has a disease when he/she does not.

Forced-response format A method of eliciting responses to a questionnaire in which there is no middle response category. This is sometimes done to avoid acquiescent response mode.

Forest plot A graph representing the outcomes of a meta-analysis. Typically, a forest plot shows the effect size and 95% confidence intervals for the individual trials and the overall or 'pooled' effect size.

Frequency distribution The way in which scores within a given sample or population are distributed.

Frequency polygon A method of graphing frequency distributions.

Grounded theory A qualitative research approach that advocates the development of theories to explain social phenomena grounded in data, following a process of induction, deduction and verification.

Hawthorne effect An effect which results in the improvement of subjects' performances through being observed and/or social contact. An example of a placebo effect.

Hermeneutics An approach to analysing the meaning of texts in the cultural contexts in which they were originally produced.

Histogram A method of graphing frequency distributions.

History A threat to the validity of studies in which unforeseen and uncontrolled events occur to the participants during the study that are outside the control of the researcher and which may be responsible for changes in the participants.

Hypothesis A proposition advanced by the researcher which is evaluated using the data collected.

Incidence rate The occurrence of new cases of a disease or condition within a specified time frame. See also *prevalence*.

Incidental sample A method of sampling in which the researcher takes the most conveniently available cases.

Independent variable In an experiment an independent variable is the variable or condition manipulated by the researcher.

Induction The process in which a set of observations is made and a general principle formed to explain them. For example, 'every human I have read about eventually dies; this is a human, therefore I expect him/her to die'.

Informed consent The situation where a competent person, in possession of all the relevant facts, has agreed to participate in a research study.

Instrumentation In a study, instrumentation may be a threat to internal validity. It refers to the situation when the instrumentation changes over the period of the study, thus invalidating comparison of measured results.

Internal validity In a study, internal validity refers to the ability of the researcher to attribute differences in the groups or participants to the independent variable.

Inter-observer reliability The extent to which observers rating a particular phenomenon agree with each other.

Interrupted time series A type of research design in which a case is repeatedly measured over time to produce a series of measurements. The series is interrupted by an intervention or event, the effects of which may then be monitored by continuing the measurement series.

Interval scale A type of measurement scale with the following properties: (i) the values are distinguishable; (ii) they are ordered; (iii) the intervals between the points on the scale are equal; (iv) the zero point is not absolute, i.e. does not represent the absence of the quantity.

Interview A conversation between one or more interviewers and interviewees with the purpose of eliciting certain information.

Intra-observer reliability The extent to which an observer rating a particular phenomenon agrees with his/her own rating when presented with the same task on two different occasions.

Likert scale A five-point response scale used in questionnaires, e.g. strongly agree, agree, undecided, disagree, strongly disagree.

Literature review This is a section of a research report in which the previous research that has been done in the area is reviewed and related to the present problem being studied.

Matching In a study, subjects may be assigned to their groups using matching or random assignment. In matching in a two-group study, pairs of similar 'matched' subjects are formed and then one member of the pair is randomly assigned to one group and the other member to the other group. This ensures that the two groups have similar characteristics.

Maturation The phenomenon where participants in a study change spontaneously over time due to natural maturational changes. For example, children may grow older or an infection may spontaneously clear up.

Mean The average of a group of scores. For example, the mean of the scores 7, 8 and 9 is $(7 + 8 + 9) \div 3 = 8$. In statistical notation the mean of a sample is represented by the symbol $\bar{X}$. The mean of a population is represented by the symbol μ.

Measurement A procedure where qualities or quantities are attributed to characteristics of objects, persons or events. Weighing a patient involves a measurement process, as does a clinical judgment about whether a symptom is present or not.

Median The 'middle' score of a group of scores. For example, the median of the scores 7, 8 and 9 is 8. The median is the 50 percentile. The median is often used in preference to the mean when a group of scores contains a small number of extremely small or large scores because it is less sensitive to extreme values.

Meta-analysis Statistical approach to combining the results extracted from several related studies. The overall, pooled statistic represents the best estimate of the effect of a factor on health-related outcomes.

Mode The mode is the most frequently occurring score in a group of scores. For example, the mode of the scores 7, 8, 8, 9, 10 is 8.

Mortality Used to describe a situation where some participants in a study are unable to continue in a study. This might be because they died or because they refuse to continue. If there is high mortality in a group in a study this can jeopardize the internal validity of the study, because differences between the groups may be caused by differential mortality.

Multiple group time series A type of research design where two groups or cases are repeatedly measured over time to produce a series of measurements. One group or case receives an intervention and the other does not. The effects of the intervention may then be studied by comparing the two series.

n The symbol used to represent the number of cases in a sample.

N The symbol used to represent the number of cases in a population.

n **= 1 design** A research design in which one subject, rather than a group of subjects, is studied.

Natural comparison study A type of study in which naturally occurring groups are compared with one another. For example, the health status of smokers versus non-smokers may be studied in a natural comparison study. The researcher does not assign the participants to the groups. These are naturally occurring. Studies of gender differences are natural comparisons.

Natural setting The normal setting of the phenomenon or people under study. Studies performed under laboratory conditions may sometimes have diminished external validity.

Negative correlation A correlation is a measure of the strength and direction of the association between two variables. A negative correlation between two variables implies that, as one variable gets bigger, the value of the other variable becomes smaller.

Negative skew A frequency distribution where there is a long tail towards the negative end of the x-axis. The figure below represents both positively and negatively skewed samples. The position of the 'tail' of the distribution determines whether the skew is positive or negative.

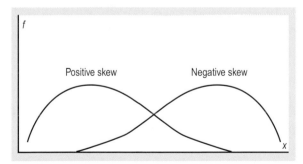

Figure G1.1 • Negative skew.

Nominal scale Measurement scales may be nominal, ordinal, interval or ratio. A nominal scale (often called a categorical scale) is one in which the values are distinct categories, e.g. male or female, Catholic or Protestant or Jewish or Muslim. It has the property of distinctiveness of values, but not ordering, equidistant intervals or an absolute zero.

Non-directional hypothesis This asserts that there are differences between groups in the data but with no direction specified. For example, the hypothesis 'smokers and non-smokers have different life expectancies' is a non-directional hypothesis.

Non-experimental study A study in which the researcher observes a situation but does not systematically manipulate or experiment with it. This may also be called a descriptive design.

Non-parametric test Statistical tests are chosen on the basis of the type of scales that are being analysed. Tests that are suitable for the analysis of ordinal or nominal data are termed non-parametric.

Normal curve A bell-shaped curve, as shown in the figure below. The normal curve is symmetrical and unimodal (has one peak).

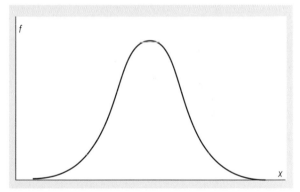

Figure G1.2 • Normal curve.

Null hypothesis The hypothesis in a study that asserts there is no difference between groups or relationship between variables. The statistician normally poses the null hypothesis and then tests it statistically. If it is rejected, the alternative hypothesis (that there is a difference between two groups or a relationship between variables) is accepted. The null hypothesis is represented by the symbol H_0.

Objective measures Measures derived from a mechanical measuring process involving a minimum amount of human interpretation, e.g. weight measurements.

Observation A situation where the researcher studies the phenomenon without deliberate intervention.

Observed frequency The actual number of occurrences of an event observed by a researcher. For example, the observed frequency of females who passed the exam in a group of students might be 37 students. See also *expected frequency*.

Observer as participant Where the researcher studies the behaviour of a group by actively participating in the group's activities and situation.

One-tailed test A statistical test where a difference between two groups is expected to occur in a particular direction. For example, it may be hypothesized that smokers will have more health problems than non-smokers. This would be tested by applying a one-tailed test of significance.

Open-ended question If a question is asked without a predefined set of responses it is an open-ended question. For example, the question 'What did you think about the programme?' is an open-ended question.

Operational definition The specific way in which a concept or variable has been measured in a study. For example, the operational definition of anxiety in a study might be scores from the Spielberger State–Trait Anxiety Inventory or a self-rating on a 1 to 10 scale.

Ordinal scale Measurement scales may be nominal, ordinal, interval or ratio. An ordinal scale has the following properties: (i) the values are distinguishable; (ii) they are ordered but the intervals between the points are not equidistant, nor is there a meaningful zero point. The values of an ordinal scale are often ranked, e.g. 1st, 3rd.

Parametric test Statistical tests are chosen on the basis of the type of data being analysed. Statistical tests that are suitable for the analysis of interval or ratio data are termed parametric.

Participation A situation where the researcher studies the phenomenon by actively participating.

Percentile The position of a score on a frequency distribution expressed in standard score units such that the 50 percentile is the median and all scores fall below the 100 percentile.

Phenomenology In qualitative research, the study and understanding of human conscious experience.

Pie diagram A graphical method of representing the frequency distribution of a set of categorical data in the shape of a pie.

Pilot study A preliminary study where the procedures and protocols are tested or 'piloted'.

Placebo effect The phenomenon where an otherwise worthless intervention in a study nevertheless induces an improvement in the patient's condition or perception of the condition, perhaps due to the expectations of the participants in the study.

Population A group of people, institutions, cases or objects defined as that under study by the researcher. Samples are drawn from populations. Examples of populations are all coronary heart disease cases in the UK, all Australian men, all 'not-for-profit' hospitals in Canada.

Population parameter A value derived from a population. For example, the average age of all the patients in a population defined by the researcher is a population parameter. In statistical notation, population parameters are represented by Greek letters.

Population validity The extent to which a sample reflects the characteristics of a population from which it is drawn.

Positive correlation A correlation is a measure of the strength and direction of the association between two variables. A positive correlation between two variables implies that, as the values of one variable get bigger, so do the values of the other variable.

Positive skew A frequency distribution where there is a long tail towards the positive end of the x-axis.

Post-test only design A type of experimental study in which measurements of the groups are taken only after an intervention has occurred. This is generally done to avoid the effects of measurement upon people's response to the interventions.

Power The probability of rejecting the null hypothesis when the alternative hypothesis is true, i.e. correctly identifying an effect when it is there.

Pre-test/post-test design A type of experimental study in which measurements of the groups are taken both prior to and following an intervention. This allows the direct comparison of pre-intervention and post-intervention results for individual subjects and groups of subjects.

Predictive validity The extent to which a test or measure can validly predict a future event. For example, a clinical test may have high predictive validity with respect to 5-year mortality of people with cancer. It is often expressed in the form of a correlation coefficient.

Prevalence The overall occurrence of a particular disease in a specific population at a specific point in time.

Probability The chance or likelihood of an event. The probability of flipping a 'heads' with a fair coin is 0.5 or 1/2. Probabilities may vary in value from 0 ('no chance') to 1 (certain).

Procedure A section in a research report that describes the protocol or procedure followed for the collection of data.

Proportion The ratio of one value to another expressed as a fraction of 1. For example, the proportion of women in the adult population is about 0.5.

Protocol deviation A deviation from the ideal procedure described as having been followed in a study by the researcher.

Qualitative methods An approach to research that emphasizes the non-numerical and interpretive analysis of social phenomena.

Quantitative methods An approach to research that emphasizes the collection of numerical data and the statistical analysis of hypotheses proposed by the researcher.

Quasi-experimental design A structured research design that is experiment-like but does not involve its full characteristics such as a control group and random assignment of subjects to treatment groups.

Questionnaire A means of collecting data from people where they provide written responses to a set of questions, either in their own words or by selecting predefined answers.

Quota sample The result of a sampling procedure in which the researcher sets quotas for the number of cases in particular categories to be included in the sample. For example, a sample of 100 might have quotas of 50 men and 50 women. The cases, however, are still selected on the basis of convenience rather than randomly. See also *stratified random sample*.

Random assignment In an experiment, subjects are assigned to their groups by using a random assignment method. In random assignment, subjects are assigned to their groups using a random procedure. For example, in a two-group study the tossing of a coin to assign subjects to groups would be a random assignment procedure.

Random sample A group of cases drawn from a population such that each member of the population has had an equal chance of selection.

Random sampling The process of selecting cases from a population such that each member of the population has had an equal chance of selection.

Range In a group of scores the range is the difference between the maximum and minimum scores.

Ratio scale Measurement scales may be nominal, ordinal, interval or ratio. A ratio scale has the following properties: the values are distinctive, ordered, equidistant and the zero point represents an absence of the quantity rather than being an arbitrary zero. Metres and kilograms are examples of ratio scales.

Refereed journal A journal in which the articles are vetted by independent referees for quality and interest. Refereed journals generally carry more highly regarded articles.

Regression to the mean The phenomenon where an individual who is measured on a test and obtains an extreme (very high or low) score and then upon re-measurement tends to move towards (regress) the average score (mean). Regression to the mean may be misinterpreted as representing a real change in score.

Relationships Associations between variables.

Reliability The extent to which a test or measurement result is reproducible.

Repeated measures The situation where a group of cases are measured on more than one occasion, for example prior to and following an intervention.

Representative sample A sample that accurately reflects the characteristics of the population from which it is drawn. Sometimes termed an 'unbiased' sample.

Reversal Reversal of the order of interventions is often used in experimental studies to control for the effects of order of administration. For example, intervention B preceded by intervention A may have a different effect than B followed by A.

Risk factors In epidemiology, a risk factor is an agent that is believed to increase the probability of a certain outcome or illness. For example, smoking may be a risk factor for the onset of coronary heart disease.

Rosenthal effect The phenomenon where the expectations of the researchers in a study influence the outcome. For example, if an observer believes that a particular intervention is effective, he/she may under-report or discount symptoms inconsistent with this belief.

Sample A group of cases selected from a population.

Sampling error Because a sample is smaller than the population from which it is drawn, there is often a discrepancy between the values obtained for the sample and those that apply to the population. For example, the average age of a sample might be 22 years and the average age of the population might be 28 years. This discrepancy is termed the sampling error.

Sampling method The method by which a sample is drawn from a population. Broadly, there are two approaches: random, in which every case in the population has an equal chance of selection, and non-random, in which cases have different chances of selection.

Scattergram A graph displaying the relationship between a set of paired scores on two variables. Also referred to as a scatterplot.

Semi-interquartile range A measure of the spread of a frequency distribution, being the distance between the first and third quartiles.

Semiotics A method of interpretation aiming to uncover the hidden, implicit meanings in texts.

Sensitivity The proportion of people who test as positive to a disease who really do have the disease. See also *true positive*.

Shared variance In the examination of relationships between variables, researchers are concerned about the extent to which when one variable changes the other also changes. Shared variance refers to the extent to which this occurs.

Skewness A characteristic of the shape of a frequency distribution. See also *negative skew*, *positive skew*.

Specificity The proportion of people who test negative to a disease who really do not have the disease. See also *true negative*.

Standard deviation A measure of the dispersion or variability of a group of scores. The standard deviation of a sample is represented by the symbol s and by the symbol σ for a population.

Standard error of the mean If a number of samples were taken from the same population and the mean calculated for each sample, the standard deviation of this distribution of means is known as the standard error of the mean. The standard error of the mean is used in statistical inferences about population means.

Standard normal curve An idealized normal or bell-shaped frequency distribution with a mean of 0 and a standard deviation of 1 unit.

Standardized test A standardized test is one that has known characteristics, especially known levels of reliability and validity. Researchers use standardized tests wherever possible in preference to unstandardized tests.

Statistic A statistic is a number with known properties derived from sample data. There are two types of statistics: inferential statistics, which are used to apply statistical tests, and descriptive statistics, which are used to describe characteristics of the sample.

Statistical significance When researchers have demonstrated statistical significance through the application of a statistical test, they have demonstrated that the result obtained is probably not due to chance but is 'real'. This does not mean the result is important or interesting. See also *clinical significance*.

Stratified random sample A type of sample in which the researcher wishes to ensure that important subgroups and their representation are preserved in the sample. For example, if a researcher randomly selected a subsample of 50 men and then 50 women, the sample has been stratified with respect to gender. See also *quota sample*.

Structured interview An interview in which the questions are generally predefined, i.e. asked in a fixed order with the answers recorded by the researcher on a response sheet.

Subjective measures Measures derived from a measurement process involving a substantial degree of human interpretation, e.g. subjective ratings of pain, clinical ratings of social skills.

Subjects Participants in a study.

Surveys A type of research design in which characteristics of the cases under study are systematically recorded without the researcher attempting actively to change the situation. A non-experimental type of study.

Systematic sample A method of drawing a sample from a population where, for example, every 10th case is selected from a population list.

Systematic review A principled approach to summarizing research in a specific area of health care. The system used is parallel to the methodology for conducting empirical research.

Test–retest reliability When a test or assessment procedure is administered twice to the same group of people, the correlation between the first score and the second score is termed the test–retest reliability. This is a measure of the reproducibility of an assessment procedure.

Time series A series of measurements taken repeatedly from the same person, or group of people, over time.

Transcript A verbatim written version of an interview.

Transformed score A score that has been altered by an arithmetic manipulation, such as a z score.

True negative The situation that occurs when a diagnostic test indicates the person being assessed does not have a disease when he/she really does not.

True positive The situation that occurs when a diagnostic test indicates the person being assessed does have a disease when he/she does.

Two-tailed test A statistical test where a difference between two groups is tested without reference to the expected direction of the difference.

Type I error When researchers, on the basis of a statistical test applied to a sample of data, wrongly conclude that there is evidence of an association between variables or difference between groups in the population, they have committed a Type I error. The probability of a Type I error is represented by the symbol α.

Type II error A 'miss'. When researchers, on the basis of a statistical test applied to a sample of data, wrongly conclude that there is no evidence of an association between variables or difference between groups in the population, they have committed a Type II error. The probability of a Type II error is represented by the symbol β.

Unstructured interview An interview in which there may be no pre-planned questions or fixed agenda. The dialogue is usually recorded in a transcript or field notes which are subsequently analysed.

Validity The extent to which a test measures what it is intended to measure.

Variability The extent to which a group of scores varies or is spread out. This is usually measured by a descriptive statistic such as the standard deviation range or semi-interquartile range.

Variable A property or attribute that varies. For example, gender, age, weight are all variables.

Variance A measure of the dispersion or variability of a group of scores. The variance of a sample is represented by the symbol s^2 and the symbol σ^2 for a population. See also *standard deviation*.

z scores Transformed scores which express how many standard deviations a specific score is above or below the mean. For instance, a corresponding z score of -2 implies that a given score is two standard deviations below the mean.

Zero correlation Correlation is used to measure the strength and direction of an association between two variables. A zero correlation implies that two variables are unrelated to one another.

References and further reading

References

Bailey K D 1987 Methods of social research. Free Press, New York

Barlow D H, Hersen M 1984 Single case experimental designs: strategies for studying behavior change, 2nd edn. Allyn and Bacon, Boston

Beaglehole R, Bonita R, Kjellstrom T 2000 Basic epidemiology. World Health Organization, Geneva

Beecher H K 1959 Measurement of subjective responses. Oxford University Press, Oxford

Bloch R 1987 Methodology in clinical pain trials. Spine 12: 430–432

Bogdan R, Taylor S 1976 The judged, not the judges: an insider's view of mental retardation. American Psychologist 31 (1): 47–52

Bowling A 1997 Measuring health. Open University Press, Philadelphia

Broad W, Wade N 1982 Betrayers of the truth. Simon & Schuster, New York

Chalmers A F 1976 What is this thing called science? Queensland University Press, St Lucia

Coates S J, Steed L G 2003 SPSS: analysis without anguish. Version 11.0 for Windows. John Wiley, Brisbane

Cochrane A L 1972 Effectiveness and efficiency. Random reflections on health services. Nuffield Provincial Hospitals Trust, London

Cohen J 1988 Statistical power analysis for the behavioural health sciences, 2nd edn. Lawrence Erlbaum, Mahwah

Cook T D, Campbell D T 1979 Quasi-experimentation: design and analysis issues for field settings. Rand McNally, Chicago

Coppleson L, Factor R, Strums S et al 1970 Observer disagreement in the classification and histology of Hodgkin's disease. Journal of the National Cancer Institute 45: 731–740

Daly J, Kellehear A, Gliksman M 1997 The health researcher: a methodological guide. Oxford University Press, Melbourne, pp 180–181

Denzin N K, Lincoln Y S 1994 Handbook of qualitative research. Sage, Newbury Park, California

Donabedian A 1990 The even pillars of quality. Archives of Pathology and Laboratory Medicine 114 (11): 1115–1118

Dooley D 1984 Social research methods. Prentice Hall, New Jersey

Doyle J, Thomas S A 2000 Capturing policy in hearing-aid decisions by audiologists. In: Connolly T, Arkes J, Hammond K (eds) Judgment and decision making, 2nd edn. Cambridge University Press, Cambridge, pp 245–258

Engel G 1977 The need for a new medical model: a challenge for biomedicine. Science 196: 129–136

Feyerabend P 1975 Against method. Verso, London

Gardner H (ed.) 1989 The politics of health: the Australian experience. Churchill Livingstone, Melbourne

Glaser B G, Strauss A 1967 The discovery of grounded theory: strategies for qualitative research. Aldine, New York

Grundy S 1987 Curriculum: product or praxis. Falmer Press, East Sussex, pp 15–19, 106–114

Guba E G, Lincoln Y S 1983 Epistemological and methodological bases of naturalistic enquiry. In: Madaus G F, Scriven M, Stufflebeam D L (eds) Evaluation models. Kluwer Nishoff, Boston, pp 311–339

Hay D, Oken D 1977 The psychological stress of intensive care unit nursing. In: Monat A, Lazarus R S (eds) Stress and coping. Columbia University Press, New York, pp 118–131

Huck S W, Cormier W H, Bounds W G 1974 Reading statistics and research. Harper & Row, New York

Krzyzowski J 1989 The historical development of electroconvulsive therapy. European Journal of Psychiatry 3 (1): 49–54

Kuhn T S 1970 The structure of scientific revolutions. Chicago University Press, Chicago

Kvale S 1996 An introduction to qualitative research interviewing. Sage, Newbury Park, California

Laing R D, Esterson A 1970 Sanity, madness and the family. Penguin, London

Lakatos I 1970 Falsification and the methodology of scientific research programmes. In: Lakatos I, Musgrave A (eds) Criticism and the growth of knowledge. Cambridge University Press, Cambridge, pp 91–196

Last A M 1988 A dictionary of epidemiology, 2nd edn. Oxford University Press, New York

Liamputtong Rice P, Ezzy D 1999 Qualitative research methods: a health focus. Oxford University Press, South Melbourne

Lincoln Y S, Guba E G 1985 Naturalistic inquiry. Sage, Newbury Park, California

Lofland J 1971 Analyzing social settings. Wadsworth, Belmont, California

McGartland M, Polgar S 1994 Paradigm collapse in psychology: the necessity for a 'two methods' approach. Australian Psychologist 29 (1): 21–28

McGinn F 1996 The plight of rural parents caring for adult children with HIV. Families in Society: The Journal of Contemporary Human Services 77: 269–278

Melzack R F, Wall P D 1965 Pain mechanisms: a new theory. Science 1250: 971

Merton R K 1946 The focused interview. American Journal of Sociology 51: 541–557

Miles M B, Huberman A M 1984 Analyzing qualitative data: a source book for new methods. Sage, Beverly Hills, California

Morse J M, Field P A 2003 Nursing research: the application of qualitative approaches, 2nd edn. Nelson Thornes, Cheltenham

Muir Gray J A 1997 Evidence-based healthcare: how to make health policy and management decisions. Churchill Livingstone, Edinburgh

Olanow C W 2004 The scientific basis for the current treatment of Parkinson's disease. Annual Review of Medicine 55: 41–60

Patton M Q 1990 Qualitative evaluation and research methods, 2nd edn. Sage, Newbury Park, California

Polgar S, Swerissen H 2000 Research methods in health 2. La Trobe University, Bundoora, Victoria

Polgar S, Morris M E, Reilly S et al 2003 Reconstructive neurosurgery for Parkinson's disease: a systematic review and preliminary meta-analysis. Brain Research Bulletin 60: 1–24

Rosenhan D L 1975 On being sane in insane places. In: Krupat E (ed.) Psychology is social. Scott Foresman, Glenview, Illinois, pp 189–200

Rosenthal R 1976 Experimenter effects in behavioural research. Irvington, New York

Sackett D, Strauss S, Richardson W et al 2000 Evidence-based medicine: how to practise and teach EBM, 2nd edn. Churchill Livingstone, Edinburgh

Schatzman L, Strauss A L 1973 Field research: strategies for a natural sociology. Prentice Hall, Englewood Cliffs, New Jersey

Schwartz M, Polgar S 2003 Statistics for evidence-based health care. Tertiary Press, Melbourne

Strauss A L 1987 Qualitative analysis for social scientists. Cambridge University Press, New York

Strauss A L, Corbin J M 1998 Basics of qualitative research: techniques and procedures for developing grounded theory, 2nd edn. Sage, Newbury Park, California

Tashakkori A, Teddlie C 1998 Mixed methodology: combining qualitative and quantitative approaches. Sage, Newbury Park, California

Taylor R 1979 Medicine out of control. Sun Books, Melbourne

Teltscher B, Polgar S 1981 Objective knowledge about Huntington's disease and attitudes towards predictive tests of persons at risk. Journal of Medical Genetics 18 (1): 31–39

Thomas S A, Henry P, McCoy A et al 1989 Why do parents stay overnight with children in hospitals? Australian Health Review 12 (2): 39–49

Thomas S A, Wearing A, Bennett M 1991 Clinical decision making for nurses and health professionals. Harcourt Brace Jovanovich, Sydney

Thomas S A, Steven I, Browning C et al 1992 Focus groups in health research: a methodological review. Annual Review of Health Social Sciences 2: 7–20

Thomas S A, Steven I, Browning C et al 1993 Patient knowledge, opinions, satisfaction and choices in primary health care provision: a progress report. In: Doessel D P (ed.) The general practice evaluation program: the 1992 work-in progress conference. Australian Government Publishing Service, Canberra

Walker Q, Langlands A 1986 The nurse of mammography in the management of breast cancer. Medical Journal of Australia 1435: 185–187

Further reading

Babbie E 1979 The practice of social research, 2nd edn. Wadsworth, Belmont, California. *This book offers a lucid theoretical account of social research methods.*

Bailey K D 1978 Methods of social research. Free Press, New York. *This is an excellent book with a very good set of chapters on survey design and execution.*

Castle W M 1976 Statistics in small doses, 2nd edn. Churchill Livingstone, Edinburgh. *This is a good little book for extra computational examples in statistics.*

Cook T D, Campbell D T 1979 Quasi-experimentation: design and analysis issues for field settings. Rand McNally, Chicago. *Following on from Campbell's earlier book with Stanley, this text offers an excellent account of design and control issues in quasi-experimental research, with an excellent chapter on philosophy of science issues.*

Hersen M, Barlow D H 1976 Single case experimental designs: strategies for studying behaviour change. Pergamon, New York. *This is a useful book for additional reading in the area of single-case experimental approaches. It is, however, rather lengthy in its descriptions of the theory rather than the practicalities of carrying out such research.*

Minichiello V, Aroni R, Timewell E et al 1991 In depth interviewing. Churchill Livingstone, Melbourne. *An excellent text for qualitative researchers who use interviews in their research.*

Moser C, Kalton G 1971 Survey methods in social investigation, 2nd edn. Heinemann, London. *An excellent book on survey methods.*

Answers to questions

Chapter 1

True or false

1. T
2. F
3. T
4. T
5. T
6. T
7. F
8. F
9. F
10. F
11. F
12. T
13. T
14. T
15. F
16. T
17. T
18. F
19. T
20. F

Multiple choice

1. d
2. b
3. b
4. a
5. c
6. a
7. c
8. d
9. b
10. c
11. a
12. d
13. c
14. d
15. c
16. a

Chapter 2

True or false

1. F
2. F
3. F
4. F
5. T
6. F
7. T
8. F
9. T
10. F
11. F
12. T
13. F
14. T
15. F
16. T
17. T
18. F
19. F
20. T
21. T
22. F
23. T
24. F
25. F
26. F
27. F
28. T

Multiple choice

1. e
2. d
3. b
4. a
5. b
6. b
7. c
8. d

9. d
10. d
11. c

Chapter 3

True or false

1. T
2. F
3. T
4. T
5. T
6. F
7. F
8. F
9. F
10. F
11. F
12. F
13. F
14. T
15. F
16. F
17. T
18. T
19. T
20. F
21. F
22. T
23. F

Multiple choice

1. a
2. d
3. a
4. c
5. d
6. a
7. d
8. b
9. a
10. c
11. b
12. c
13. c

Chapter 4

True or false

1. F
2. F
3. T
4. F
5. F
6. T
7. F
8. F
9. T
10. T

Multiple choice

1. a
2. b
3. c
4. d
5. c
6. a
7. a
8. d

Chapter 5

True or false

1. T
2. T
3. F
4. F
5. F
6. F
7. T
8. F
9. F
10. T
11. T
12. T
13. F
14. T
15. T
16. F

Multiple choice

1. d
2. c
3. b
4. c
5. d
6. c
7. e
8. a
9. d
10. a
11. d
12. c
13. a
14. c
15. a
16. d
17. b
18. a
19. d
20. d

Chapter 6

True or false

1. T
2. F
3. T
4. T
5. T
6. F
7. T
8. T
9. T
10. T
11. F
12. T
13. F
14. F
15. F
16. T
17. T
18. F
19. T
20. F

21. F
22. T

Multiple choice

1. d
2. b
3. d
4. a
5. d
6. d
7. a
8. b
9. d
10. b
11. d
12. a
13. c
14. d

Chapter 7

True or false

1. F
2. T
3. F
4. F
5. F
6. T
7. F
8. T
9. F
10. T
11. F
12. F
13. T
14. T
15. F
16. T

Multiple choice

1. c
2. b
3. c
4. a

5. a
6. c
7. c
8. c
9. c
10. c

Chapter 8

True or false

1. T
2. F
3. T
4. F
5. F
6. F
7. F
8. T
9. T
10. T
11. F
12. T

Multiple choice

1. b
2. d
3. d
4. b
5. a
6. a
7. c

Chapter 9

True or false

1. F
2. T
3. F
4. F
5. F
6. F
7. F
8. T
9. F

10. T

Multiple choice

1. a
2. a
3. d
4. c
5. c
6. d
7. b
8. b
9. c

Chapter 10

True or false

1. F
2. F
3. F
4. T
5. T
6. F
7. F
8. T

Multiple choice

1. a
2. b
3. d
4. c
5. c
6. d
7. c
8. a

Chapter 11

True or false

1. T
2. F
3. T
4. T
5. F

6. F
7. T
8. F
9. F
10. T

Multiple choice

1. b
2. a
3. c
4. c
5. d
6. c
7. a
8. c

Chapter 12

True or false

1. T
2. T
3. T
4. Г
5. F
6. T
7. T
8. F
9. T
10. T
11. F
12. F
13. F
14. F
15. T
16. F
17. F
18. T
19. T
20. T
21. T
22. F
23. F
24. T
25. F
26. F

27. T
28. T
29. F
30. T

Multiple choice

1. a
2. e
3. b
4. e
5. c
6. d
7. b
8. a
9. b
10. b
11. a
12. c
13. a
14. a
15. d
16. a
17. c
18. d
19. c
20. a

Chapter 13

True or false

1. T
2. F
3. T
4. T
5. F
6. T
7. F
8. F
9. F
10. F
11. T
12. T
13. T
14. F
15. T

16. T
17. F
18. T
19. F
20. F
21. F
22. F

Multiple choice

1. b
2. e
3. c
4. e
5. d
6. d
7. c
8. b
9. d
10. c
11. d
12. c
13. a
14. a
15. a
16. a
17. c
18. c
19. b
20. a
21. a
22. c
23. c
24. b
25. a
26. d
27. d
28. b
29. d
30. b

Chapter 14

True or false

1. F
2. F
3. T

4. F
5. T
6. F
7. T
8. T
9. T
10. T
11. F
12. F
13. T
14. T
15. T
16. T
17. T
18. T
19. T
20. T
21. T
22. F
23. T
24. F
25. F

Multiple choice

1. b
2. d
3. a
4. d
5. c
6. b
7. a
8. d
9. b
10. c
11. a
12. d
13. d
14. c
15. d
16. a
17. c
18. b
19. a
20. b
21. c
22. b
23. d

24. b
25. a
26. d
27. a
28. c

Chapter 15

True or false

1. T
2. F
3. F
4. F
5. T
6. T
7. F
8. F
9. T
10. F
11. F
12. F
13. T
14. F
15. T
16. F
17. T
18. T
19. F
20. T

Multiple choice

1. d
2. c
3. c
4. d
5. a
6. b
7. d
8. e
9. a
10. c
11. b
12. c
13. d
14. d

15. b
16. d
17. c
18. a
19. b
20. c
21. d
22. c
23. b
24. a
25. d

Chapter 16

True or false

1. F
2. T
3. T
4. T
5. F
6. T
7. T
8. F
9. F
10. T
11. F
12. T
13. F
14. T
15. F
16. T
17. T
18. F
19. T
20. T
21. F
22. F
23. F
24. T
25. F
26. F
27. F
28. F
29. T
30. F

Multiple choice

1. a
2. d
3. e
4. b
5. c
6. d
7. a
8. b
9. c
10. b
11. c
12. c
13. d
14. c
15. b
16. e
17. a
18. b
19. d
20. e
21. c
22. b
23. a
24. a

Chapter 17

True or false

1. F
2. T
3. F
4. T
5. F
6. T
7. T
8. F
9. T
10. T
11. F
12. T
13. T
14. F
15. F
16. T
17. T
18. F
19. F
20. T

Multiple choice

1. a
2. c
3. a
4. a
5. d
6. c
7. a
8. b
9. c
10. c
11. b
12. a
13. b
14. d
15. a
16. b
17. c
18. b
19. d
20. c
21. a
22. b
23. d
24. a
25. c
26. c
27. b
28. c
29. c
30. c
31. b
32. d
33. b
34. a
35. a

Chapter 18

True or false

1. T
2. F
3. T
4. T

5. T
6. T
7. F
8. T
9. T
10. T
11. F
12. F
13. T
14. T
15. T
16. T
17. T
18. T
19. F
20. T

Multiple choice

1. a
2. d
3. a
4. e
5. c
6. b
7. a
8. d
9. a
10. d
11. d
12. d
13. e
14. d
15. a
16. a
17. d
18. c
19. a
20. d
21. a
22. b
23. e
24. c

Chapter 19

True or false

1. T
2. F

3. F
4. T
5. F
6. T
7. F
8. T
9. T
10. F
11. T
12. T
13. T
14. T
15. F
16. T
17. T
18. T
19. T
20. F

Multiple choice

1. d
2. b
3. d
4. c
5. c
6. f
7. c
8. c
9. a
10. d
11. b
12. c
13. b
14. a
15. b
16. c
17. a
18. a
19. b
20. c
21. c
22. a
23. d
24. a
25. b
26. a
27. d

28. a
29. a
30. b
31. a

Chapter 20

True or false

1. F
2. F
3. T
4. F
5. F
6. T
7. F
8. T
9. T
10. F

Multiple choice

1. c
2. c
3. a
4. a
5. a
6. a
7. c
8. a
9. a
10. b

Chapter 21

True or false

1. T
2. F
3. T
4. T
5. F
6. F
7. T
8. T
9. F
10. T

11. F
12. F
13. T
14. F
15. T
16. T
17. F
18. F
19. F
20. T

Multiple choice

1. c
2. d
3. d
4. d
5. a
6. b
7. d
8. b
9. a
10. a
11. b
12. c

Chapter 22

True or false

1. F
2. T
3. T
4. F
5. F
6. T
7. F
8. T
9. T
10. T
11. F
12. T
13. F
14. F
15. F
16. T
17. T

18. F
19. F

Multiple choice

1. b
2. b
3. b
4. a
5. c
6. d
7. b
8. d
9. a
10. d

Chapter 23

True or false

1. T
2. F
3. F
4. T
5. F
6. T
7. F
8. T
9. F
10. F
11. T
12. F
13. T
14. T
15. F
16. T

Multiple choice

1. d
2. c
3. d
4. d
5. d
6. b
7. a

8. d
9. b
10. c
11. d
12. d
13. d
14. b

Chapter 24

True or false

1. F
2. T
3. F
4. F
5. T
6. T
7. T
8. F
9. F
10. F
11. T
12. F
13. T
14. F
15. T
16. T

Multiple choice

1. b
2. c
3. d
4. a
5. a
6. d
7. a
8. d
9. a
10. e
11. d
12. c
13. c
14. a

Appendix A

z scores and associated areas between z and mean and beyond

z	Area between mean and z	Area beyond z	z	Area between mean and z	Area beyond z	z	Area between mean and z	Area beyond z
0.00	0.0000	0.5000	0.18	0.0714	0.4286	0.36	0.1406	0.3594
0.01	0.0040	0.4960	0.19	0.0753	0.4247	0.37	0.1443	0.3557
0.02	0.0080	0.4920	0.20	0.0793	0.4207	0.38	0.1480	0.3520
0.03	0.0120	0.4880	0.21	0.0832	0.4168	0.39	0.1517	0.3483
0.04	0.0160	0.4840	0.22	0.0871	0.4129	0.40	0.1554	0.3446
0.05	0.0199	0.4801	0.23	0.0910	0.4090	0.41	0.1591	0.3409
0.06	0.0239	0.4761	0.24	0.0948	0.4052	0.42	0.1628	0.3372
0.07	0.0279	0.4721	0.25	0.0987	0.4013	0.43	0.1664	0.3336
0.08	0.0319	0.4681	0.26	0.1026	0.3974	0.44	0.1700	0.3300
0.09	0.0359	0.4641	0.27	0.1064	0.3936	0.45	0.1736	0.3264
0.10	0.0398	0.4602	0.28	0.1103	0.3897	0.46	0.1772	0.3228
0.11	0.0438	0.4562	0.29	0.1141	0.3859	0.47	0.1808	0.3192
0.12	0.0478	0.4522	0.30	0.1179	0.3821	0.48	0.1844	0.3156
0.13	0.0517	0.4483	0.31	0.1217	0.3783	0.49	0.1879	0.3121
0.14	0.0557	0.4443	0.32	0.1255	0.3745	0.50	0.1915	0.3085
0.15	0.0596	0.4404	0.33	0.1293	0.3707	0.51	0.1950	0.3050
0.16	0.0636	0.4364	0.34	0.1331	0.3669	0.52	0.1985	0.3015
0.17	0.0675	0.4325	0.35	0.1368	0.3632	0.53	0.2019	0.2981

(*Continued*)

z	Area between mean and z	Area beyond z	z	Area between mean and z	Area beyond z	z	Area between mean and z	Area beyond z
0.54	0.2054	0.2946	0.81	0.2910	0.2090	1.08	0.3599	0.1401
0.55	0.2088	0.2912	0.82	0.2939	0.2061	1.09	0.3621	0.1379
0.56	0.2123	0.2877	0.83	0.2967	0.2033	1.10	0.3643	0.1357
0.57	0.2157	0.2843	0.84	0.2995	0.2005	1.11	0.3665	0.1335
0.58	0.2190	0.2810	0.85	0.3023	0.1977	1.12	0.3686	0.1314
0.59	0.2224	0.2776	0.86	0.3051	0.1949	1.13	0.3708	0.1292
0.60	0.2257	0.2743	0.87	0.3078	0.1922	1.14	0.3729	0.1271
0.61	0.2291	0.2709	0.88	0.3106	0.1894	1.15	0.3749	0.1251
0.62	0.2324	0.2676	0.89	0.3133	0.1867	1.16	0.3770	0.1230
0.63	0.2357	0.2643	0.90	0.3159	0.1841	1.17	0.3790	0.1210
0.64	0.2389	0.2611	0.91	0.3186	0.1814	1.18	0.3810	0.1190
0.65	0.2422	0.2578	0.92	0.3212	0.1788	1.19	0.3830	0.1170
0.66	0.2454	0.2546	0.93	0.3238	0.1762	1.20	0.3849	0.1151
0.67	0.2486	0.2514	0.94	0.3264	0.1736	1.21	0.3869	0.1131
0.68	0.2517	0.2483	0.95	0.3289	0.1711	1.22	0.3888	0.1112
0.69	0.2549	0.2451	0.96	0.3315	0.1685	1.23	0.3907	0.1093
0.70	0.2580	0.2420	0.97	0.3340	0.1660	1.24	0.3925	0.1075
0.71	0.2611	0.2389	0.98	0.3365	0.1635	1.25	0.3944	0.1056
0.72	0.2642	0.2358	0.99	0.3389	0.1611	1.26	0.3962	0.1038
0.73	0.2673	0.2327	1.00	0.3413	0.1587	1.27	0.3980	0.1020
0.74	0.2704	0.2296	1.01	0.3438	0.1562	1.28	0.3997	0.1003
0.75	0.2734	0.2266	1.02	0.3461	0.1539	1.29	0.4015	0.0985
0.76	0.2764	0.2236	1.03	0.3485	0.1515	1.30	0.4032	0.0968
0.77	0.2794	0.2206	1.04	0.3508	0.1492	1.31	0.4049	0.0951
0.78	0.2823	0.2177	1.05	0.3531	0.1469	1.32	0.4066	0.0934
0.79	0.2852	0.2148	1.06	0.3554	0.1446	1.33	0.4082	0.0918
0.80	0.2881	0.2119	1.07	0.3577	0.1423	1.34	0.4099	0.0901

(Continued)

z	Area between mean and z	Area beyond z	z	Area between mean and z	Area beyond z	z	Area between mean and z	Area beyond z
1.35	0.4115	0.0885	1.62	0.4474	0.0526	1.89	0.4706	0.0294
1.36	0.4131	0.0869	1.63	0.4484	0.0516	1.90	0.4713	0.0287
1.37	0.4147	0.0853	1.64	0.4495	0.0505	1.91	0.4719	0.0281
1.38	0.4162	0.0838	1.65	0.4505	0.0495	1.92	0.4726	0.0274
1.39	0.4177	0.0823	1.66	0.4515	0.0485	1.93	0.4732	0.0268
1.40	0.4192	0.0808	1.67	0.4525	0.0475	1.94	0.4738	0.0262
1.41	0.4207	0.0793	1.68	0.4535	0.0465	1.95	0.4744	0.0256
1.42	0.4222	0.0778	1.69	0.4545	0.0455	1.96	0.4750	0.0250
1.43	0.4236	0.0764	1.70	0.4554	0.0446	1.97	0.4756	0.0244
1.44	0.4251	0.0749	1.71	0.4564	0.0436	1.98	0.4761	0.0239
1.45	0.4265	0.0735	1.72	0.4573	0.0427	1.99	0.4767	0.0233
1.46	0.4279	0.0721	1.73	0.4582	0.0418	2.00	0.4772	0.0228
1.47	0.4292	0.0708	1.74	0.4591	0.0409	2.01	0.4778	0.0222
1.48	0.4306	0.0694	1.75	0.4599	0.0401	2.02	0.4783	0.0217
1.49	0.4319	0.0681	1.76	0.4608	0.0392	2.03	0.4788	0.0212
1.50	0.4332	0.0668	1.77	0.4616	0.0384	2.04	0.4793	0.0207
1.51	0.4345	0.0655	1.78	0.4625	0.0375	2.05	0.4798	0.0202
1.52	0.4357	0.0643	1.79	0.4633	0.0367	2.06	0.4803	0.0197
1.53	0.4370	0.0630	1.80	0.4641	0.0359	2.07	0.4808	0.0192
1.54	0.4382	0.0618	1.81	0.4649	0.0351	2.08	0.4812	0.0188
1.55	0.4394	0.0606	1.82	0.4656	0.0344	2.09	0.4817	0.0183
1.56	0.4406	0.0594	1.83	0.4664	0.0336	2.10	0.4821	0.0179
1.57	0.4418	0.0582	1.84	0.4671	0.0329	2.11	0.4826	0.0174
1.58	0.4429	0.0571	1.85	0.4678	0.0322	2.12	0.4830	0.0170
1.59	0.4441	0.0559	1.86	0.4686	0.0314	2.13	0.4834	0.0166
1.60	0.4452	0.0548	1.87	0.4693	0.0307	2.14	0.4838	0.0162
1.61	0.4463	0.0537	1.88	0.4699	0.0301	2.15	0.4842	0.0158

(*Continued*)

z	Area between mean and z	Area beyond z	z	Area between mean and z	Area beyond z	z	Area between mean and z	Area beyond z
2.16	0.4846	0.0154	2.43	0.4925	0.0075	2.70	0.4965	0.0035
2.17	0.4850	0.0150	2.44	0.4927	0.0073	2.71	0.4966	0.0034
2.18	0.4854	0.0146	2.45	0.4929	0.0071	2.72	0.4967	0.0033
2.19	0.4857	0.0143	2.46	0.4931	0.0069	2.73	0.4968	0.0032
2.20	0.4861	0.0139	2.47	0.4932	0.0068	2.74	0.4969	0.0031
2.21	0.4864	0.0136	2.48	0.4934	0.0066	2.75	0.4970	0.0030
2.22	0.4868	0.0132	2.49	0.4936	0.0064	2.76	0.4971	0.0029
2.23	0.4871	0.0129	2.50	0.4938	0.0062	2.77	0.4972	0.0028
2.24	0.4875	0.0125	2.51	0.4940	0.0060	2.78	0.4973	0.0027
2.25	0.4878	0.0122	2.52	0.4941	0.0059	2.79	0.4974	0.0026
2.26	0.4881	0.0119	2.53	0.4943	0.0057	2.80	0.4974	0.0026
2.27	0.4884	0.0116	2.54	0.4945	0.0055	2.81	0.4975	0.0025
2.28	0.4887	0.0113	2.55	0.4946	0.0054	2.82	0.4976	0.0024
2.29	0.4890	0.0110	2.56	0.4948	0.0052	2.83	0.4977	0.0023
2.30	0.4893	0.0107	2.57	0.4949	0.0051	2.84	0.4977	0.0023
2.31	0.4896	0.0104	2.58	0.4951	0.0049	2.85	0.4978	0.0022
2.32	0.4898	0.0102	2.59	0.4952	0.0048	2.86	0.4979	0.0021
2.33	0.4901	0.0099	2.60	0.4953	0.0047	2.87	0.4979	0.0021
2.34	0.4904	0.0096	2.61	0.4955	0.0045	2.88	0.4980	0.0020
2.35	0.4906	0.0094	2.62	0.4956	0.0044	2.89	0.4981	0.0019
2.36	0.4909	0.0091	2.63	0.4957	0.0043	2.90	0.4981	0.0019
2.37	0.4911	0.0089	2.64	0.4959	0.0041	2.91	0.4982	0.0018
2.38	0.4913	0.0087	2.65	0.4960	0.0040	2.92	0.4982	0.0018
2.39	0.4916	0.0084	2.66	0.4961	0.0039	2.93	0.4983	0.0017
2.40	0.4918	0.0082	2.67	0.4962	0.0038	2.94	0.4984	0.0016
2.41	0.4920	0.0080	2.68	0.4963	0.0037	2.95	0.4984	0.0016
2.42	0.4922	0.0078	2.69	0.4964	0.0036	2.96	0.4985	0.0015

(*Continued*)

z	Area between mean and z	Area beyond z	z	Area between mean and z	Area beyond z	z	Area between mean and z	Area beyond z
2.97	0.4985	0.0015	3.10	0.4990	0.0010	3.23	0.4994	0.0006
2.98	0.4986	0.0014	3.11	0.4991	0.0009	3.24	0.4994	0.0006
2.99	0.4986	0.0014	3.12	0.4991	0.0009	3.25	0.4994	0.0006
3.00	0.4987	0.0013	3.13	0.4991	0.0009	3.30	0.4995	0.0005
3.01	0.4987	0.0013	3.14	0.4992	0.0008	3.35	0.4996	0.0004
3.02	0.4987	0.0013	3.15	0.4992	0.0008	3.40	0.4997	0.0003
3.03	0.4988	0.0012	3.16	0.4992	0.0008	3.45	0.4997	0.0003
3.04	0.4988	0.0012	3.17	0.4992	0.0008	3.50	0.4998	0.0002
3.05	0.4989	0.0011	3.18	0.4993	0.0007	3.60	0.4998	0.0002
3.06	0.4989	0.0011	3.19	0.4993	0.0007	3.70	0.4999	0.0001
3.07	0.4989	0.0011	3.20	0.4993	0.0007	3.80	0.4999	0.0001
3.08	0.4990	0.0010	3.21	0.4993	0.0007	3.90	0.49995	0.00005
3.09	0.4990	0.0010	3.22	0.4994	0.0006	4.00	0.49997	0.00003

Appendix B

t distribution

Directional *p*	0.4	0.25	0.1	0.05	0.025	0.01	0.005	0.001
Non-directional *p*	0.8	0.5	0.2	0.1	0.05	0.02	0.01	0.002
Degrees of freedom								
1	0.325	1.000	3.078	6.314	12.706	31.821	63.657	318.31
2	0.289	0.816	1.886	2.920	4.303	6.965	9.925	22.326
3	0.277	0.765	1.638	2.353	3.182	4.541	5.841	10.213
4	0.271	0.741	1.533	2.132	2.776	3.747	4.604	7.173
5	0.267	0.727	1.476	2.015	2.571	3.365	4.032	5.893
6	0.265	0.718	1.440	1.943	2.447	3.143	3.707	5.208
7	0.263	0.711	1.415	1.895	2.365	2.998	3.499	4.785
8	0.262	0.706	1.397	1.860	2.306	2.896	3.355	4.501
9	0.261	0.703	1.383	1.833	2.262	2.821	3.250	4.297
10	0.260	0.700	1.372	1.812	2.228	2.764	3.169	4.144
11	0.260	0.697	1.363	1.796	2.201	2.718	3.106	4.025
12	0.259	0.695	1.356	1.782	2.179	2.681	3.055	3.930
13	0.259	0.694	1.350	1.771	2.160	2.650	3.012	3.852
14	0.258	0.692	1.345	1.761	2.145	2.624	2.977	3.787
15	0.258	0.691	1.341	1.753	2.131	2.602	2.947	3.733
16	0.258	0.690	1.337	1.746	2.120	2.583	2.921	3.686
17	0.257	0.689	1.333	1.740	2.110	2.567	2.898	3.646
18	0.257	0.688	1.330	1.734	2.101	2.552	2.878	3.610
19	0.257	0.688	1.328	1.729	2.093	2.539	2.861	3.579

(*Continued*)

Directional p	0.4	0.25	0.1	0.05	0.025	0.01	0.005	0.001
Non-directional p	0.8	0.5	0.2	0.1	0.05	0.02	0.01	0.002
Degrees of freedom								
20	0.257	0.687	1.325	1.725	2.086	2.528	2.845	3.552
21	0.257	0.686	1.323	1.721	2.080	2.518	2.831	3.527
22	0.256	0.686	1.321	1.717	2.074	2.508	2.819	3.505
23	0.256	0.685	1.319	1.714	2.069	2.500	2.807	3.485
24	0.256	0.685	1.318	1.711	2.064	2.492	2.797	3.467
25	0.256	0.684	1.316	1.708	2.060	2.485	2.787	3.450
26	0.256	0.684	1.315	1.706	2.056	2.479	2.779	3.435
27	0.256	0.684	1.314	1.703	2.052	2.473	2.771	3.421
28	0.256	0.683	1.313	1.701	2.048	2.467	2.763	3.408
29	0.256	0.683	1.311	1.699	2.045	2.462	2.756	3.396
30	0.256	0.683	1.310	1.697	2.042	2.457	2.750	3.385
40	0.255	0.681	1.303	1.684	2.021	2.423	2.704	3.307
60	0.254	0.679	1.296	1.671	2.000	2.390	2.660	3.232
120	0.254	0.677	1.289	1.658	1.980	2.358	2.617	3.160
∞	0.253	0.674	1.282	1.645	1.960	2.326	2.576	3.090

Appendix C

Chi-square (χ^2)

df	0.99	0.98	0.95	0.90	0.80	0.70	0.50	0.30	0.20	0.10	0.05	0.02	0.01	0.001
1	0.00016	0.00063	0.0039	0.016	0.064	0.15	0.46	1.07	1.64	2.71	3.84	5.41	6.64	10.83
2	0.02	0.04	0.10	0.21	0.45	0.71	1.39	2.41	3.22	4.60	5.99	7.82	9.21	13.82
3	0.12	0.18	0.35	0.58	1.00	1.42	2.37	3.66	4.64	6.25	7.82	9.84	11.34	16.27
4	0.30	0.43	0.71	1.06	1.65	2.20	3.36	4.88	5.99	7.78	9.49	11.67	13.28	18.46
5	0.55	0.75	1.14	1.61	2.34	3.00	4.35	6.06	7.29	9.24	11.07	13.39	15.09	20.52
6	0.87	1.13	1.64	2.20	3.07	3.83	5.35	7.23	8.56	10.64	12.59	15.03	16.81	22.46
7	1.24	1.56	2.17	2.83	3.82	4.67	6.35	8.38	9.80	12.02	14.07	16.62	18.48	24.32
8	1.65	2.03	2.73	3.49	4.59	5.53	7.34	9.52	11.03	13.36	15.51	18.17	20.09	26.12
9	2.09	2.53	3.32	4.17	5.38	6.39	8.34	10.66	12.24	14.68	16.92	19.68	21.67	27.88
10	2.56	3.06	3.94	4.86	6.18	7.27	9.34	11.78	13.44	15.99	18.31	21.16	23.21	29.59
11	3.05	3.61	4.58	5.58	6.99	8.15	10.34	12.90	14.63	17.28	19.68	22.62	24.72	31.26
12	3.57	4.18	5.23	6.30	7.81	9.03	11.34	14.01	15.81	18.55	21.03	24.05	26.22	32.91
13	4.11	4.76	5.89	7.04	8.63	9.93	12.34	15.12	16.98	19.81	22.36	25.47	27.69	34.53
14	4.66	5.37	6.57	7.79	9.47	10.82	13.34	16.22	18.15	21.06	23.68	26.87	29.14	36.12
15	5.23	5.98	7.26	8.55	10.31	11.72	14.34	17.32	19.31	22.31	25.00	28.26	30.58	37.70
16	5.81	6.61	7.96	9.31	11.15	12.62	15.34	18.42	20.46	23.54	26.30	29.63	32.00	39.29
17	6.41	7.26	8.67	10.08	12.00	13.53	16.34	19.51	21.62	24.77	27.59	31.00	33.41	40.75
18	7.02	7.91	9.39	10.86	12.86	14.44	17.34	20.60	22.76	25.99	28.87	32.35	34.80	42.31
19	7.63	8.57	10.12	11.65	13.72	15.35	18.34	21.69	23.90	27.20	30.14	33.69	36.19	43.82
20	8.26	9.24	10.85	12.44	14.58	16.27	19.34	22.78	25.04	28.41	31.41	35.02	37.57	45.32
21	8.90	9.92	11.59	13.24	15.44	17.18	20.34	23.86	26.17	29.62	32.67	36.34	38.93	46.80

(Continued)

df	0.99	0.98	0.95	0.90	0.80	0.70	0.50	0.30	0.20	0.10	0.05	0.02	0.01	0.001
22	9.54	10.60	12.34	14.04	16.31	18.10	21.34	24.94	27.30	30.81	33.92	37.66	40.29	48.27
23	10.20	11.29	13.09	14.85	17.19	19.02	22.34	26.02	28.43	32.01	35.17	38.97	41.64	49.73
24	10.86	11.99	13.85	15.66	18.06	19.94	23.34	27.10	29.55	33.20	36.42	40.27	42.98	51.18
25	11.52	12.70	14.61	16.47	18.94	20.87	24.34	28.17	30.68	34.38	37.65	41.57	44.31	52.62
26	12.20	13.41	15.38	17.29	19.82	21.79	25.34	29.25	31.80	35.56	38.88	42.86	45.64	54.05
27	12.88	14.12	16.15	18.11	20.70	22.72	26.34	30.32	32.91	36.74	40.11	44.14	46.96	55.48
28	13.56	14.85	16.93	18.94	21.59	23.65	27.34	31.39	34.03	37.92	41.34	45.42	48.28	56.89
29	14.26	15.57	17.71	19.77	22.48	24.58	28.34	32.46	35.14	39.09	42.56	46.69	49.59	58.30
30	14.95	16.31	18.49	20.60	23.36	25.51	29.34	33.53	36.25	40.26	43.77	47.96	50.89	59.70

Index

Page numbers in **bold** refer to an explanation of terms in the glossary.